# 病理生理学学习指导

## （汉英对照）

主　编　赵　颖

**副主编**　赵丽梅　孙丽娜

苏州大学出版社

**图书在版编目（CIP）数据**

病理生理学学习指导：汉英对照／赵颖主编. —苏州：
苏州大学出版社，2022.6
ISBN 978-7-5672-3946-3

Ⅰ. ①病… Ⅱ. ①赵… Ⅲ. ①病理生理学－医学院校
－教学参考资料 Ⅳ. ①R363

中国版本图书馆 CIP 数据核字（2022）第 083750 号

Bingli Shenglixue Xuexi Zhidao
**病理生理学学习指导**
（汉英对照）

赵 颖 主编

责任编辑 吴 钰

助理编辑 何 睿

苏 州 大 学 出 版 社 出 版 发 行
（地址：苏州市十梓街 1 号 邮编：215006）
苏 州 市 深 广 印 刷 有 限 公 司 印 装
（地址：苏州市高新区浒关工业园青花路 6 号 2 号楼 邮编：215151）

开本 787 mm×1 092 mm 1/16 印张 20.75 字数 493 千
2022 年 6 月第 1 版 2022 年 6 月第 1 次印刷
ISBN 978-7-5672-3946-3 定价：58.00 元

若有印装错误，本社负责调换
苏州大学出版社营销部 电话：0512-67481020
苏州大学出版社网址 http://www.sudapress.com
苏州大学出版邮箱 sdcbs@suda.edu.cn

# 《病理生理学学习指导》编写组

主　编　赵　颖（苏州大学苏州医学院）

副主编　赵丽梅（苏州大学苏州医学院）

　　　　孙丽娜（苏州大学苏州医学院）

编　委　（按姓氏笔画排序）

　　　　刘立民（苏州大学苏州医学院）

　　　　孙晓东（苏州大学苏州医学院）

　　　　李　明（苏州大学附属第一医院）

　　　　李　晖（苏州大学附属第二医院）

　　　　郑　栋（苏州大学苏州医学院）

　　　　单立冬（苏州大学苏州医学院）

　　　　盛　瑞（苏州大学苏州医学院）

主　审　余卫平教授（东南大学医学院）

　　　　邓秀玲教授（西安交通大学基础医学院）

　　　　庞天庆教授（江南大学无锡医学院）

　　　　李俐教授（徐州医科大学）

　　　　夏天娇副教授（南京大学医学院）

　　　　刘霞副教授（南通大学医学院）

　　　　胡亚娥副教授（南通大学医学院）

　　　　张霞副教授（苏州大学附属第二医院）

　　　　张艳青讲师（扬州大学医学院）

　　　　丁红群讲师（江苏大学医学院）

# 前　言

　　病理生理学是一门研究疾病发生、发展机制,以及机体相关机能、代谢变化的学科。作为连接基础医学与临床医学的桥梁,病理生理学对医学生尤为重要。病理生理学与其他医学基础课程及临床疾病联系紧密,知识量大,覆盖面广,逻辑性强,学习难度大。本书旨在系统搭建病理生理学知识框架,帮助学生提升分析与解决问题的能力,培养学生的临床与科研思维。

　　本书是以国家卫生健康委员会"十三五"规划教材《病理生理学》(第9版)为依据编写的中英文双语学习辅导教材,涵盖疾病概论、疾病的基本病理生理学和器官系统病理生理学相关章节内容。全书分三大部分:学习目标与思维导图、案例分析题和实验拓展与思考。学习目标与思维导图部分系统地归纳总结了各章节的重点与难点。案例分析题部分主要包括A3型选择题和临床案例分析问答题。实验拓展与思考部分提供了实验相关的科研文献与讨论问题。本双语教材可供医学各相关专业学生包括留学生使用,也可作为教师备课及相关考生备考的参考书。

　　本书是在江苏高校省级外国留学生精品课程基金资助下,由苏州大学苏州医学院病理生理学、神经生物学和药理学教研室的多位老师共同编写完成。感谢来自南京大学医学院、东南大学医学院、江南大学无锡医学院、江苏大学医学院、扬州大学医学院、南通大学医学院、徐州医科大学、西安交通大学基础医学院和苏州大学附属第二医院的多位专家为本书提出宝贵意见。鉴于我们的能力水平有限,书中难免存在错误、疏漏和不妥之处,敬请广大读者不吝指正。

编　者

2022 年 4 月

# 目 录

中文版

## English Version

中文版

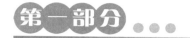

# 学习目标与思维导图

## 第一章 疾病概论

### 学习目标

（1）掌握疾病、健康与亚健康的概念。

（2）掌握病因学中病因、条件、诱因、危险因素的概念。

（3）熟悉病因的分类。

（4）掌握发病学的基本原理与机制。

（5）熟悉疾病的转归。

（6）掌握脑死亡的概念与标准。

## 思维导图

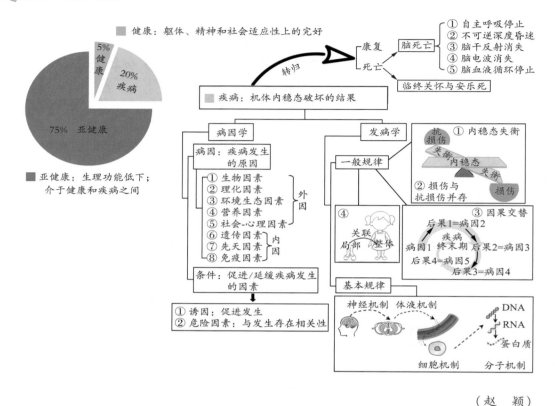

（赵　颖）

# 第二章　水、电解质代谢紊乱

## 学习目标

（1）了解水、钠、钾、镁、钙及磷的正常代谢与调节。

（2）掌握低渗/高渗性脱水的概念、病因、发病机制及对机体的影响。

（3）熟悉水/盐中毒的概念、病因、发病机制及对机体的影响。

（4）掌握水肿的概念与发病机制，并熟悉水肿液的分类、特点及对机体的影响。

（5）掌握低/高钾血症的概念、病因、发病机制及对机体的影响。

（6）熟悉低/高镁血症的概念、病因、发病机制及对机体的影响。

（7）熟悉低/高钙血症和低/高磷血症的概念、病因、发病机制及对机体的影响。

（8）熟悉各类水、电解质紊乱的防治原理。

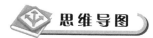

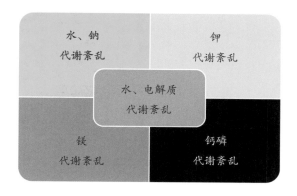

## ◇ 水、钠代谢紊乱

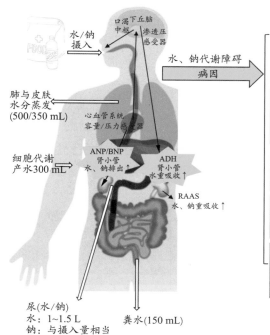

① 水摄入减少结合水丢失过多→失水＞失钠→高渗性脱水
　胃肠：呕吐、腹泻
　皮肤：大量出汗
　呼吸：呼吸增快
　肾脏：ADH不足性尿崩，高渗性利尿

② 失钠＞失水→低渗性脱水
　肾脏：长期使用排钠性利尿药(呋塞米/噻嗪类)；肾小管酸中毒和髓袢升支病变；肾上腺皮质不全导致的醛固酮↓
　胃肠/皮肤：丢失水分合并单纯性补水
　第三间隙：炎症引发的大量胸腔积液与腹水

③ 水摄入过多或排出减少→水中毒
　摄入过多：灌肠；静脉输入过快
　排出减少：急性肾衰，外伤或休克等导致ADH的过度分泌

④ 钠摄入过多或排出减少→盐中毒
　摄入过多：高渗盐溶液或高浓度碳酸氢钠静脉输入过多
　排出减少：醛固酮增多引发的钠潴留

⑤ 水肿
　水钠潴留：肾脏疾病、心力衰竭
　血管内外液体交换失衡：高血压、肝硬化、肾病综合征、恶性肿瘤、炎症、丝虫病等

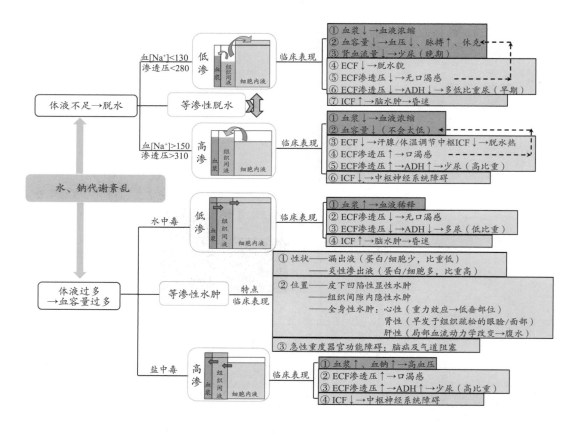

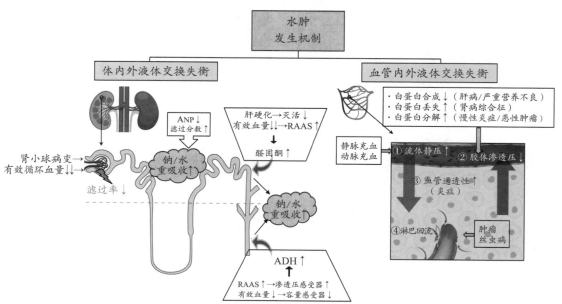

（ADH:抗利尿激素；ANP/BNP：心房/脑钠尿肽；ECF:细胞外液；ICF:细胞内液；RAAS:肾素-血管紧张素-醛固酮系统）

## ◇ 钾代谢紊乱

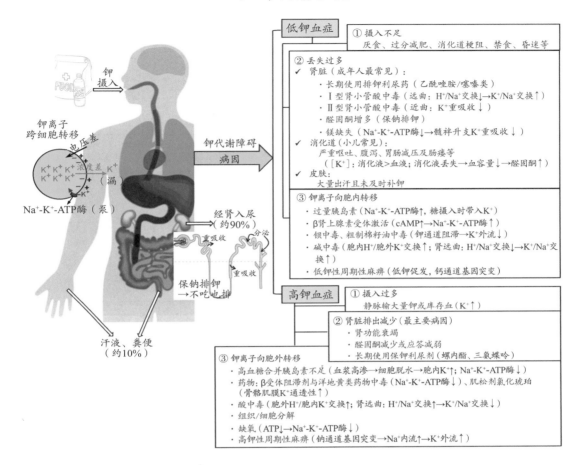

**低钾血症**

**① 摄入不足**
厌食、过分减肥、消化道梗阻、禁食、昏迷等

**② 丢失过多**
✓ 肾脏（成年人最常见）：
· 长期使用排钾利尿药（乙酰唑胺/噻嗪类）
· Ⅰ型肾小管酸中毒（远曲：$H^+/Na^+$交换↓→$K^+/Na^+$交换↑）
· Ⅱ型肾小管酸中毒（近曲：$K^+$重吸收↓）
· 醛固酮增多（保钠排钾）
· 镁缺失（$Na^+-K^+-ATP$酶↓→髓袢升支$K^+$重吸收↓）
✓ 消化道（小儿常见）：
严重呕吐、腹泻、胃肠减压及肠瘘等
（$[K^+]$：消化液>血液；消化液丢失→血容量↓→醛固酮↑）
✓ 皮肤
大量出汗且未及时补钾

**③ 钾离子向胞内转移**
· 过量胰岛素（$Na^+-K^+-ATP$酶↑，糖摄入时带入$K^+$）
· β肾上腺素受体激活（cAMP↑→$Na^+-K^+-ATP$酶↑）
· 钡中毒、粗制棉籽油中毒（钾通道阻滞→$K^+$外流↓）
· 碱中毒（胞内$H^+$/胞外$K^+$交换↑；肾远曲：$H^+/Na^+$交换↓→$K^+/Na^+$交换↑）
· 低钾性周期性麻痹（低钾促发，钙通道基因突变）

**高钾血症**

**① 摄入过多**
静脉输大量钾或库存血（$K^+$↑）

**② 肾脏排出减少**（最主要病因）
· 肾功能衰竭
· 醛固酮减少或应答减弱
· 长期使用保钾利尿剂（螺内酯、三氨蝶呤）

**③ 钾离子向胞外转移**
· 高血糖合并胰岛素不足（血浆高渗→细胞脱水→胞内$K^+$↑；$Na^+-K^+-ATP$酶↓）
· 药物：β受体阻滞剂与洋地黄类药物中毒（$Na^+-K^+-ATP$酶）、肌松剂氯化琥珀（骨骼肌膜$K^+$通透性↑）
· 酸中毒（胞外$H^+$/胞内$K^+$交换↑；肾远曲：$H^+/Na^+$交换↑→$K^+/Na^+$交换↓）
· 组织/细胞分解
· 缺氧（ATP↓→$Na^+-K^+-ATP$酶↓）
· 高钾性周期性麻痹（钠通道基因突变→$Na^+$内流↑→$K^+$外流↑）

钾
摄入

钾离子
跨细胞转移

电压差
$K^+$
$K^+$ $K^+$ $K^+$ 浓度差 $K^+$
$K^+$ $K^+$ $K^+$ （漏）
$K^+$
$Na^+-K^+-ATP$酶（泵）

钾代谢障碍
病因

经肾入尿
（约90%）
重吸收　分泌
重吸收

保钠排钾
→不吃也排

汗液、粪便
（约10%）

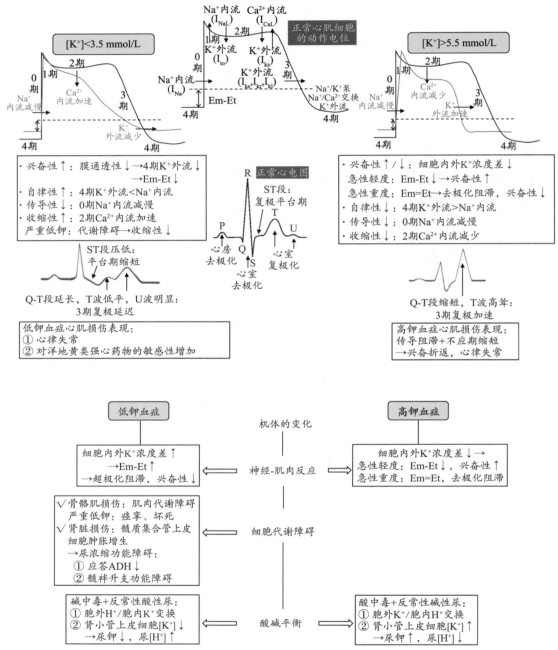

（ADH:抗利尿激素;Em：静息电位;Et:阈电位）

# ◇ 镁代谢紊乱

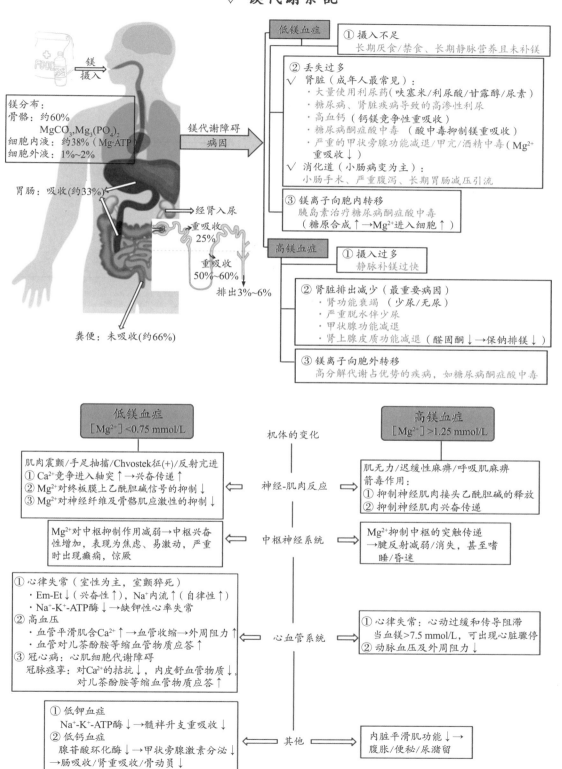

**低镁血症**

① 摄入不足
长期厌食/禁食、长期静脉营养且未补镁

② 丢失过多
√ 肾脏（成年人最常见）：
· 大量使用利尿药（呋塞米/利尿酸/甘露醇/尿素）
· 糖尿病、肾脏疾病导致的高渗性利尿
· 高血钙（钙镁竞争性重吸收）
· 糖尿病酮症酸中毒（酸中毒抑制镁重吸收）
· 严重的甲状旁腺功能减退/甲亢/酒精中毒（$Mg^{2+}$重吸收↓）
√ 消化道（小肠病变为主）：
小肠手术、严重腹泻、长期胃肠减压引流

③ 镁离子向胞内转移
胰岛素治疗糖尿病酮症酸中毒
（糖原合成↑→$Mg^{2+}$进入细胞↑）

**高镁血症**

① 摄入过多
静脉补镁过快

② 肾脏排出减少（最重要病因）
· 肾功能衰竭（少尿/无尿）
· 严重脱水伴少尿
· 甲状腺功能减退
· 肾上腺皮质功能减退（醛固酮↓→保钠排镁↓）

③ 镁离子向胞外转移
高分解代谢占优势的疾病，如糖尿病酮症酸中毒

镁摄入

镁分布：
骨骼：约60%
$MgCO_3,Mg_3(PO_4)_2$
细胞内液：约38%（Mg·ATP）
细胞外液：1%~2%

镁代谢障碍病因

胃肠：吸收（约33%）

经肾入尿
重吸收25%
重吸收50%~60%
排出3%~6%

粪便：未吸收(约66%)

---

**低镁血症**
$[Mg^{2+}] < 0.75$ mmol/L

机体的变化

**高镁血症**
$[Mg^{2+}] > 1.25$ mmol/L

---

肌肉震颤/手足抽搐/Chvostek征(+)/反射亢进
① $Ca^{2+}$竞争进入轴突↑→兴奋传递↑
② $Mg^{2+}$对终板膜上乙酰胆碱信号的抑制↓
③ $Mg^{2+}$对神经纤维及骨骼肌应激性的抑制↓

← 神经-肌肉反应 →

肌无力/迟缓性麻痹/呼吸肌麻痹
箭毒作用：
① 抑制神经肌肉接头乙酰胆碱的释放
② 抑制神经肌肉兴奋传递

---

$Mg^{2+}$对中枢抑制作用减弱→中枢兴奋性增加，表现为焦虑、易激动，严重时出现癫痫，惊厥

← 中枢神经系统 →

$Mg^{2+}$抑制中枢的突触传递→腱反射减弱/消失，甚至嗜睡/昏迷

---

① 心律失常（室性为主，室颤猝死）
· Em-Et↓（兴奋性↑），$Na^+$内流↑（自律性↑）
· $Na^+$-$K^+$-ATP酶↓→缺钾性心率失常
② 高血压
· 血管平滑肌含$Ca^{2+}$↑→血管收缩→外周阻力↑
· 血管对儿茶酚胺等缩血管物质应答↑
③ 冠心病：心肌细胞代谢障碍
冠脉痉挛：对$Ca^{2+}$的拮抗，内皮舒血管物质↓，
对儿茶酚胺等缩血管物质应答↑

← 心血管系统 →

① 心律失常：心动过缓和传导阻滞
当血镁>7.5 mmol/L，可出现心脏骤停
② 动脉血压及外周阻力↓

---

① 低钾血症
$Na^+$-$K^+$-ATP酶↓→髓袢升支重吸收↓
② 低钙血症
腺苷酸环化酶↓→甲状旁腺激素分泌↓
→肠吸收/肾重吸收/骨动员↓

← 其他 →

内脏平滑肌功能↓→腹胀/便秘/尿潴留

# ◇ 钙磷代谢紊乱

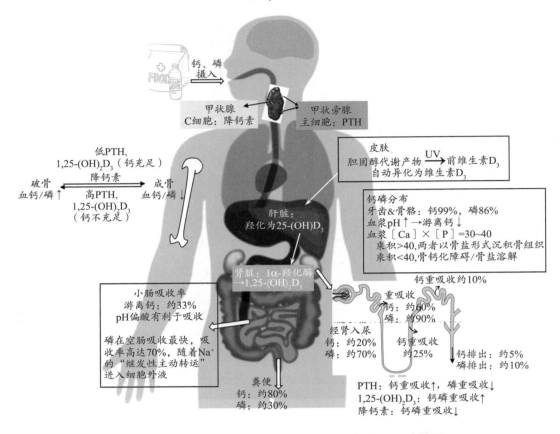

钙、磷摄入

甲状腺
C细胞：降钙素

甲状旁腺
主细胞：PTH

皮肤
胆固醇代谢产物 $\xrightarrow{UV}$ 前维生素$D_3$
自动异化为维生素$D_3$

低PTH，
$1,25-(OH)_2D_3$（钙充足）
降钙素

高PTH，
$1,25-(OH)_2D_3$
（钙不充足）

破骨 ⇄ 成骨
血钙/磷↑ 血钙/磷↓

肝脏：
羟化为$25-(OH)D_3$

钙磷分布
牙齿&骨骼：钙99%，磷86%
血浆pH↑→游离钙↓
血浆$[Ca] \times [P] = 30\sim40$
乘积>40，两者以骨盐形式沉积骨组织
乘积<40，骨钙化障碍/骨盐溶解

肾脏：$1\alpha$-羟化酶
$\to 1,25-(OH)_2D_3$

钙重吸收约10%

重吸收
钙：约60%
磷：约90%

钙重吸收
约25%

钙排出：约5%
磷排出：约10%

小肠吸收率
游离钙：约33%
pH偏酸有利于吸收

磷在空肠吸收最快，吸收率高达70%，随着$Na^+$的"继发性主动转运"进入细胞外液

经肾入尿
钙：约20%
磷：约70%

PTH：钙重吸收↑，磷重吸收↓
$1,25-(OH)_2D_3$：钙磷重吸收↑
降钙素：钙磷重吸收↓

粪便
钙：约80%
磷：约30%

## 低钙血症
$[Ca^{2+}] < 1.0$ mmol/L

病因：
① UV/肠吸收不足：维生素D代谢障碍、肝/肾病时羟化障碍
② PTH缺乏/抵抗：甲状旁腺功能退化
③ 肠吸收↓，PTH敏感性↓：慢性肾衰、急性胰腺炎
④ PTH↓，骨盐的钙镁交换障碍：低镁血症

机体表现：
① 神经肌肉：肌肉痉挛、手足抽搐、喉鸣、惊厥
② 心肌：
  · $Na^+$内流↑→兴奋性/传导性↑
  · 平台期$Ca^{2+}$内流↓→QT/ST段延长，T波低平/倒置
③ 骨骼：佝偻病（儿童）/骨质疏松（成人）
④ 婴幼儿：免疫力↓、皮肤干燥、指甲易脆

## 高钙血症
$[Ca^{2+}] > 1.4$ mmol/L

病因：
① 溶骨↑：
  · 甲状旁腺功能亢进：
    原发性：甲状旁腺腺瘤/增生/腺癌
    继发性：维生素D缺乏、慢性肾衰
  · 恶性肿瘤的骨转移、甲亢
② 肠吸收↑：维生素D中毒
③ 肾重吸收↑：Addison病、维生素A摄入过多、噻嗪类药物

机体表现：
① 神经肌肉：兴奋性↓→乏力/腱反射↓/精神障碍
② 心肌：
  · $Na^+$内流↓→兴奋性/传导性↓
  · 平台期$Ca^{2+}$内流↑→QT缩短
③ 肾脏：肾小管损伤，早期浓缩功能↓
④ 血管/脏器：异位钙化形成

低磷血症
[Pi] <0.8 mmol/L

病因:
① 小肠吸收障碍:饥饿、呕吐、吸收不良综合征、1,25-$(OH)_2D_3$缺乏、结合磷酸的制酸剂
② 尿磷排泄↑:利尿剂、急性酒精中毒、维生素D抵抗、甲状旁腺功能亢进、肾小管与代谢性酸中毒
③ 磷向细胞内转移:人工胰岛素、糖、雄性激素、恢复进食综合征、呼吸性碱中毒(糖磷酸化↑)

机体表现(无特异性症状):
① ATP合成不足→肌无力、精神障碍
② 2,3-DPG减少→红细胞与氧的亲和力增加

高磷血症
[Pi] >1.6/1.9 mmol/L(成人/儿童)

病因:
① 尿磷排泄↓:急/慢性肾功能不全、甲状旁腺功能低下、肢端肥大症(生长激素↑→尿磷↓)
② 溶骨↑:甲亢
③ 肠吸收与肾重吸收↑:维生素D中毒
④ 磷向细胞外转移:急性酸中毒、骨骼肌破坏、高热、淋巴性白血病、恶性肿瘤(化疗)
⑤ 磷摄入过多:含磷缓泻剂、磷酸盐注射液

机体表现:
① 低钙血症:$1\alpha$-羟化酶↓,骨重吸收↓
② 血管/脏器:异位钙化形成

(2,3-DPG:2,3-二磷酸甘油酸;ATP:三磷酸腺苷;PTH:甲状旁腺激素;UV:紫外线)

(赵丽梅 赵 颖)

# 第三章 酸碱平衡紊乱

## 学习目标

(1)掌握酸碱平衡紊乱的概念、反映酸碱平衡状况的常用指标及其意义。

(2)熟悉体液酸碱物质的来源和酸碱平衡的调节。

(3)掌握代谢性酸中毒、呼吸性酸中毒、代谢性碱中毒和呼吸性碱中毒的概念、发病机制、机体的代偿调节及对机体的主要影响。

(4)熟悉代谢性酸中毒、呼吸性酸中毒、代谢性碱中毒和呼吸性碱中毒的病因分类。

(5)掌握混合型酸碱平衡紊乱的类型、原因、特点,以及分析判断酸碱平衡紊乱的方法。

(6)了解防治代谢性酸中毒、呼吸性酸中毒、代谢性碱中毒和呼吸性碱中毒的病理生理学基础。

**思维导图**

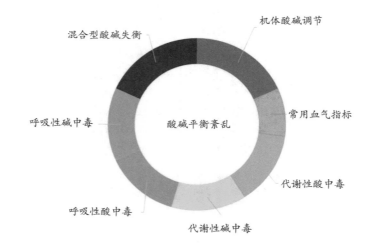

机体酸碱调节

常用血气指标

代谢性酸中毒

代谢性碱中毒

呼吸性酸中毒

呼吸性碱中毒

混合型酸碱失衡

酸碱平衡紊乱

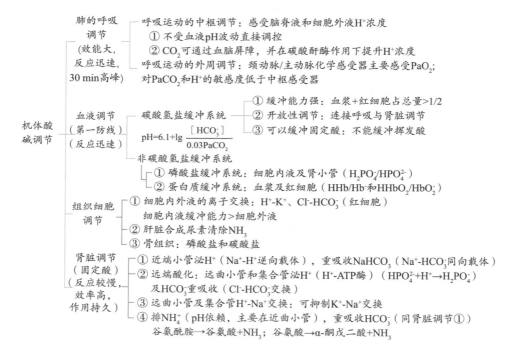

机体酸碱调节

肺的呼吸调节（效能大，反应迅速，30 min高峰）

呼吸运动的中枢调节：感受脑脊液和细胞外液$H^+$浓度
① 不受血液pH波动直接调控
② $CO_2$可通过血脑屏障，并在碳酸酐酶作用下提升$H^+$浓度
呼吸运动的外周调节：颈动脉/主动脉化学感受器主要感受$PaO_2$；对$PaCO_2$和$H^+$的敏感度低于中枢感受器

血液调节（第一防线）（反应迅速）

碳酸氢盐缓冲系统
① 缓冲能力强：血浆+红细胞占总量>1/2
② 开放性调节：连接呼吸与肾脏调节
③ 可以缓冲固定酸；不能缓冲挥发酸
$$pH=6.1+\lg\frac{[HCO_3^-]}{0.03PaCO_2}$$
非碳酸氢盐缓冲系统
① 磷酸盐缓冲系统：细胞内液及肾小管（$H_2PO_4^-/HPO_4^{2-}$）
② 蛋白质缓冲系统：血浆及红细胞（$HHb/Hb^-$和$HHbO_2/HbO_2^-$）

组织细胞调节

① 细胞内外液的离子交换：$H^+-K^+$、$Cl^--HCO_3^-$（红细胞）
细胞内液缓冲能力>细胞外液
② 肝脏合成尿素清除$NH_3$
③ 骨组织：磷酸盐和碳酸盐

肾脏调节（固定酸）（反应较慢，效率高，作用持久）

① 近端小管泌$H^+$（$Na^+-H^+$逆向载体），重吸收$NaHCO_3$（$Na^+-HCO_3^-$同向载体）
② 远端酸化：远曲小管和集合管泌$H^+$（$H^+-ATP$酶）（$HPO_4^{2-}+H^+\rightarrow H_2PO_4^-$）
及$HCO_3^-$重吸收（$Cl^--HCO_3^-$交换）
③ 远曲小管及集合管$H^+-Na^+$交换：可抑制$K^+-Na^+$交换
④ 排$NH_4^+$（pH依赖，主要在近曲小管），重吸收$HCO_3^-$（同肾脏调节①）
谷氨酰胺→谷氨酸+$NH_3$；谷氨酸→α-酮戊二酸+$NH_3$

常用血气指标

pH
- <7.35：失代偿性酸中毒
- >7.45：失代偿性碱中毒

PaCO₂（呼吸性指标）
- <33 mmHg（通气过度）：呼碱或代偿后代酸
- >46 mmHg（通气不足）：呼酸或代偿后代碱

标准碳酸氢盐SB（代谢性指标）—— 标准条件：T38 ℃，PaCO₂40 mmHg，SO₂100%

实际碳酸氢盐AB
- ① AB≈SB
  - <22 mmol/L：代酸
  - >27 mmol/L：代碱
- ② AB>SB：呼酸
- ③ AB<SB：呼碱
- ④ 肾脏代偿继发性变化：慢性呼酸—SB↑；慢性呼碱—SB↓

缓冲碱BB（代谢性指标）
- 标准条件下，负离子碱总和
- 代酸：BB↓；代碱：BB↑

碱剩余BE（BE=BB-48；代谢性指标）
- 代酸：BE负值↑
- 代碱：BE正值↑

阴离子间隙 AG=Na⁺−(HCO₃⁻+Cl⁻)
- >16 mmol/L，AG增高型代酸，多见于固定酸增多

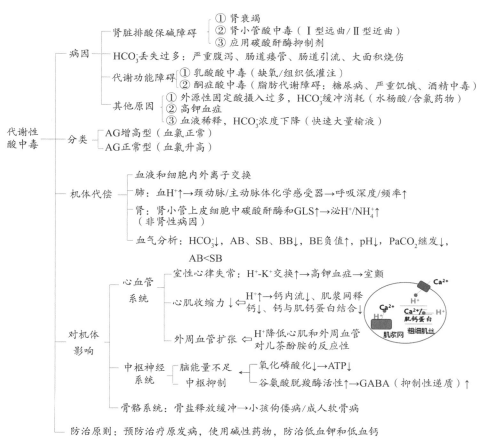

代谢性酸中毒

病因
- 肾脏排酸保碱障碍
  - ① 肾衰竭
  - ② 肾小管酸中毒（Ⅰ型远曲/Ⅱ型近曲）
  - ③ 应用碳酸酐酶抑制剂
- HCO₃⁻丢失过多：严重腹泻、肠道瘘管、肠道引流、大面积烧伤
- 代谢功能障碍
  - ① 乳酸酸中毒（缺氧/组织低灌注）
  - ② 酮症酸中毒（脂肪代谢障碍：糖尿病、严重饥饿、酒精中毒）
- 其他原因
  - ① 外源性固定酸摄入过多，HCO₃⁻缓冲消耗（水杨酸/含氯药物）
  - ② 高钾血症
  - ③ 血液稀释，HCO₃⁻浓度下降（快速大量输液）

分类
- AG增高型（血氯正常）
- AG正常型（血氯升高）

机体代偿
- 血液和细胞内外离子交换
- 肺：血H⁺↑→颈动脉/主动脉体化学感受器→呼吸深度/频率↑
- 肾：肾小管上皮细胞中碳酸酐酶和GLS↑→泌H⁺/NH₄⁺↑（非肾性病因）
- 血气分析：HCO₃⁻↓，AB、SB、BB↓，BE负值↑，pH↓，PaCO₂继发↓，AB<SB

对机体影响
- 心血管系统
  - 室性心律失常：H⁺-K⁺交换↑→高钾血症→室颤
  - 心肌收缩力↓←H⁺↑→钙内流↓、肌浆网释钙↓、钙与肌钙蛋白结合↓
  - 外周血管扩张←H⁺降低心肌和外周血管对儿茶酚胺的反应性
- 中枢神经系统
  - 脑能量不足
  - 中枢抑制
  - ←氧化磷酸化↓→ATP↓
  - ←谷氨酸脱羧酶活性↑→GABA（抑制性递质）↑
- 骨骼系统：骨盐释放缓冲→小孩佝偻病/成人软骨病

防治原则：预防治疗原发病，使用碱性药物，防治低血钾和低血钙

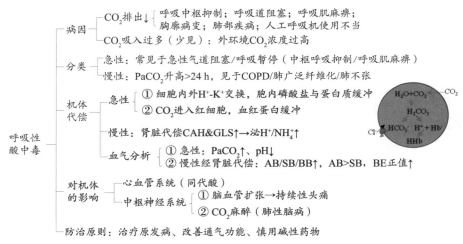

呼吸性酸中毒
- 病因
  - CO₂排出↓：呼吸中枢抑制；呼吸道阻塞；呼吸肌麻痹；胸廓病变；肺部疾病；人工呼吸机使用不当
  - CO₂吸入过多（少见）：外环境CO₂浓度过高
- 分类
  - 急性：常见于急性气道阻塞/呼吸暂停（中枢呼吸抑制/呼吸肌麻痹）
  - 慢性：PaCO₂升高>24 h，见于COPD/肺广泛纤维化/肺不张
- 机体代偿
  - 急性
    - ① 细胞内外H⁺-K⁺交换，胞内磷酸盐与蛋白质缓冲
    - ② CO₂进入红细胞，血红蛋白缓冲
  - 慢性：肾脏代偿CAH&GLS↑→泌H⁺/NH₄⁺↑
  - 血气分析
    - ① 急性：PaCO₂↑、pH↓
    - ② 慢性经肾脏代偿：AB/SB/BB↑，AB>SB，BE正值↑
- 对机体的影响
  - 心血管系统（同代酸）
  - 中枢神经系统
    - ① 脑血管扩张→持续性头痛
    - ② CO₂麻醉（肺性脑病）
- 防治原则：治疗原发病、改善通气功能、慎用碱性药物

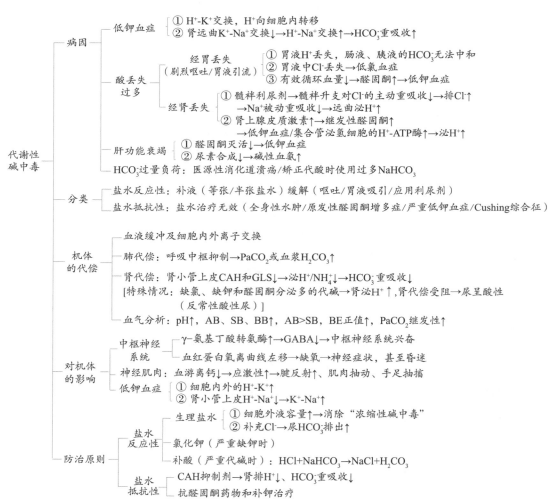

代谢性碱中毒
- 病因
  - 低钾血症
    - ① H⁺-K⁺交换，H⁺向细胞内转移
    - ② 肾远曲K⁺-Na⁺交换↓→H⁺-Na⁺交换↑→HCO₃⁻重吸收↑
  - 酸丢失过多
    - 经胃丢失（剧烈呕吐/胃液引流）
      - ① 胃液H⁺丢失，肠液、胰液的HCO₃⁻无法中和
      - ② 胃液中Cl⁻丢失→低氯血症
      - ③ 有效循环血量↓→醛固酮↑→低钾血症
    - 经肾丢失
      - ① 髓袢利尿剂→髓袢升支对Cl⁻的主动重吸收↓→排Cl↑→Na⁺被动重吸收↓→远曲泌H⁺↑
      - ② 肾上腺皮质激素↑→继发性醛固酮↑→低钾血症/集合管泌氢细胞的H⁺-ATP酶↑→泌H⁺↑
  - 肝功能衰竭
    - ① 醛固酮灭活↓→低钾血症
    - ② 尿素合成↓→碱性血氨↑
  - HCO₃⁻过量负荷：医源性消化道溃疡/矫正代酸时使用过多NaHCO₃
- 分类
  - 盐水反应性：补液（等张/半张盐水）缓解（呕吐/胃液吸引/应用利尿剂）
  - 盐水抵抗性：盐水治疗无效（全身性水肿/原发性醛固酮增多症/严重低钾血症/Cushing综合征）
- 机体的代偿
  - 血液缓冲及细胞内外离子交换
  - 肺代偿：呼吸中枢抑制→PaCO₂或血浆H₂CO₃↑
  - 肾代偿：肾小管上皮CAH和GLS↓→泌H⁺/NH₄⁺↓→HCO₃⁻重吸收↓
  - [特殊情况：缺氯、缺钾和醛固酮分泌多的代碱→肾泌H⁺↑,肾代偿受阻→尿呈酸性（反常性酸性尿）]
  - 血气分析：pH↑，AB、SB、BB↑，AB>SB，BE正值↑，PaCO₂继发性↑
- 对机体的影响
  - 中枢神经系统
    - γ-氨基丁酸转氨酶↑→GABA↓→中枢神经系统兴奋
    - 血红蛋白氧离曲线左移→缺氧→神经症状，甚至昏迷
  - 神经肌肉：血游离钙↓→应激性↑→腱反射↑、肌肉抽动、手足抽搐
  - 低钾血症
    - ① 细胞内外的H⁺-K⁺↑
    - ② 肾小管上皮H⁺-Na⁺↓→K⁺-Na⁺↑
- 防治原则
  - 盐水反应性
    - 生理盐水
      - ① 细胞外液容量↑→消除"浓缩性碱中毒"
      - ② 补充Cl⁻→尿HCO₃⁻排出↑
    - 氯化钾（严重缺钾时）
    - 补酸（严重代碱时）：HCl+NaHCO₃→NaCl+H₂CO₃
  - 盐水抵抗性
    - CAH抑制剂→肾排H⁺↓、HCO₃⁻重吸收↓
    - 抗醛固酮药物和补钾治疗

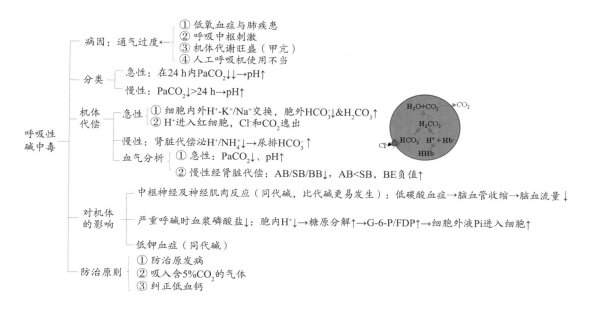

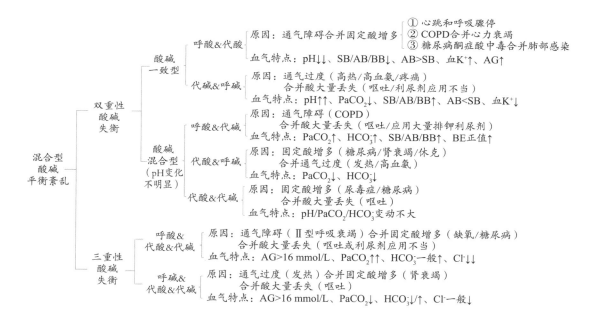

（ATP：三磷酸腺苷；CAH：碳酸酐酶；COPD：慢性阻塞性肺疾病；GABA：γ-氨基丁酸；GLS：谷氨酰胺酶；Pi：磷酸盐）

（郑　栋　赵　颖）

# 第四章　发　热

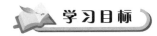

（1）掌握发热、过热、发热激活物、内生致热原和热限的概念。

（2）掌握发热的病因和发病机制。

（3）熟悉体温升高的分类;熟悉发热激活物、内生致热原和中枢正（负）调节介质的分类及作用。

（4）熟悉发热时机体代谢与功能的改变。

（5）熟悉发热的时相及各时相的热代谢特点。

（6）了解体温调定点学说。

（7）了解发热防治的病理生理学基础。

## 思维导图

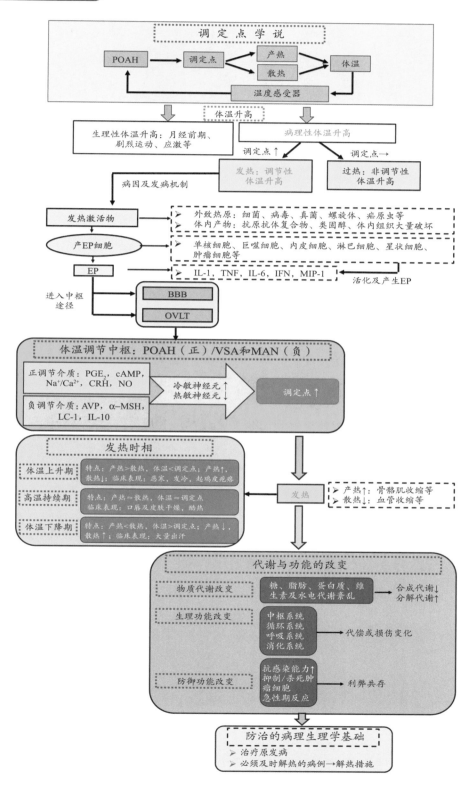

（AVP：精氨酸升压素；BBB：血脑屏障；cAMP：环磷酸腺苷；CRH：促肾上腺皮质激素释放激素；EP：内源性致热原；IFN：干扰素；IL-1：白介素-1；IL-6：白介素-6；IL-10：白介素-10；LC-1：脂皮质蛋白-1；LPS：脂多糖；MAN：中杏仁核；MIP-1：巨噬细胞炎症蛋白-1；NO：一氧化氮；OVLT：终板血管器；PGE：前列腺素 E；POAH：视前区下丘脑前部；TNF：肿瘤坏死因子；VSA：腹中隔；α-MSH：α-黑素细胞刺激素）

（孙丽娜）

# 第五章　应　激

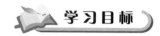

（1）掌握应激和应激原的概念；掌握全身适应反应综合征的概念和分期。

（2）掌握应激的神经内分泌反应及机制、急性期反应和急性期反应蛋白、细胞的热休克反应和热休克蛋白。

（3）掌握应激性溃疡的概念及发病机制。

（4）熟悉应激反应的分类；熟悉应激时机体的代谢及功能变化。

（5）熟悉应激的心理行为反应。

（6）熟悉应激与心血管疾病、精神神经疾病、免疫相关疾病及内分泌和代谢性疾病的关系。

（7）了解应激时其他内分泌反应和免疫反应；了解氧化应激的概念及机制。

（8）了解病理性应激的防治原则。

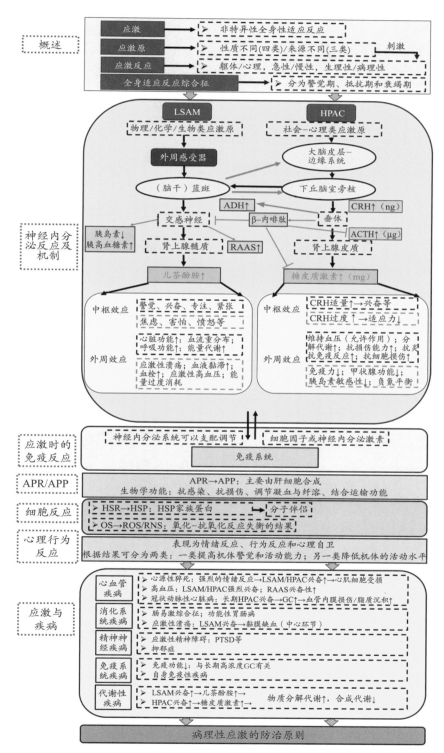

（ACTH:促肾上腺皮质激素;ADH:抗利尿激素;APP:急性期反应蛋白;APR:急性期反应;CA:儿茶酚胺;CHD:冠状动脉性心脏病;CRH:促肾上腺皮质激素释放激素;FGID:功能性胃肠病;GAS:全身适应综合征;GC:糖皮质激素;HPAC:下丘脑-垂体-肾上腺皮质系统;HSP:热休克蛋白;HSR:热休克反应;IBS:肠易激综合征;LC:蓝斑;LSAM:蓝斑-交感-肾上腺髓质系统;PTSD:创伤后应激障碍;PVN:下丘脑室旁核;RAAS:肾素-血管紧张素-醛固酮系统;SCD:心源性猝死）

（孙丽娜）

# 第六章　缺　氧

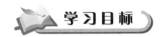

（1）掌握缺氧、发绀和肠源性发绀的概念。

（2）掌握常用血氧指标,包括血氧分压($PO_2$)、血氧容量($CO_2max$)、血氧含量($CO_2$)和血氧饱和度($SO_2$)的概念;掌握血氧指标的正常值、影响因素及数值变化的含义。

（3）掌握缺氧的分类、不同类型缺氧的病因和发病机制。

（4）掌握不同类型缺氧时血氧指标的变化。

（5）掌握缺氧时呼吸系统、循环系统和血液系统的代偿及损伤性变化。

（6）熟悉缺氧时中枢神经系统和组织、细胞的代偿反应及损伤性变化。

（7）了解缺氧治疗的病理生理学基础。

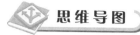

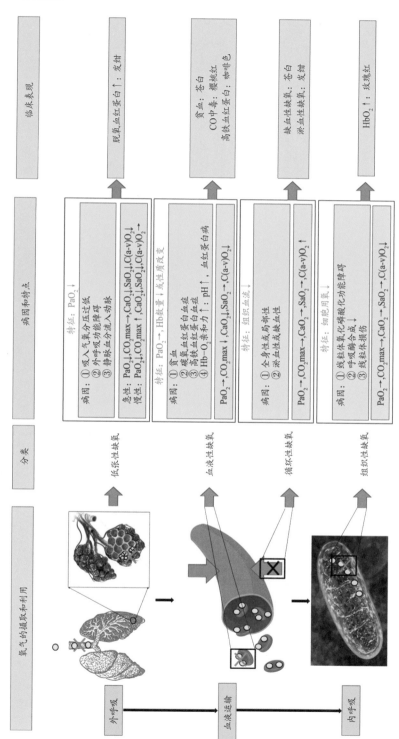

| 氧气的摄取和利用 | | 分类 | 病因和特点 | 临床表现 |

**氧气的摄取和利用**

**外呼吸** → **血液运输** → **内呼吸**

**低张性缺氧**

特征：$PaO_2\downarrow$
病因：①吸入气氧分压过低
②外呼吸功能障碍
③静脉血分流入动脉
急性：$PaO_2\downarrow,CO_2max\rightarrow,CaO_2\downarrow,SaO_2\downarrow,C(a-v)O_2\downarrow$
慢性：$PaO_2\downarrow,CO_2max\uparrow,CaO_2\downarrow,SaO_2\downarrow,C(a-v)O_2\rightarrow$

脱氧血红蛋白↑：发绀

**血液性缺氧**

特征：$PaO_2\rightarrow$，Hb数量↓或性质改变
病因：①贫血
②碳氧血红蛋白血症
③高铁血红蛋白血症
④$Hb-O_2$亲和力↑：$pH\uparrow$，血红蛋白病
$PaO_2\rightarrow,CO_2max\uparrow,CaO_2\downarrow,SaO_2\rightarrow,C(a-v)O_2\downarrow$

贫血：苍白
CO中毒：樱桃红
高铁血红蛋白：咖啡色

**循环性缺氧**

特征：组织血流↓
病因：①全身性或局部性
②淤血性或缺血性
$PaO_2\rightarrow,CO_2max\rightarrow,CaO_2\rightarrow,SaO_2\rightarrow,C(a-v)O_2\uparrow$

缺血性缺氧：苍白
淤血性缺氧：发绀

**组织性缺氧**

特征：细胞用氧
病因：①线粒体氧化磷酸化功能障碍
②呼吸酶合成↓
③线粒体损伤
$PaO_2\rightarrow,CO_2max\rightarrow,CaO_2\rightarrow,SaO_2\rightarrow,C(a-v)O_2\downarrow$

$HbO_2\uparrow$：玫瑰红

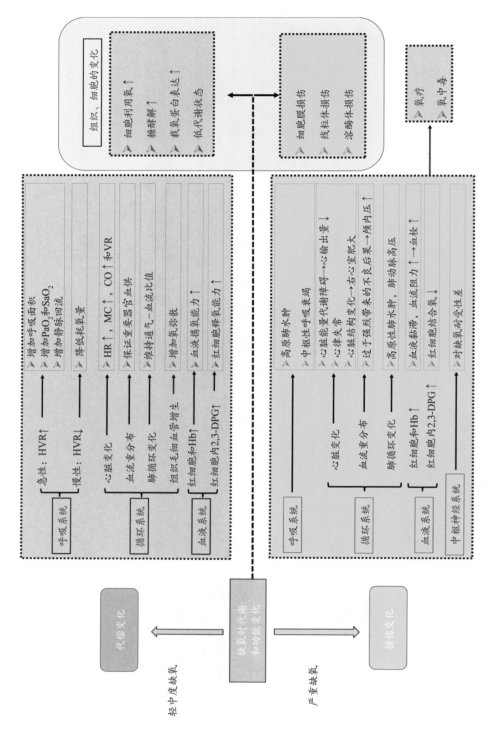

[C(a-v)O₂:动脉-静脉血氧含量差;CaO₂:动脉血氧含量;CNS:中枢神经系统;CO:心输出量;CO₂:血氧含量;CO₂max:血氧容量;Hb:血红蛋白;HR:心率;MC:心肌收缩力;PaO₂:动脉血氧分压;PO₂:血氧分压;SO₂:血氧饱和度;VR:心室重塑]

（孙丽娜）

# 第七章　休　克

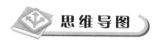

（1）掌握休克的概念及休克发生的始动环节。
（2）掌握休克的分期及各期微循环障碍的发生机制及对机体的影响。
（3）熟悉休克常见的病因及常见的分类。
（4）熟悉休克的细胞分子机制。
（5）熟悉休克时机体功能与代谢变化。
（6）了解失血性休克、感染性休克、过敏性休克和心源性休克的特点及发生机制。
（7）了解休克防治的病理生理学基础。

## 思维导图

### 1.休克的病因及始动环节

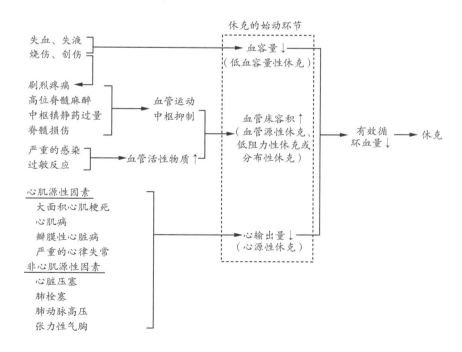

### 2. 休克各期微循环变化的机制

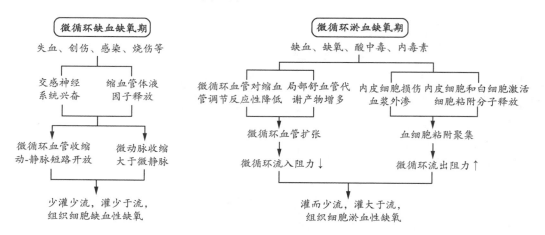

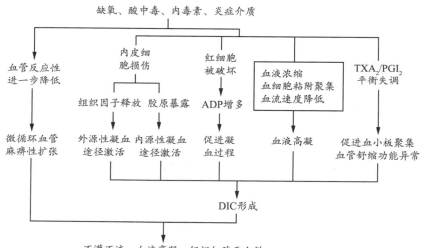

（ADP：二磷酸腺苷；DIC：弥散性血管内凝血；PGI$_2$：前列环素；TXA$_2$：血栓素 A$_2$）

## 3. 休克各期微循环变化对机体的影响

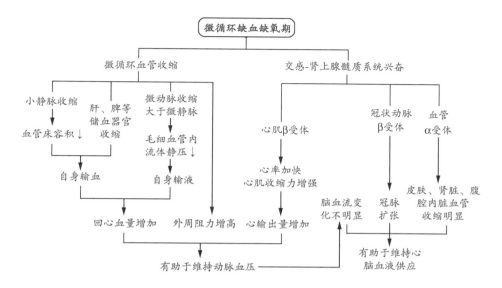

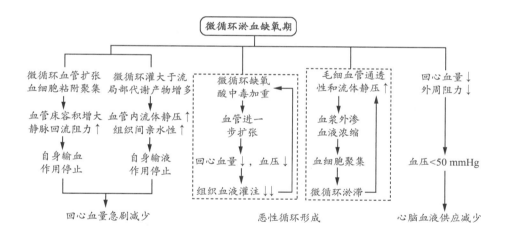

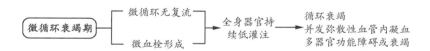

（赵丽梅）

# 第八章　凝血与抗凝血平衡紊乱

## 学习目标

（1）掌握弥散性血管内凝血（DIC）的基本概念、发病机制、功能代谢变化。

（2）熟悉 DIC 的常见病因及影响 DIC 发生、发展的因素。

（3）熟悉机体凝血、抗凝和纤溶系统功能及其平衡紊乱的原因。

（4）了解 DIC 的分型、分期及 DIC 防治的病理生理学基础。

## 思维导图

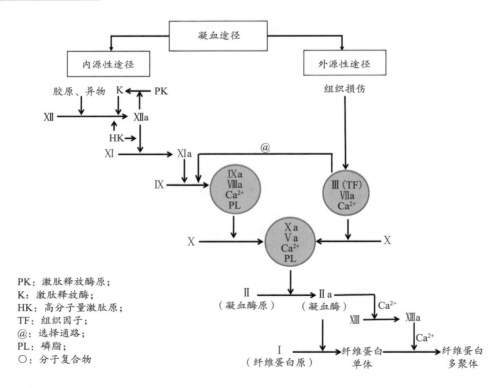

PK：激肽释放酶原；
K：激肽释放酶；
HK：高分子量激肽原；
TF：组织因子；
@：选择通路；
PL：磷脂；
○：分子复合物

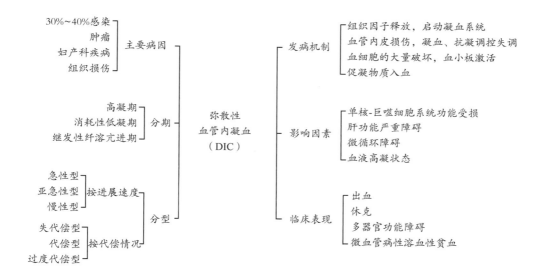

（刘立民　赵丽梅）

# 第九章　缺血-再灌注损伤

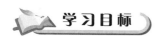

（1）掌握缺血-再灌注损伤的概念及发病机制。

（2）熟悉缺血-再灌注损伤的原因及影响因素。

（3）熟悉缺血-再灌注损伤时机体各器官功能代谢的变化。

（4）了解防治缺血-再灌注损伤的病理生理学基础。

**思维导图**

组织器官缺血后恢复血供
休克微循环疏通和心肺复苏
断肢再植和器官移植 —— 病因
血管再通
体外循环下心、肺手术

缺血时间、侧支循环
需氧程度、再灌注条件 —— 条件

病因及条件

再灌注性心律失常
心肌顿抑 —— 心肌
结构变化

酸中毒
脑细胞水肿、脑水肿
细胞坏死 —— 脑
神经元功能障碍

肺、肝、肾、肠 —— 其他

功能代谢变化

最易受攻击

缺血-再灌注损伤

发生机制

自由基增多

线粒体受损
黄嘌呤氧化酶增多
中性粒细胞呼吸爆发
儿茶酚胺增加和氧化

脂质过氧化增强
蛋白质功能抑制
核酸破坏与DNA断裂

细胞内钙超载

$Na^+/Ca^{2+}$交换异常
儿茶酚胺增多
生物膜损伤

能量代谢障碍
生物膜及蛋白结构分解
加重酸中毒

炎症反应过度激活

趋化因子生成增多
粘附分子表达增加

细胞损伤←炎症细胞释放活性物质
微血管损伤←流变学改变、通透性↑

$Na^+/Ca^{2+}$交换异常

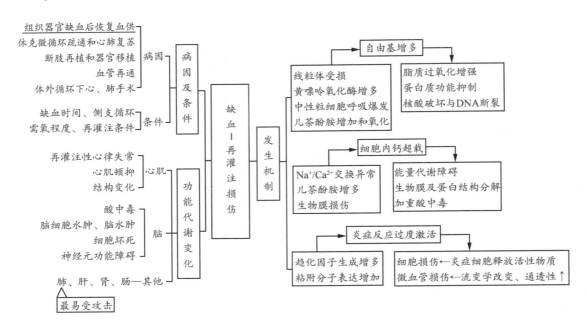

"Forward mode"　　"Reverse mode"

① 直接激活——细胞内高$Na^+$的作用
② 间接激活——细胞内高$H^+$的作用
　　（通过$Na^+/H^+$交换蛋白）

（刘立民　赵丽梅）

# 第十章 心功能不全

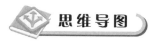 学习目标

（1）掌握心功能不全和心力衰竭的概念。
（2）掌握心功能不全的发生机制,心功能不全时心脏的代偿反应和心外代偿反应。
（3）掌握心功能不全临床表现的病理生理学基础。
（4）熟悉心功能不全的病因、诱因和分类。
（5）熟悉心功能不全时神经体液等的代偿反应。
（6）了解防治心功能不全的病理生理学基础。

思维导图

## 1.心功能不全的病因及诱因

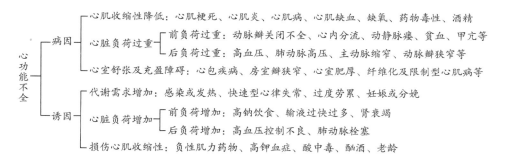

## 2．心功能不全机体的代偿反应

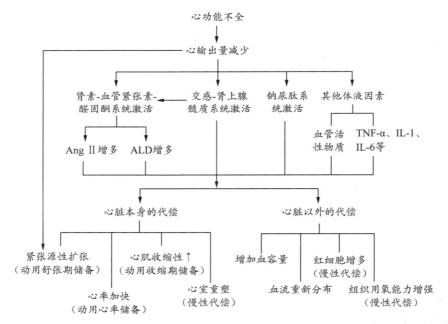

（ALD：醛固酮；Ang Ⅱ：血管紧张素Ⅱ；IL-1：白介素-1；IL-6：白介素-6；TNF-α：肿瘤坏死因子α）

有利作用：一定程度上增加心输出量，维持血压，保证重要器官血液供应，增加组织供氧和用氧。

不利影响：心脏负荷↑，心肌耗氧量↑，冠脉灌流↓，心室充盈↓，心律失常，外周组织缺血，长期心功能失代偿。

## 3．心功能不全的发生机制

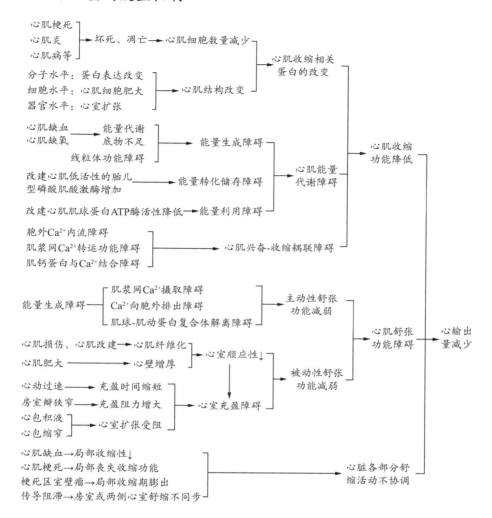

## 4．心功能不全临床表现的病理生理学基础

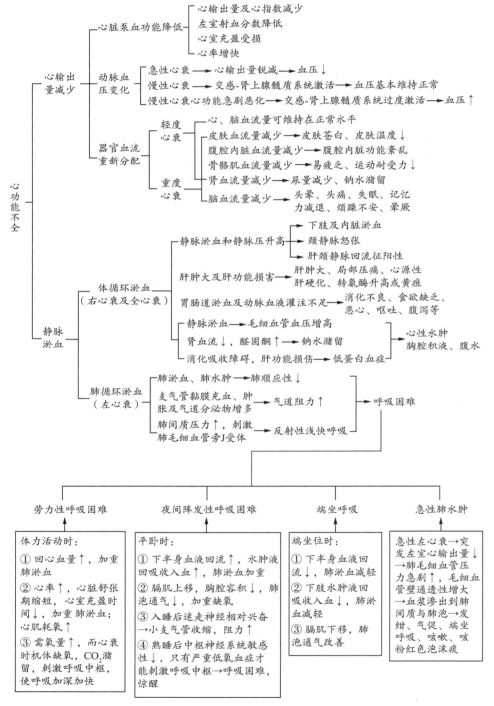

```
心功能不全
├─ 心输出量减少
│   ├─ 心脏泵血功能降低
│   │   ├─ 心输出量及心指数减少
│   │   ├─ 左室射血分数降低
│   │   ├─ 心室充盈受损
│   │   └─ 心率增快
│   ├─ 动脉血压变化
│   │   ├─ 急性心衰 → 心输出量锐减 → 血压↓
│   │   ├─ 慢性心衰 → 交感-肾上腺髓质系统激活 → 血压基本维持正常
│   │   └─ 慢性心衰心功能急剧恶化 → 交感-肾上腺髓质系统过度激活 → 血压↑
│   └─ 器官血流重新分配
│       ├─ 轻度心衰
│       │   ├─ 心、脑血流量可维持在正常水平
│       │   ├─ 皮肤血流量减少 → 皮肤苍白、皮肤温度↓
│       │   ├─ 腹腔内脏血流量减少 → 腹腔内脏功能紊乱
│       │   └─ 骨骼肌血流量减少 → 易疲乏、运动耐受力↓
│       └─ 重度心衰
│           ├─ 肾血流量减少 → 尿量减少、钠水潴留
│           └─ 脑血流量减少 → 头晕、头痛、失眠、记忆力减退、烦躁不安、晕厥
└─ 静脉淤血
    ├─ 体循环淤血（右心衰及全心衰）
    │   ├─ 静脉淤血和静脉压升高
    │   │   ├─ 下肢及内脏淤血
    │   │   ├─ 颈静脉怒张
    │   │   └─ 肝颈静脉回流征阳性
    │   ├─ 肝肿大及肝功能损害 → 肝肿大、局部压痛、心源性肝硬化、转氨酶升高或黄疸
    │   ├─ 胃肠道淤血及动脉血液灌注不足 → 消化不良、食欲缺乏、恶心、呕吐、腹泻等
    │   ├─ 静脉淤血 → 毛细血管血压增高 ┐
    │   ├─ 肾血流↓，醛固酮↑ → 钠水潴留 ┤→ 心性水肿、胸腔积液、腹水
    │   └─ 消化吸收障碍，肝功能损伤 → 低蛋白血症 ┘
    └─ 肺循环淤血（左心衰）
        ├─ 肺淤血、肺水肿 → 肺顺应性↓ ┐
        ├─ 支气管黏膜充血、肿胀及气道分泌物增多 → 气道阻力↑ ┤→ 呼吸困难
        └─ 肺间质压力↑，刺激肺毛细血管旁J受体 → 反射性浅快呼吸 ┘
```

| 劳力性呼吸困难 | 夜间阵发性呼吸困难 | 端坐呼吸 | 急性肺水肿 |
|---|---|---|---|
| 体力活动时：<br><br>①回心血量↑，加重肺淤血<br><br>②心率↑，心脏舒张期缩短，心室充盈时间↓，加重肺淤血；心肌耗氧↑<br><br>③需氧量↑，而心衰时机体缺氧，$CO_2$潴留，刺激呼吸中枢，使呼吸加深加快 | 平卧时：<br><br>①下半身血液回流↑，水肿液回吸收入血↑，肺淤血加重<br><br>②膈肌上移，胸腔容积↓，肺泡通气↓，加重缺氧<br><br>③入睡后迷走神经相对兴奋→小支气管收缩，阻力↑<br><br>④熟睡后中枢神经系统敏感性↓，只有严重低氧血症才能刺激呼吸中枢→呼吸困难，惊醒 | 端坐位时：<br><br>①下半身血液回流↓，肺淤血减轻<br><br>②下肢水肿液回吸收入血↓，肺淤血减轻<br><br>③膈肌下移，肺泡通气改善 | 急性左心衰→突发左室心输出量↓→肺毛细血管压力急剧↑，毛细血管壁通透性增大→血浆渗出到肺间质与肺泡→发绀、气促、端坐呼吸、咳嗽、咳粉红色泡沫痰 |

（赵丽梅）

# 第十一章 肺功能不全

## 学习目标

（1）掌握呼吸衰竭的概念、病因、基本发病机制与机体功能代谢变化。
（2）熟悉呼吸衰竭时的血氧变化。
（3）熟悉急性呼吸窘迫综合征的概念、病因和发病机制。
（4）熟悉慢性阻塞性肺疾病的概念、病因和发病机制。
（5）了解呼吸衰竭防治的病理生理学基础。

## 思维导图

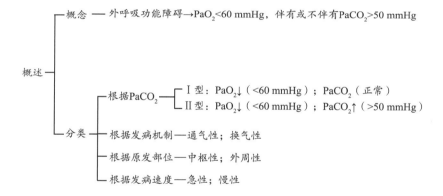

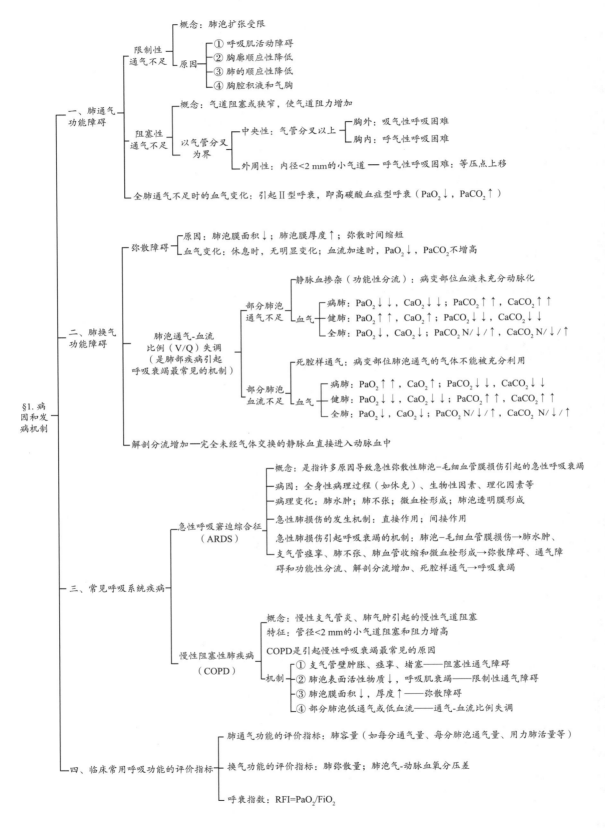

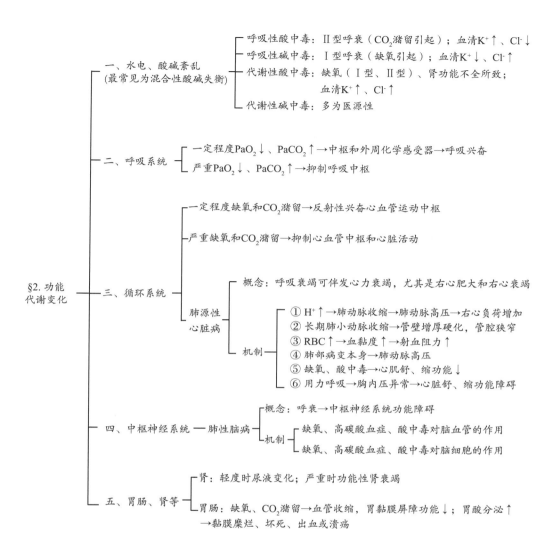

§2. 功能代谢变化

一、水电、酸碱紊乱 (最常见为混合性酸碱失衡)
- 呼吸性酸中毒：Ⅱ型呼衰（$CO_2$潴留引起）；血清$K^+$↑、$Cl^-$↓
- 呼吸性碱中毒：Ⅰ型呼衰（缺氧引起）；血清$K^+$↓、$Cl^-$↑
- 代谢性酸中毒：缺氧（Ⅰ型、Ⅱ型）、肾功能不全所致；血清$K^+$↑、$Cl^-$↑
- 代谢性碱中毒：多为医源性

二、呼吸系统
- 一定程度$PaO_2$↓、$PaCO_2$↑→中枢和外周化学感受器→呼吸兴奋
- 严重$PaO_2$↓、$PaCO_2$↑→抑制呼吸中枢

三、循环系统
- 一定程度缺氧和$CO_2$潴留→反射性兴奋心血管运动中枢
- 严重缺氧和$CO_2$潴留→抑制心血管中枢和心脏活动
- 肺源性心脏病
  - 概念：呼吸衰竭可伴发心力衰竭，尤其是右心肥大和右心衰竭
  - 机制
    - ① $H^+$↑→肺动脉收缩→肺动脉高压→右心负荷增加
    - ② 长期肺小动脉收缩→管壁增厚硬化，管腔狭窄
    - ③ RBC↑→血黏度↑→射血阻力↑
    - ④ 肺部病变本身→肺动脉高压
    - ⑤ 缺氧、酸中毒→心肌舒、缩功能↓
    - ⑥ 用力呼吸→胸内压异常→心脏舒、缩功能障碍

四、中枢神经系统 — 肺性脑病
- 概念：呼衰→中枢神经系统功能障碍
- 机制
  - 缺氧、高碳酸血症、酸中毒对脑血管的作用
  - 缺氧、高碳酸血症、酸中毒对脑细胞的作用

五、胃肠、肾等
- 肾：轻度时尿液变化；严重时功能性肾衰竭
- 胃肠：缺氧、$CO_2$潴留→血管收缩，胃黏膜屏障功能↓；胃酸分泌↑→黏膜糜烂、坏死、出血或溃疡

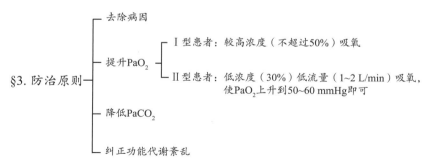

§3. 防治原则
- 去除病因
- 提升$PaO_2$
  - Ⅰ型患者：较高浓度（不超过50%）吸氧
  - Ⅱ型患者：低浓度（30%）低流量（1~2 L/min）吸氧，使$PaO_2$上升到50~60 mmHg即可
- 降低$PaCO_2$
- 纠正功能代谢紊乱

（孙晓东　赵　颖）

# 第十二章　肝功能不全

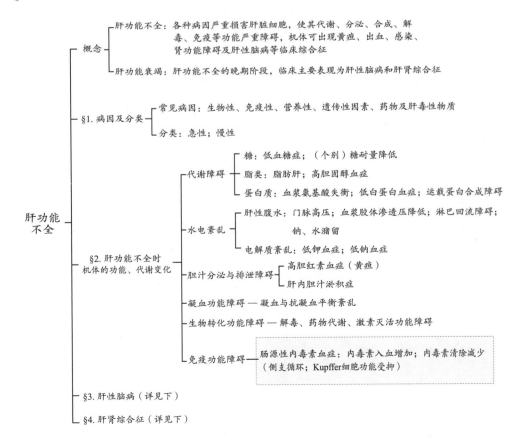

**学习目标**

（1）掌握肝功能不全的概念、肝功能不全时机体功能与代谢变化。
（2）掌握肝性脑病的概念、发病机制及诱因。
（3）熟悉肝功能不全的病因与分类。
（4）熟悉肝性脑病的分期与临床表现。
（5）熟悉肝肾综合征的概念、病因和发病机制。
（6）了解防治肝功能不全的病理生理学基础。

**思维导图**

肝功能不全

- 概念
  - 肝功能不全：各种病因严重损害肝脏细胞，使其代谢、分泌、合成、解毒、免疫等功能严重障碍，机体可出现黄疸、出血、感染、肾功能障碍及肝性脑病等临床综合征
  - 肝功能衰竭：肝功能不全的晚期阶段，临床主要表现为肝性脑病和肝肾综合征
- §1.病因及分类
  - 常见病因：生物性、免疫性、营养性、遗传性因素、药物及肝毒性物质
  - 分类：急性；慢性
- §2.肝功能不全时机体的功能、代谢变化
  - 代谢障碍
    - 糖：低血糖症；（个别）糖耐量降低
    - 脂类：脂肪肝；高胆固醇血症
    - 蛋白质：血浆氨基酸失衡；低白蛋白血症；运载蛋白合成障碍
  - 水电紊乱
    - 肝性腹水：门脉高压；血浆胶体渗透压降低；淋巴回流障碍；钠、水潴留
    - 电解质紊乱：低钾血症；低钠血症
  - 胆汁分泌与排泄障碍
    - 高胆红素血症（黄疸）
    - 肝内胆汁淤积症
  - 凝血功能障碍——凝血与抗凝血平衡紊乱
  - 生物转化功能障碍——解毒、药物代谢、激素灭活功能障碍
  - 免疫功能障碍
    - 肠源性内毒素血症：内毒素入血增加；内毒素清除减少（侧支循环；Kupffer细胞功能受抑）
- §3.肝性脑病（详见下）
- §4.肝肾综合征（详见下）

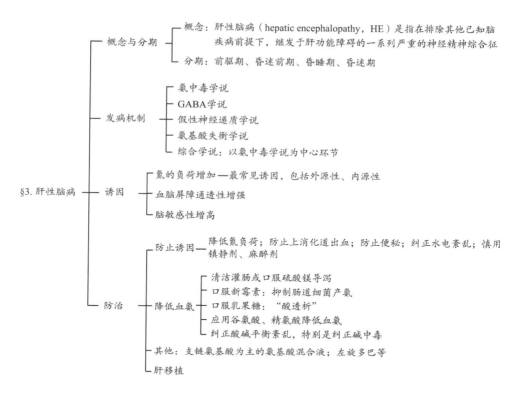

§3.肝性脑病

概念与分期
- 概念：肝性脑病（hepatic encephalopathy，HE）是指在排除其他已知脑疾病前提下，继发于肝功能障碍的一系列严重的神经精神综合征
- 分期：前驱期、昏迷前期、昏睡期、昏迷期

发病机制
- 氨中毒学说
- GABA学说
- 假性神经递质学说
- 氨基酸失衡学说
- 综合学说：以氨中毒学说为中心环节

诱因
- 氨的负荷增加——最常见诱因，包括外源性、内源性
- 血脑屏障通透性增强
- 脑敏感性增高

防治
- 防止诱因——降低氮负荷；防止上消化道出血；防止便秘；纠正水电紊乱；慎用镇静剂、麻醉剂
- 降低血氨
  - 清洁灌肠或口服硫酸镁导泻
  - 口服新霉素：抑制肠道细菌产氨
  - 口服乳果糖："酸透析"
  - 应用谷氨酸、精氨酸降低血氨
  - 纠正酸碱平衡紊乱，特别是纠正碱中毒
- 其他：支链氨基酸为主的氨基酸混合液；左旋多巴等
- 肝移植

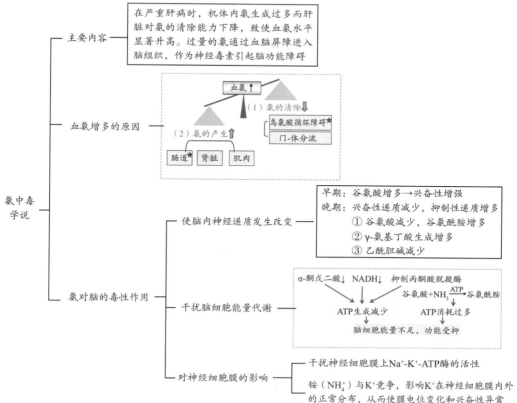

氨中毒学说

主要内容
在严重肝病时，机体内氨生成过多而肝脏对氨的清除能力下降，致使血氨水平显著升高。过量的氨通过血脑屏障进入脑组织，作为神经毒素引起脑功能障碍

血氨增多的原因

血氨↑
- （1）氨的清除↓
  - 鸟氨酸循环障碍★
  - 门-体分流
- （2）氨的产生↑
  - 肠道★　肾脏　肌肉

氨对脑的毒性作用

使脑内神经递质发生改变
早期：谷氨酸增多→兴奋性增强
晚期：兴奋性递质减少，抑制性递质增多
① 谷氨酸减少，谷氨酰胺增多
② γ-氨基丁酸生成增多
③ 乙酰胆碱减少

干扰脑细胞能量代谢
α-酮戊二酸↓　NADH↓　抑制丙酮酸脱羧酶　谷氨酸+NH₃ →ATP→ 谷氨酰胺
ATP生成减少　　　　ATP消耗过多
脑细胞能量不足，功能受抑

对神经细胞膜的影响
- 干扰神经细胞膜上Na⁺-K⁺-ATP酶的活性
- 铵（NH₄⁺）与K⁺竞争，影响K⁺在神经细胞膜内外的正常分布，从而使膜电位变化和兴奋性异常

GABA学说
- GABA是脑内最主要的一种抑制性神经递质

- 突触后抑制
  突触前神经元兴奋，GABA从囊泡内释放，与突触后神经元GABA-R结合，使突触后膜对Cl⁻的通透性增大，Cl⁻内流增加，产生超极化阻滞

- 突触前抑制
  GABA作用于突触前的轴突末梢时，也可使轴突膜对Cl⁻通透性增高，但由于轴浆内Cl⁻浓度高于轴突外，Cl⁻外流，产生去极化，使神经冲动到达神经末梢时，释放神经递质的量减少

- 肝性脑病时，GABA能神经元抑制性活动增强
  血中GABA增高
  脑突触后膜GABA-A受体活性↑，结合能力增强

假性神经递质学说
- 意识维持的基础
  结构基础：脑干网状结构上行激动系统
  物质基础：多巴胺和去甲肾上腺素等神经递质

- 假性神经递质
  苯乙醇胺和羟苯乙醇胺（鳝胺），化学结构和正常神经递质相似，但作用极弱，不能推持正常唤醒功能

- 肝衰竭时假性神经递质增多的原因
  正常时：胺类物质从肠道吸收，经门静脉到达肝脏，经肝脏单胺氧化酶的作用氧化分解而被清除
  肝衰竭时：食物腐败↑→产苯乙胺、酪胺↑，肝解毒功能↓；门-体分流，绕过肝脏→体循环中苯乙胺、酪胺↑，入脑，使脑中苯乙胺、酪胺增多→在β-羟化酶作用下，在侧链β位置上被羟化，生成苯乙醇胺、羟苯乙醇胺↑

- 假性神经递质的毒性作用

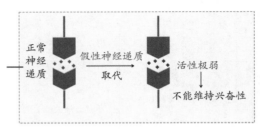

血浆氨基酸失衡的表现
① 芳香族氨基酸（AAA）（苯丙氨酸、酪氨酸、色氨酸）增多
② 支链氨基酸（BCAA）（缬氨酸、亮氨酸、异亮氨酸）减少

氨基酸失衡学说

血浆氨基酸失衡的发生机制

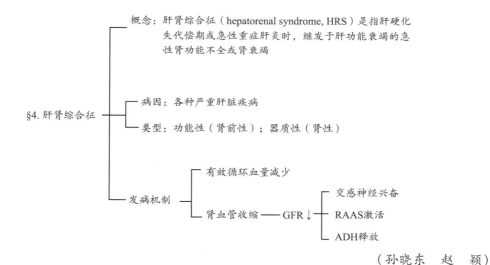

血浆氨基酸失衡导致肝性脑病的机制
由AAA入脑增多引起
① 生成假性神经递质苯乙醇胺和羟苯乙醇胺（鳝胺）增多
② 多巴胺和去甲肾上腺素生成减少
③ 抑制性递质5-羟色胺增多

§4.肝肾综合征

概念：肝肾综合征（hepatorenal syndrome, HRS）是指肝硬化失代偿期或急性重症肝炎时，继发于肝功能衰竭的急性肾功能不全或肾衰竭

病因：各种严重肝脏疾病

类型：功能性（肾前性）；器质性（肾性）

发病机制

有效循环血量减少

肾血管收缩 —— GFR↓

交感神经兴奋

RAAS激活

ADH释放

（孙晓东 赵 颖）

# 第十三章　肾功能不全

## 学习目标

（1）掌握急性肾功能衰竭的概念、分类、病因、发病机制、发病过程及功能代谢变化。

（2）掌握慢性肾功能衰竭的概念、病因、发病机制及功能代谢变化。

（3）熟悉肾功能不全的基本发病环节，慢性肾功能不全发展过程及分期，尿毒症的概念、尿毒症毒素。

（4）了解急、慢性肾功能不全防治的病理生理学基础。

（5）了解尿毒症的功能代谢变化及其防治的病理生理学基础。

## 思维导图

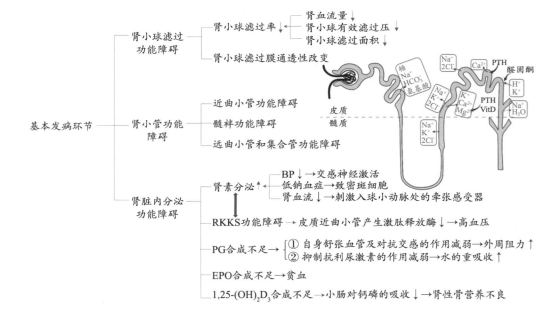

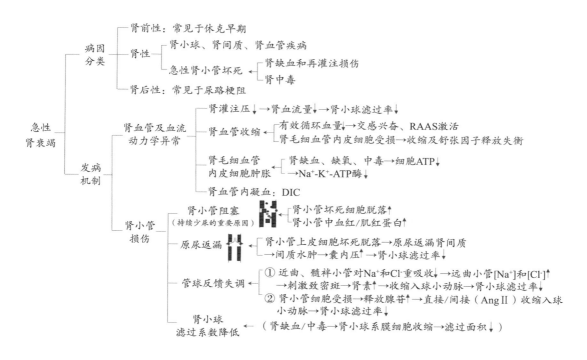

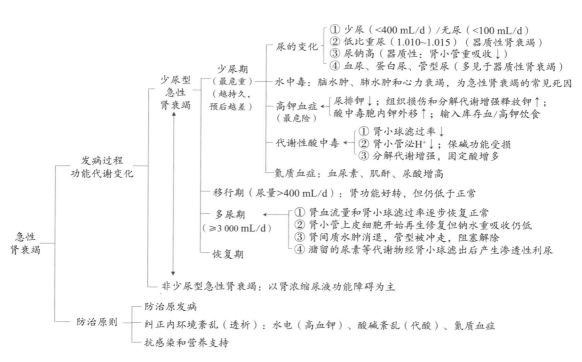

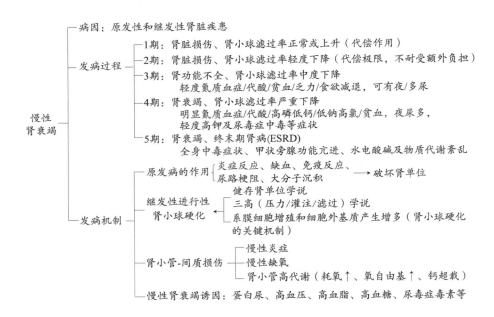

```
                    ┌─ 病因：原发性和继发性肾脏疾患
                    │                 ┌─ 1期：肾脏损伤、肾小球滤过率正常或上升（代偿作用）
                    │                 ├─ 2期：肾脏损伤、肾小球滤过率轻度下降（代偿极限，不耐受额外负担）
                    │                 ├─ 3期：肾功能不全、肾小球滤过率中度下降
                    │                 │       轻度氮质血症/代酸/贫血/乏力/食欲减退，可有夜/多尿
                    ├─ 发病过程 ───────┤
                    │                 ├─ 4期：肾衰竭、肾小球滤过率严重下降
                    │                 │       明显氮质血症/代酸/高磷低钙/低钠高氯/贫血，夜尿多，
                    │                 │       轻度高钾及尿毒症中毒等症状
          慢性      │                 └─ 5期：肾衰竭、终末期肾病(ESRD)
          肾衰竭 ───┤                         全身中毒症状、甲状旁腺功能亢进、水电酸碱及物质代谢紊乱
                    │                 ┌─ 原发病的作用 ┬ 炎症反应、缺血、免疫反应 ──→ 破坏肾单位
                    │                 │               └ 尿路梗阻、大分子沉积
                    │                 │                   ┌ 健存肾单位学说
                    │                 ├─ 继发性进行性 ────┤ 三高（压力/灌注/滤过）学说
                    │                 │   肾小球硬化      └ 系膜细胞增殖和细胞外基质产生增多（肾小球硬化
                    └─ 发病机制 ──────┤                                                   的关键机制）
                                      │                   ┌ 慢性炎症
                                      ├─ 肾小管-间质损伤 ─┤ 慢性缺氧
                                      │                   └ 肾小管高代谢（耗氧↑、氧自由基↑、钙超载）
                                      └─ 慢性肾衰竭诱因：蛋白尿、高血压、高血脂、高血糖、尿毒症毒素等
```

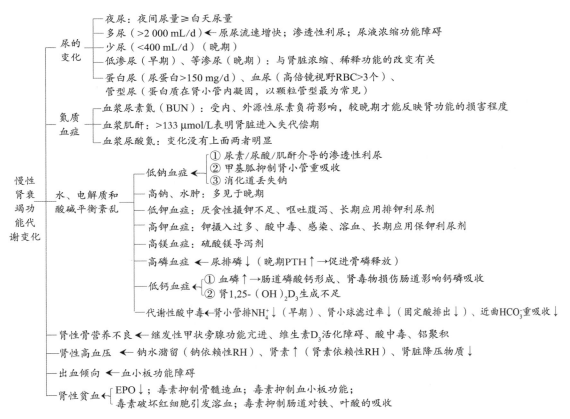

```
                    ┌─ 夜尿：夜间尿量≥白天尿量
                    │       ┌─ 多尿（>2 000 mL/d）←原尿流速增快；渗透性利尿；尿液浓缩功能障碍
                    ├─ 尿的 ┤  少尿（<400 mL/d）（晚期）
                    │  变化 │  低渗尿（早期）、等渗尿（晚期）：与肾脏浓缩、稀释功能的改变有关
                    │       └─ 蛋白尿（尿蛋白>150 mg/d）、血尿（高倍镜视野RBC>3个）、
                    │          管型尿（蛋白质在肾小管内凝固，以颗粒管型最为常见）
                    │       ┌─ 血浆尿素氮（BUN）：受内、外源性尿素负荷影响，较晚期才能反映肾功能的损害程度
                    ├─ 氮质 ┤  血浆肌酐：>133 μmol/L表明肾脏进入失代偿期
                    │  血症 └─ 血浆尿酸氮：变化没有上面两者明显
                    │                         ┌ ① 尿素/尿酸/肌酐介导的渗透性利尿
                    │              ┌─ 低钠血症 ┤ ② 甲基胍抑制肾小管重吸收
                    │              │           └ ③ 消化道丢失钠
          慢性      │              ├─ 高钠、水肿：多见于晚期
          肾衰      │  水、电解质和├─ 低钾血症：厌食性摄钾不足、呕吐腹泻、长期应用排钾利尿剂
          竭功 ─────┤  酸碱平衡紊乱├─ 高钾血症：钾摄入过多、酸中毒、感染、溶血、长期应用保钾利尿剂
          能代      │              ├─ 高镁血症：硫酸镁导泻剂
          谢变化    │              ├─ 高磷血症 ←尿排磷↓（晚期PTH↑→促进骨磷释放）
                    │              │           ┌ ① 血磷↑→肠道磷酸钙形成、肾毒物损伤肠道影响钙磷吸收
                    │              ├─ 低钙血症 ┤ ② 肾1,25-(OH)₂D₃生成不足
                    │              └─ 代谢性酸中毒←肾小管排NH₄⁺↓（早期）、肾小球滤过率↓（固定酸排出↓）、近曲HCO₃⁻重吸收↓
                    ├─ 肾性骨营养不良 ←继发性甲状旁腺功能亢进、维生素D₃活化障碍、酸中毒、铝聚积
                    ├─ 肾性高血压 ← 钠水潴留（钠依赖性RH）、肾素↑（肾素依赖性RH）、肾脏降压物质↓
                    ├─ 出血倾向 ←血小板功能障碍
                    └─ 肾性贫血 ←┬ EPO↓；毒素抑制骨髓造血；毒素抑制血小板功能；
                                 └ 毒素破坏红细胞引发溶血；毒素抑制肠道对铁、叶酸的吸收
```

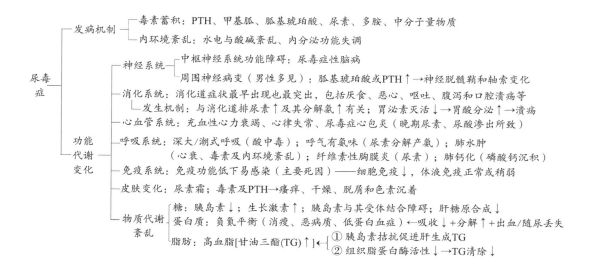

尿毒症
　　├─ 发病机制
　　│　　├─ 毒素蓄积：PTH、甲基胍、胍基琥珀酸、尿素、多胺、中分子量物质
　　│　　└─ 内环境紊乱：水电与酸碱紊乱、内分泌功能失调
　　└─ 功能代谢变化
　　　　├─ 神经系统
　　　　│　　├─ 中枢神经系统功能障碍：尿毒症性脑病
　　　　│　　└─ 周围神经病变（男性多见）：胍基琥珀酸或PTH↑→神经脱髓鞘和轴索变化
　　　　├─ 消化系统：消化道症状最早出现也最突出，包括厌食、恶心、呕吐、腹泻和口腔溃疡等
　　　　│　　└─ 发生机制：与消化道排尿素↑及其分解氨↑有关；胃泌素灭活↓→胃酸分泌↑→溃疡
　　　　├─ 心血管系统：充血性心力衰竭、心律失常、尿毒症心包炎（晚期尿素、尿酸渗出所致）
　　　　├─ 呼吸系统：深大/潮式呼吸（酸中毒）；呼气有氨味（尿素分解产氨）；肺水肿（心衰、毒素及内环境紊乱）；纤维素性胸膜炎（尿素）；肺钙化（磷酸钙沉积）
　　　　├─ 免疫系统：免疫功能低下易感染（主要死因）——细胞免疫↓，体液免疫正常或稍弱
　　　　├─ 皮肤变化：尿素霜；毒素及PTH→瘙痒、干燥、脱屑和色素沉着
　　　　└─ 物质代谢紊乱
　　　　　　├─ 糖：胰岛素↓；生长激素↑；胰岛素与其受体结合障碍；肝糖原合成↓
　　　　　　├─ 蛋白质：负氮平衡（消瘦、恶病质、低蛋白血症）←吸收↓+分解↑+出血/随尿丢失
　　　　　　└─ 脂肪：高血脂[甘油三酯(TG)↑]←① 胰岛素拮抗促进肝生成TG　② 组织脂蛋白酶活性↓→TG清除↓

慢性肾衰竭和尿毒症的防治原则
　　├─ ① 治疗原发病，改善肾功能
　　├─ ② 消除加重肾损伤的因素
　　├─ ③ 饮食与营养治疗：优质低蛋白高热量，控制磷、钾、嘌呤及脂质的摄入
　　├─ ④ 透析治疗（血液透析、腹膜透析）
　　└─ ⑤ 肾移植

（AngⅡ：血管紧张素Ⅱ；BP：血压；DIC：弥散性血管内凝血；EPO：促红细胞生成素；PG：前列腺素；PTH：甲状旁腺激素；RH：肾性高血压；RKKS：肾激肽释放酶-激肽系统）

（郑　栋　赵　颖）

# 第十四章　脑功能不全

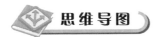

（1）掌握脑功能不全、认知与意识障碍的概念。

（2）掌握学习记忆障碍的发病机制。

（3）掌握意识障碍的发病机制。

（4）熟悉认知障碍的病因、临床表现及其对机体的影响。

（5）熟悉意识障碍的病因、临床表现及其对机体的影响。

（6）了解防治认知与意识障碍的病理生理学基础。

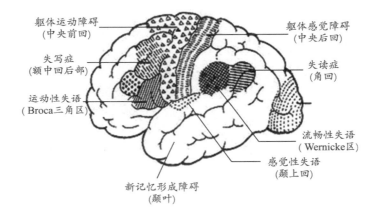

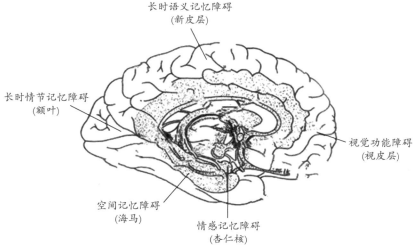

长时语义记忆障碍
(新皮层)

长时情节记忆障碍
(额叶)

视觉功能障碍
(视皮层)

空间记忆障碍
(海马)

情感记忆障碍
(杏仁核)

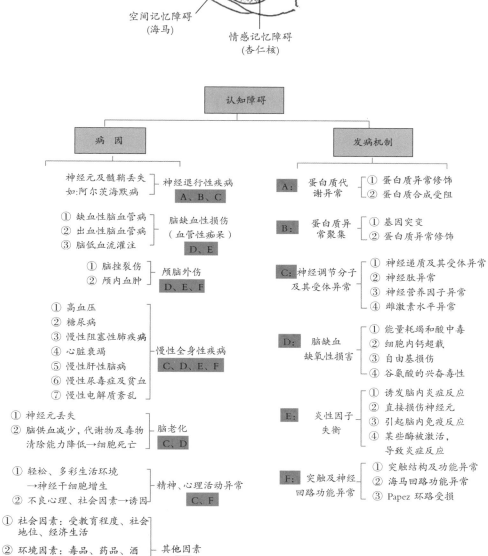

认知障碍

病 因

神经元及髓鞘丢失
如:阿尔茨海默病 — 神经退行性疾病
A、B、C

① 缺血性脑血管病
② 出血性脑血管病 — 脑缺血性损伤
③ 脑低血流灌注 (血管性痴呆)
D、E

① 脑挫裂伤
② 颅内血肿 — 颅脑外伤
D、E、F

① 高血压
② 糖尿病
③ 慢性阻塞性肺疾病
④ 心脏衰竭 — 慢性全身性疾病
⑤ 慢性肝性脑病 C、D、E、F
⑥ 慢性尿毒症及贫血
⑦ 慢性电解质紊乱

① 神经元丢失
② 脑供血减少,代谢物及毒物 — 脑老化
清除能力降低→细胞死亡 C、D

① 轻松、多彩生活环境
→神经干细胞增生 — 精神、心理活动异常
② 不良心理、社会因素→诱因 C、F

① 社会因素:受教育程度、社会
地位、经济生活
② 环境因素:毒品、药品、酒 — 其他因素
精、重金属 C
③ 性别:慢性病、雌激素

发病机制

A: 蛋白质代谢异常 — ① 蛋白质异常修饰
② 蛋白质合成受阻

B: 蛋白质异常聚集 — ① 基因突变
② 蛋白质异常修饰

C: 神经调节分子及其受体异常
① 神经递质及其受体异常
② 神经肽异常
③ 神经营养因子异常
④ 雌激素水平异常

D: 脑缺血缺氧性损害
① 能量耗竭和酸中毒
② 细胞内钙超载
③ 自由基损伤
④ 谷氨酸的兴奋毒性

E: 炎性因子失衡
① 诱发脑内炎症反应
② 直接损伤神经元
③ 引起脑内免疫反应
④ 某些酶被激活,导致炎症反应

F: 突触及神经回路功能异常
① 突触结构及功能异常
② 海马回路功能异常
③ Papez 环路受损

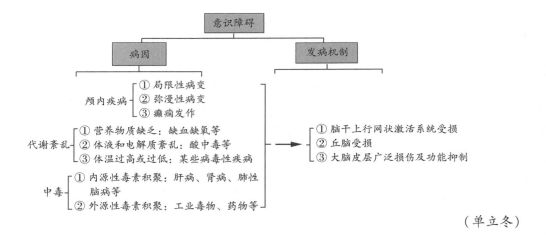

（单立冬）

# 第十五章　多器官功能障碍

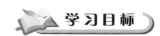 **学习目标**

（1）掌握多器官功能障碍综合征（MODS）的概念及基本发病机制。

（2）熟悉 MODS 的病因、分类及各系统器官的功能代谢变化。

（3）了解 MODS 防治的病理生理基础。

**思维导图**

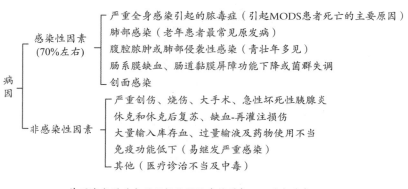

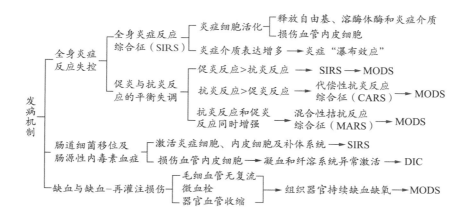

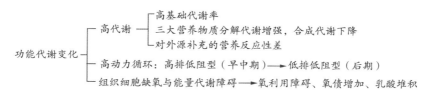

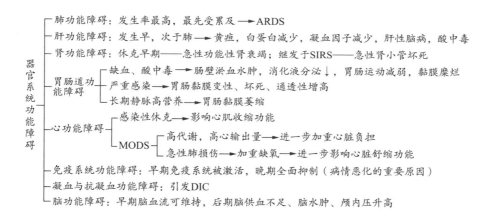

（ARDS：急性呼吸窘迫综合征；CARS：代偿性抗炎反应综合征；DIC：弥散性血管内凝血；MARS：混合性拮抗反应综合征；MODS：多器官功能障碍综合征；SIRS：全身炎症反应综合征）

（赵丽梅）

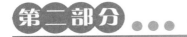

# 案例分析题

## 第一章　疾病概论

### 案例分析选择题（多选一）

1. 患者,60 岁男性,因肺炎住院治疗,已吸烟 40 年。

（1）下列哪项是该患者的致病因素？

    A. 理化因素　　　　　　　　　　B. 生物因素

    C. 营养因素　　　　　　　　　　D. 先天因素

    E. 遗传因素

（2）下列哪项是该患者发病的条件？

    A. 细菌感染　　　　　　　　　　B. 病毒感染

    C. 吸烟　　　　　　　　　　　　D. 血压升高

    E. 心律失常

（3）该疾病体现了下列哪种发病规律？

    A. 损伤与抗损伤失衡　　　　　　B. 整体与局部

    C. 恶性循环　　　　　　　　　　D. 相互联系

    E. 相互转化

（4）该患者年龄对疾病的影响不包括下列哪项？

    A. 机体储备的下降　　　　　　　B. 机体内稳态调控能力的下降

    C. 年龄导致的反应迟钝　　　　　D. 机体对外环境适应能力的下降

    E. 机体免疫力的持续

（5）下列哪项是该患者体内疾病的转归？

    A. 康复　　　　　　　　　　　　B. 健康

    C. 疾病　　　　　　　　　　　　D. 康复/死亡

    E. 死亡

2. 患者,60 岁女性,肥胖、高血压、高血脂,多年前患急性心肌梗死,后发展为慢性心力衰竭。

（1）下列哪项是该患者的致病因素？

  A. 理化因素         B. 生物因素

  C. 营养因素         D. 先天因素

  E. 遗传因素

（2）下列哪项是该患者发病的病因？

  A. 肥胖           B. 高血压

  C. 心肌梗死         D. 高血脂

  E. 衰老

（3）肥胖、高血压、高血脂不是发生急性心肌梗死的_____。

  A. 病因           B. 条件

  C. 诱因           D. 危险因素

  E. 结果

（4）本案例中,心肌梗死是该患者发生慢性心力衰竭的_____。

  A. 病因           B. 条件

  C. 诱因           D. 一般条件

  E. 结果

（5）该疾病的发生机制不包括下列哪项？

  A. 软组织机制        B. 神经机制

  C. 体液机制         D. 细胞机制

  E. 分子机制

3. 35 岁女性,长期吸烟饮酒,意外怀孕产下一名单纯唇裂的女婴。

（1）导致该患儿发生唇裂的因素为下列哪项？

  A. 社会-心理因素      B. 免疫因素

  C. 营养因素         D. 先天因素

  E. 遗传因素

（2）研究发现,吸烟(包括二手烟)导致胎儿发生唇裂的概率提升了 1 倍。吸烟是该患儿出现唇裂的_____。

  A. 病因           B. 条件

  C. 诱因           D. 危险因素

  E. 结果

（3）动物模型研究发现,成纤维细胞因子与骨形态发生蛋白通路可能参与了唇腭裂的发生。这些研究揭示了该疾病的哪种机制？

  A. 免疫机制         B. 神经机制

  C. 体液机制         D. 细胞机制

  E. 分子机制

4. 15 岁女孩,因 β-珠蛋白基因突变引发的地中海贫血接受骨髓移植配型半相合的脐带血干细胞治疗。在骨髓移植后 1 个月突发移植排斥与感染而不幸离世。

(1) 导致该患儿发生地中海贫血的因素为下列哪项?

    A. 社会-心理因素          B. 免疫因素

    C. 营养因素              D. 先天因素

    E. 遗传因素

(2) 导致该患儿发生地中海贫血的发病规律是下列哪项?

    A. 损伤与抗损伤        B. 整体与局部

    C. 恶性循环             D. 内稳态失衡

    E. 相互转化

(3) 导致该患儿发生移植排斥的因素为下列哪项?

    A. 理化因素             B. 生物因素

    C. 免疫因素             D. 环境生态因素

    E. 社会-心理因素

(4) 导致该患儿骨髓移植后发生移植排斥与感染的发病规律是下列哪项?

    A. 损伤与抗损伤        B. 整体与局部

    C. 因果交替             D. 相互转化

    E. 以上都不是

5. 已婚中年女性,因严重烫伤入院。该患者出现局部感染及白细胞计数升高,并有高烧表现,经治疗后恢复。但其毁容后性情大变,离异后患上抑郁症。

(1) 该患者脸部烫伤后出现高烧体现了下列哪个发病规律?

    A. 相互转化             B. 内稳态失衡

    C. 局部与整体关联       D. 因果交替

    E. 以上都不是

(2) "离异"是该患者发生抑郁的_____。

    A. 原因                B. 结果

    C. 致病因素             D. 病因

    E. 诱因

(3) 导致该患者患上抑郁症的因素是下列哪项?

    A. 社会-心理因素        B. 免疫因素

    C. 营养因素             D. 先天因素

    E. 生物因素

**参考答案**

**案例分析选择题(多选一)**

1. BCAED; 2. CCEAA; 3. DDE; 4. EDCC; 5. CEA

(赵 颖)

# 第二章 水、电解质代谢紊乱

## ◇ 水、钠代谢紊乱

### 案例分析选择题（多选一）

1. 患儿2岁,轮状病毒感染,高烧,上吐下泻,未进食,仅补充了少量葡萄糖水。

（1）该患儿最易发生何种水、电解质代谢紊乱?

  A. 高渗性脱水      B. 低渗性脱水

  C. 等渗性脱水      D. 水中毒

  E. 盐中毒

（2）患儿体液可能发生的变化是下列哪项?

  A. 细胞内液减少     B. 细胞外液减少

  C. 血浆不变       D. 细胞内液不变

  E. 以上都不对

（3）患儿的何种症状可帮助判断其是否发生了水、电解质代谢紊乱?

  A. 面部潮红       B. 呼吸急促

  C. 口渴,尿少      D. 眼窝内陷,皮肤无弹性

  E. 下肢水肿

（4）该患儿最易发生何种危险病症?

  A. 休克        B. 心力衰竭

  C. 肾衰竭       D. 肝衰竭

  E. 内出血

（5）医生应该如何纠正此水、电解质代谢紊乱?

  A. 补充5%葡萄糖    B. 补充2.5%葡萄糖

  C. 补充0.9%生理盐水   D. 补充0.5%生理盐水

  E. 单纯补充水分

2. 中年男性,职业为快递员,平时身体健康,夏天某日忘记带水杯,工作时大量出汗,有明显的口渴感。

（1）该男性最易发生何种水、电解质代谢紊乱?

  A. 高渗性脱水      B. 低渗性脱水

  C. 等渗性脱水      D. 高血钾

  E. 代谢性酸中毒

（2）该男性体液可能发生的变化是下列哪项？

    A．细胞内液减少            B．细胞外液减少

    C．血浆减少               D．细胞内液不变

    E．以上都不对

（3）该男性的何种症状可帮助判断其是否发生了水、电解质代谢紊乱？

    A．面部潮红             B．呼吸急促

    C．尿少                D．眼窝内陷，皮肤无弹性

    E．下肢水肿

（4）下列哪项检测结果最可能是该男子的？

    A．血［$Na^+$］160 mmol/L       B．血［$K^+$］5.8 mmol/L

    C．心率 120 次/min         D．血压 100/70 mmHg

    E．无尿钠

（5）医生应该如何纠正此水、电解质代谢紊乱？

    A．仅补充 5% 葡萄糖        B．仅补充 2.5% 葡萄糖

    C．仅补充 0.9% 生理盐水     D．仅补充 0.5% 生理盐水

    E．口服补水，糖盐并用

3. 出生后尚未足月的男婴，尽管饮食正常却精神不振并出现明显的脱水貌。血检结合尿检确诊为高血钾型肾小管酸中毒。

（1）该婴儿不会出现下列哪种疾病状态？

    A．代谢性酸中毒          B．高氯血症

    C．低渗性脱水            D．高渗性脱水

    E．高血钾

（2）该婴儿的血浆检测结果不可能是下列哪项？

    A．［$Na^+$］151 mmol/L       B．［$Na^+$］139 mmol/L

    C．［$Na^+$］130 mmol/L       D．渗透压 295 mmol/L

    E．渗透压 285 mmol/L

（3）下列哪个机制可能参与该婴儿脱水的发生？

    A．摄入不足            B．经皮肤丢失

    C．经肾远曲小管及集合管钠水重吸收减少

    D．经肾近曲小管钠水重吸收减少     E．体液分布改变

（4）该婴儿出现病症可能是下列哪个神经体液因子分泌不足的结果？

    A．醛固酮              B．去甲肾上腺素

    C．肾素                D．血管紧张素

    E．抗利尿激素

4. 患儿 5 岁,因恶心、呕吐、全身乏力去医院就诊。患儿 10 天前患上呼吸道感染。尿检发现血尿与蛋白尿,诊断为急性肾小球肾炎。

（1）该患儿如果出现水肿,最早出现在身体的哪个部位?

　　A. 眼睑或面部　　　　　　　　　B. 上肢

　　C. 肺部　　　　　　　　　　　　D. 腿部

　　E. 腹部

（2）该患儿如果出现水肿,下列哪项变化参与了水肿的发生?

　　A. 毛细血管流体静压增高　　　　B. 微血管壁通透性增加

　　C. 淋巴回流受阻　　　　　　　　D. 血浆胶体渗透压降低

　　E. 以上都不是

（3）下列哪个机制是该患儿发生水肿的机制?

　　A. 肾血流量下降　　　　　　　　B. 肾小球滤过率下降

　　C. 肾近曲小管钠水重吸收增加　　D. 肾远曲小管钠水重吸收增加

　　E. 以上都是

（4）该患儿如果出现水肿,下列有关此水肿的说法哪项不正确?

　　A. 水肿液为漏出液　　　　　　　B. 该水肿为显性水肿

　　C. 该水肿为凹陷性水肿　　　　　D. 患者的水肿可能为全身性水肿

　　E. 以上都不是

5. 中年女性,因尿路感染服用抗生素与镇痛剂并大量饮水。随后患者出现进行性的颤抖与神志恍惚,呕吐数次,并出现明显的语言障碍。

（1）该患者发生了何种水、电解质代谢紊乱?

　　A. 高渗性脱水　　　　　　　　　B. 低渗性脱水

　　C. 等渗性脱水　　　　　　　　　D. 水中毒

　　E. 盐中毒

（2）该患者体液可能发生的变化是下列哪项?

　　A. 细胞内液增多　　　　　　　　B. 细胞外液减少

　　C. 血浆减少　　　　　　　　　　D. 细胞内液不变

　　E. 细胞内液减少

（3）导致该患者出现精神恍惚、呕吐并出现语言障碍的原因是下列哪项?

　　A. 脑细胞脱水　　　　　　　　　B. 脑脊液压力减少

　　C. 颅内压降低　　　　　　　　　D. 脑细胞与组织水肿

　　E. 以上都不是

（4）下列哪个机制不会导致该患者出现精神恍惚、呕吐及语言障碍?

　　A. 摄盐不足　　　　　　　　　　B. 水摄入过多

　　C. 肾脏排水减少　　　　　　　　D. 细胞外液低渗

　　E. 细胞外液高渗

(5) 该患者可能发生何种危险病症?

    A. 心跳呼吸停止            B. 腹水

    C. 肾衰竭                 D. 肝衰竭

    E. 内出血

(6) 下列哪项措施可有效改善该患者的症状?

    A. 输入葡萄糖            B. 输入碳酸氢钠

    C. 使用钙剂               D. 给予甘露醇

    E. 输入盐水

## 案例分析问答题

[案例]

37 岁未孕女性,因车祸后背部疼痛入院做腰椎融合术。患者有多囊卵巢综合征和抑郁症。其日常服用的药物包括:氢氯噻嗪(25 mg/d)、度洛西汀(60 mg,每日 2 次)、阿立哌唑(10 mg/d)、氯硝西泮(0.25 mg/d)。手术前实验室检测一切正常。手术在全身麻醉下顺利完成。手术中一直以 75 mL/h 的速度输注 0.45% NaCl 和 5% 葡萄糖。手术后 1 天,患者出现激动与精神混乱并伴有严重口渴。体格检查:体温(T)36.4 ℃,心率(HR)105 次/min,血压(BP)135/80 mmHg,呼吸频率(R)15 次/min,血氧饱和度(SO₂)100%,黏膜干燥。心脏检查仅发现心动过速,肺音清晰,腹部柔软,四肢无水肿。手术切口吻合良好,无红斑与扭曲。血钠浓度升至153 mmol/L,尿排出量很多但没有具体记录,尿检显示尿比重为 1.005,尿渗透压129 mOsm/kg。静脉给予患者 4 μg 去氨加压素,患者在 2 小时内继续大量排尿,且尿渗透压为 155 mOsm/kg,继而诊断患者发生了肾源性尿崩症。

问题:

(1) 该患者发生了何种水、电解质代谢紊乱? 发生该紊乱的机制是什么?

(2) 患者出现激动、精神混乱与口渴现象的原因是什么?

(3) 患者心率与血压发生变化的机制是什么?

(4) 医生应做出的正确处理是什么?

### 参考答案

**案例分析选择题(多选一)**

**1.** BBDAC;**2.** AACAE;**3.** DACA;**4.** ADEE;**5.** DADEAD

**案例分析问答题**

(1) 该患者发生了何种水、电解质代谢紊乱? 发生该紊乱的机制是什么?

基于患者血[Na⁺]>145 mmol/L 以及尿崩症的诊断结果,患者一定是发生了高渗性脱水,这主要是尿崩症时丢失水多于丢失钠所造成的。

(2) 患者出现激动、精神混乱与口渴现象的原因是什么?

患者出现激动、精神混乱是脑细胞脱水的结果,而血渗透压升高作用于下丘脑口渴中枢引发口渴。

(3) 患者心率与血压发生变化的机制是什么?

大量失水导致患者有效循环血量减少,通过压力感受器与容量感受器激活交感系统导致心率加快。血压变化则是肾素-血管紧张素-醛固酮系统(RAAS)激活升高血管紧张素Ⅱ的结果。

（4）医生应做出的正确处理是什么？

及时纠正高渗状态,可静脉输注5%葡萄糖,待患者神志清醒后改为口服。另外,还需寻找尿崩症的病因以积极根治尿崩症。

# ◇ 钾代谢紊乱

## 案例分析选择题（多选一）

1. 患者,男,60岁,因呕吐、心慌入院。血检结果:[$Na^+$] 138 mmol/L,[$K^+$] 2.9 mmol/L, [$Mg^{2+}$] 0.95 mmol/L。

（1）该患者有哪种电解质紊乱？

    A. 高钾血症　　　　　　　　　　B. 低钾血症

    C. 低镁血症　　　　　　　　　　D. 低钠血症

    E. 高镁血症

（2）下列哪项原因导致了该患者出现电解质紊乱？

    A. 经消化道失钠　　　　　　　　B. 经消化道失镁

    C. 经消化道失水与钠　　　　　　D. 经肾失水与钠

    E. 经消化道失钾

（3）该患者可能出现下列哪项心脏功能的改变？

    A. 心肌兴奋性降低,自律性增加　　B. 心肌传导性增加,自律性增加

    C. 心肌兴奋性降低,传导性增加　　D. 心肌兴奋性降低,自律性降低

    E. 心肌自律性增加,传导性降低

（4）下列哪项是该患者心电图的典型改变？

    A. QT 间期缩短　　　　　　　　B. ST 段抬高

    C. T 波高耸　　　　　　　　　　D. U 波明显

    E. PR 间期缩短

（5）下列哪项是该患者可能出现的肌肉变化？

    A. 兴奋性增强　　　　　　　　　B. 兴奋性减弱

    C. 收缩力增强　　　　　　　　　D. 收缩力减弱

    E. 无变化

（6）该患者可能出现下列哪种变化？

    A. 代谢性酸中毒　　　　　　　　B. 低血糖

    C. 代谢性碱中毒　　　　　　　　D. 少尿

    E. 反常性碱性尿

（7）下列哪种治疗方法能安全有效地纠正患者的电解质紊乱？

    A. 静脉输入生理盐水　　　　　　B. 静脉补充钾

    C. 口服补充钾　　　　　　　　　D. 口服补充生理盐水

    E. 口服补充镁

2. 患者,女,30岁,因地震房屋坍塌被困10小时,获救后发现双下肢肿胀,无尿。血检结果:[Na$^+$]136 mmol/L,[K$^+$]6.6 mmol/L,[Cl$^-$]95 mmol/L。

(1) 该患者有下列哪种电解质紊乱?

    A. 高钾血症            B. 低钾血症

    C. 高氯血症            D. 低钠血症

    E. 高钠血症

(2) 下列哪项是该患者出现电解质异常的可能病因?

    A. 缺氧                B. 脱水

    C. 肾小球滤过减少       D. 肾小球滤过增多

    E. 盐皮质激素缺乏

(3) 下列哪项是该患者心电图的典型改变?

    A. QT 间期延长          B. T 波高耸

    C. ST 段压低            D. U 波明显

    E. T 波低平

(4) 该患者可能出现下列哪项心脏功能的改变?

    A. 心肌兴奋性降低,自律性增加    B. 心肌传导性增加,自律性增加

    C. 心肌兴奋性降低,传导性增加    D. 心肌传导性降低,自律性增加

    E. 心肌自律性降低,传导性降低

(5) 该患者不可能出现下列哪种代谢改变?

    A. 心律失常            B. 反常性碱性尿

    C. 四肢软弱无力        D. 腱反射亢进

    E. 代谢性酸中毒

(6) 该患者可能出现下列哪种致命的病症?

    A. 心室骤停            B. 反常性碱性尿

    C. 四肢软弱无力        D. 腱反射消失

    E. 代谢性酸中毒

(7) 一旦该患者出现心脏功能异常,医生不应选用以下哪项措施?

    A. 输入葡萄糖加胰岛素      B. 输入碳酸氢钠

    C. 使用钙剂            D. 使用氯化钾溶液

    E. 血液透析

## 案例分析问答题

[案例一]

一位30岁的女性,15年Ⅰ型糖尿病史。因高血压、糖尿病肾病合并慢性肾衰竭入院做肾移植手术。手术前2天她进行了透析。手术前血糖一直没有控制得很好,在60~600 mg/dL间波动。手术8小时前午夜的血糖为64 mg/dL。术前1天的动脉血气分析显示:pH 7.45,PaCO$_2$ 32 mmHg。手术当天早上5点,血糖为129 mg/dL,[Na$^+$]128 mEq/L,[K$^+$]

5.2 mEq/L，[Cl⁻]94 mEq/L。术前药物包括口服安定 10 mg 和静脉注射甲基强的松 750 mg。手术前并未给予胰岛素。手术中一直给予含 5% 葡萄糖的 0.45% NaCl 溶液，麻醉过程中通过心电图监控发现一切正常。手术的前 4 个小时，患者血糖从 150 mg/dL 升至 250 mg/dL，这期间并未给予胰岛素。血压则在 120/80 ~ 180/100 mmHg 间波动。5 个小时后，在进行手术缝合时，心电图显示 QRS 波变宽与 T 波高耸。3 分钟后，患者出现心脏停搏。血检发现：[K⁺]7.9 mEq/L，PaCO₂ 37 mmHg，pH 7.21。在给予患者纯氧、静脉滴注碳酸氢钠、胰岛素、氯化钙、利多卡因和 50% 葡萄糖后，通过心脏按压成功将患者救回。患者心跳恢复后的血检显示：[K⁺]6.8 mEq/L，PaCO₂ 34 mmHg，pH 7.31。1 小时后患者苏醒，血检显示：[K⁺]6.1 mEq/L、PaCO₂ 34 mmHg，pH 7.41。

**问题：**

（1）该患者术中出现血糖升高的原因是什么？

（2）患者肾移植手术中心电图改变的原因是什么？

（3）患者术中出现哪些疾病状态？它们的发生机制分别是什么？

（4）该患者手术中心脏功能发生了哪些改变？其机制是什么？

（5）请解释医生在抢救患者心脏骤停时使用碳酸氢钠、胰岛素和氯化钙的原理。

**［案例二］**

一位 35 岁男性因为肌肉疼痛及全身无力入院。2 周前，他出现腹痛、饮食不佳，恶心并呕吐，但无腹泻。1 周前，他感觉到肌肉无力，而且不断恶化到无法独自下床。最近数月他因颈痛每日服用布洛芬 2.4 ~ 3.2 g，并不嗜酒。入院体格检查时，他的神智与生命体征都很正常。但是，他无法抬起胳膊和腿。他的腱反射减弱但体表触觉正常。其他的检查也并未见任何异常。血检发现：血细胞计数正常，[Na⁺] 142 mEq/L，[K⁺] 1.8 mEq/L，代谢性酸中毒并排除自身免疫性疾病。尿检发现 24 小时尿钠排出 466 mEq，尿钾排出 112 mEq，尿肌酐 2.25 g，尿 pH 7.0。最终诊断为布洛芬引发的 I 型肾小管酸中毒，因为在停用布洛芬后患者的各项指标与症状都显著改善。

**问题：**

（1）该患者出现哪种水、电解质代谢紊乱？

（2）患者出现水、电解质代谢紊乱与 I 型肾小管酸中毒有何关系？

（3）患者出现肌无力的机制是什么？

（4）如果给该患者检测心电图，可能发现哪些变化？其机制是什么？

（5）医生在看到血检结果后，可以立即采取什么措施帮助患者？

**参考答案**

**案例分析选择题（多选一）**

**1**．BEEDBCC；**2**．ACBEDAD

**案例分析问答题**

**［案例一］**

（1）该患者术中出现血糖升高的原因是什么？

患者因为Ⅰ型糖尿病无法产生胰岛素,而且手术前也没有给予胰岛素。手术中不停地输注5%葡萄糖加上胰岛素缺乏导致了血糖升高。

(2)患者肾移植手术中心电图改变的原因是什么?

患者血钾升高(7.9 mEq/L > 5.5 mEq/L)引发了典型的高血钾心电图变化——QRS波变宽与T波高耸。

(3)患者术中出现哪些疾病状态?它们的发生机制分别是什么?

基于血钾7.9 mEq/L和pH 7.21,患者出现了高血钾和代谢性酸中毒。胰岛素的缺乏与高血糖导致了细胞内钾离子外流。代谢性酸中毒时,胞外$H^+$/胞内$K^+$交换也促进了高血钾的发生。代谢性酸中毒可能源于慢性肾衰竭、糖尿病的酮症或者乳酸酸中毒。

(4)该患者手术中心脏功能发生了哪些改变?其机制是什么?

急性高血钾因为去极化阻滞显著地降低了心肌的兴奋性。动作电位4期钠离子内流的减缓导致其自律性下降。去极化时,电压依赖性钠离子通道失活导致心肌传导性降低。平台期钙离子内流的减少导致了心肌收缩性的减弱。

(5)请解释医生在抢救患者心脏骤停时使用碳酸氢钠、胰岛素和氯化钙的原理。

碳酸氢钠用于纠正酸中毒。胰岛素用于降糖并诱导细胞外液中的钾离子内流入细胞而降血钾。血钾的降低可有效提高心肌的兴奋性、自律性与传导性。增加钙离子浓度及其内流增强了心肌的兴奋性和收缩性。

[案例二]

(1)该患者出现哪种水、电解质代谢紊乱?

低钾血症(1.8 mEq/L < 3.5 mEq/L)。

(2)患者出现水、电解质代谢紊乱与Ⅰ型肾小管酸中毒有何关系?

Ⅰ型肾小管酸中毒是由于远曲小管泌$H^+$障碍,导致$K^+$-$Na^+$交换增加,尿钾排出增多。与此一致,患者24小时尿钾排出(112 mEq)远大于正常水平(30 mEq)。

(3)患者出现肌无力的机制是什么?

患者因为低钾血症,细胞外液中钾离子浓度骤降。细胞外钾离子浓度与胞内钾离子浓度差值增加,导致静息电位负值增大,与阈电位间的距离拉大,引起超极化。因此,细胞的兴奋性降低。

(4)如果给该患者检测心电图,可能发现哪些变化?其机制是什么?

① 2期ST段压低:因为钙离子内流加速。

② T波低平:4期钾离子外流减慢。

③ U波增高:钾离子外流减慢,心肌动作电位超长期延长。

(5)医生在看到血检结果后,可以立即采取什么措施帮助患者?

口服补钾,同时检测血钾与心电图。

## ◇ 镁代谢紊乱

### 案例分析选择题(多选一)

1. 患者,女,因严重腹泻入院,血检结果:[$Na^+$] 142 mmol/L, [$K^+$] 3.3 mmol/L, [$Mg^{2+}$] 0.25 mmol/L, [$Ca^{2+}$] 2.28 mmol/L。

(1)此患者患有下列哪种电解质紊乱?

    A. 低钠/高钾血症        B. 低钠/低钾血症

    C. 低钾/低钙血症        D. 低镁/低钾血症

    E. 低钾/高钙血症

（2）患者心脏功能可能发生的改变是下列哪项？

    A. 心肌兴奋性降低，自律性增加    B. 心肌传导性增加，自律性增加

    C. 心肌兴奋性降低，传导性增加    D. 心肌兴奋性增加，自律性增加

    E. 心肌自律性降低，传导性降低

（3）该患者易出现下列哪项变化？

    A. 肌肉应激性降低    B. 高血压

    C. 厌食    D. 心率减低

    E. 嗜睡

（4）应该选择下列哪项方案来纠正该患者的电解质异常？

    A. 及时补钾/钠    B. 及时补钠/镁

    C. 及时补镁/钾    D. 及时补钾/钙

    E. 及时补钙/镁

2. 中年女性被诊断出甲状腺功能减退，并出现黏液性水肿。

（1）下列哪项最可能是此患者的血检结果？

    A. [$K^+$] 3.3 mmol/L    B. [$Na^+$] 155 mmol/L

    C. [$Ca^{2+}$] 1.85 mmol/L    D. [$Mg^{2+}$] 0.55 mmol/L

    E. [$Mg^{2+}$] 3.25 mmol/L

（2）该患者易出现下列哪项变化？

    A. 神经-肌肉兴奋性增高    B. 动脉血压下降

    C. 多尿    D. 心率过快

    E. 焦虑/易怒

## 案例分析问答题

[案例]

69 岁女性，因头疼 3 天出现昏迷入院。她 50 岁后一直被 Ⅱ 型糖尿病、类风湿性关节炎和偏头痛折磨着，但却从来没有过癫痫或一过性的缺血性中风。她一直服用格列苯脲、强的松龙和速尿。

入院当天，她有至少 12 次约 2 分钟的无意识的头与眼睛向左侧的转动。她的丈夫也确认这样的情况在两天前才开始出现。血液检测发现：血糖 14.7 mmol/L，糖化血红蛋白 HbA1c 18.3%（正常范围 5% ~8%），[Ca] 2.25 mmol/L（正常范围 2.2 ~2.62 mmol/L），[Pi] 1.03 mmol/L，[$K^+$] 3.8 mEq/L，血浆中的尿素、钠、碳酸氢根浓度和心肌酶活力都正常。脑 CT 无异常，脑电图显示右脑有癫痫电活动。

患者在使用胰岛素后血糖得以控制，首次 24 小时胰岛素 1 g，随后每天 300 mg。抗惊厥药物无法抑制癫痫。胰岛素治疗 48 小时后血镁浓度仅为 0.29 mmol/L，给予静脉滴注 3 g 硫酸镁后的 12 小时，她的癫痫症状好转并在再次给予 2 g 硫酸镁后完全消失。在此之后，她的血镁浓度也稳定在了 0.63 mmol/L。

问题：

（1）该患者昏迷入院的原因是什么？

（2）患者低镁血症是如何发生的？

（3）患者癫痫发作的病因与机制分别是什么？

（4）如未及时纠正患者的低镁血症,患者还会出现哪些机能代谢的改变？ 这些变化的发生机制是什么？

**参考答案**

**案例分析选择题（多选一）**

1. DDBC；2. EB

**案例分析问答题**

（1）该患者昏迷入院的原因是什么？

Ⅱ型糖尿病血糖控制不佳合并低镁血症。

（2）患者低镁血症是如何发生的？

糖尿病病人的高渗糖尿本身就会促进肾脏排镁,加上患者还服用速尿,该利尿剂可抑制肾小管髓袢升支粗段对镁离子的重吸收,这些都可导致低镁血症。而治疗高血糖中胰岛素的应用则促进镁离子过多地转入细胞内,引发严重的低镁血症。

（3）患者癫痫发作的病因与机制分别是什么？

低镁血症时,镁离子对中枢神经系统抑制作用减弱导致患者癫痫的发作。其机制可能包括：

① 低镁血症时,镁离子抑制中枢兴奋性 N-甲基-D 天冬氨酸受体作用减弱。

② 低镁血症时,$Na^+$-$K^+$-ATP 酶活力减弱,cAMP 水平异常。

（4）如未及时纠正患者的低镁血症,患者还会出现哪些机能代谢的改变？ 这些变化的发生机制是什么？

① 心律失常:是心肌兴奋性、自律性增高的结果,心肌细胞 $Na^+$-$K^+$-ATP 酶活力减弱所致胞内缺钾也可导致心律失常。

② 高血压:源于外周血管收缩性增强。

③ 冠心病:是心肌代谢异常与冠脉痉挛的结果。

④ 低钾血症:肾小管髓袢升支 $Na^+$-$K^+$-ATP 酶活力下降抑制钾离子的重吸收所致。

⑤ 低钙血症:是 PTH 分泌减少与作用减弱的结果。

## ◇ 钙磷代谢紊乱

### 案例分析选择题（多选一）

1. **婴儿自出生后闭门不出,头发疏松。**

（1）下列哪项最可能是此患儿的血检结果？

A. ［$K^+$］6.3 mmol/L　　　　B. ［$Na^+$］155 mmol/L

C. ［$Ca^{2+}$］0.8 mmol/L　　　D. ［$Ca^{2+}$］1.35 mmol/L

E. ［$Mg^{2+}$］3.25 mmol/L

（2）该患儿不易出现下列哪项变化？

A. 肌肉痉挛　　　　　　　　B. 指甲过软

C. 鸡胸　　　　　　　　　　D. O 形腿

E. 囟门闭合过快

（3）以下哪项是该患者心电图的典型改变？

    A．QT 间期延长　　　　　　　　　B．T 波高耸

    C．ST 段缩短　　　　　　　　　　D．U 波明显

    E．ST 段抬高

（4）患儿心脏功能可能发生下列哪项改变？

    A．心肌兴奋性降低,自律性增加　　B．心肌兴奋性降低,收缩性增加

    C．心肌兴奋性降低,传导性增加　　D．心肌兴奋性增加,传导性增加

    E．心肌兴奋性增加,传导性降低

**2．中年男性,白血病骨转移。**

（1）下列哪项最可能是该患者的血检结果？

    A．$[K^+]$ 3.3 mmol/L　　　　　　　B．$[Na^+]$ 155 mmol/L

    C．$[Ca^{2+}]$ 1.85 mmol/L　　　　　D．$[Ca^{2+}]$ 0.6 mmol/L

    E．$[Mg^{2+}]$ 3.25 mmol/L

（2）该患者易出现以下哪项改变？

    A．神经-肌肉兴奋性增高　　　　　B．异位钙化

    C．肌肉痉挛　　　　　　　　　　D．腱反射增强

    E．焦虑/易怒

（3）下列哪项是该患者心电图的典型改变？

    A．QT 间期缩短　　　　　　　　　B．T 波高耸

    C．ST 段压低　　　　　　　　　　D．U 波明显

    E．T 波倒置

（4）该患者的心脏功能可能出现下列哪种改变？

    A．心肌兴奋性降低,传导性降低　　B．心肌传导性增加,自律性增加

    C．心肌兴奋性降低,传导性增加　　D．心肌兴奋性增加,自律性增加

    E．心肌自律性降低,传导性增加

**3．中年男性,急性酒精中毒并伴有呼吸性碱中毒。**

（1）下列哪项最可能是此患者的血检结果？

    A．$[Na^+]$ 130 mmol/L　　　　　　B．$[Na^+]$ 155 mmol/L

    C．$[K^+]$ 3.25 mmol/L　　　　　　D．$[Pi]$ 0.5 mmol/L

    E．$[Pi]$ 1.85 mmol/L

（2）该患者不会出现以下哪种变化？

    A．肌无力　　　　　　　　　　　B．鸭态步

    C．肌肉痉挛　　　　　　　　　　D．骨痛

    E．焦虑/易怒

**4. 5 岁男童,维生素 D 中毒。**

(1) 下列哪项最可能是此患者的血检结果?

    A. [Na$^+$] 130 mmol/L           B. [Na$^+$] 155 mmol/L

    C. [K$^+$] 3.25 mmol/L           D. [Pi] 0.5 mmol/L

    E. [Pi] 2.05 mmol/L

(2) 该患者不易出现下列哪项变化?

    A. 神经-肌肉兴奋性增高         B. 异位钙化

    C. 肌肉痉挛                    D. 心脏房室传导阻滞

    E. 鸡胸

## 案例分析问答题

**[案例]**

一位 3 岁的男孩,呼吸道感染 1 周且 1 天前出现尿量减少。因为便秘,医生给予了儿童剂量的磷酸钠盐灌肠液,并在操作的前几分钟最大限度地阻止了液体的回流。随后的 2~3 小时内,该患儿有过 3 次大便和 3 次呕吐,继而变得虚弱无力,脸色发白。体检显示: T 38 ℃,脉搏(P)144 次/min,R 16 次/min,BP 96/68 mmHg,体重(BW)8.4 kg。黏膜干燥且皮肤张力差。腱反射正常但肌肉张力增加。血红蛋白 13.4 mg/dL,血细胞比容 40%,血浆中 [Na$^+$] 152 mEq/L,[K$^+$] 3.4 mEq/L,[Cl$^-$] 108 mEq/L,[Ca$^{2+}$] 0.58 mmol/L,[Pi] 6.78 mmol/L,尿素氮 3.93 mmol/L,静脉补液 12 小时后恢复。

**问题:**

(1) 该患者发生何种水、电解质代谢紊乱? 发生该紊乱的机制是什么?

(2) 患者肌张力增强的原因是什么?

(3) 如果患者此时检测心电图,会发现哪些异常?

(4) 医生为什么运用输液来纠正患者的电解质紊乱?

### 参考答案

**案例分析选择题(多选一)**

**1.** CEAD;**2.** CBAA;**3.** DC;**4.** ED

**案例分析问答题**

(1) 该患者发生何种水、电解质代谢紊乱? 发生该紊乱的机制是什么?

① 因为 2~3 小时内 3 次呕吐而发生脱水。

② 高磷血症:[Pi] 6.78 mmol/L > 1.9 mmol/L,因为使用含磷的灌肠剂合并脱水。

③ 低钙血症:[Ca$^{2+}$] 0.58 mmol/L < 1 mmol/L,高磷血症所导致。

(2) 患者肌张力增强的原因是什么?

低钙血症时,神经-肌肉兴奋性增加导致患者肌张力增强。

(3) 如果患者此时检测心电图,会发现哪些异常?

低钙血症时,钠离子内流加速,故心肌兴奋性和传导性升高;但平台期由于钙离子内流减少,平台期延长,因此会出现 ST 和 QT 段延长,T 波低平或倒置。

（4）医生为什么运用输液来纠正患者的电解质紊乱？

补液不仅降低血磷浓度，还有助于磷的排泄。而高磷血症的纠正有助于 $1,25-(OH)_2D_3$ 的生成及钙的重吸收，这些将有利于血钙水平的恢复。

（赵丽梅　赵　颖）

# 第三章　酸碱平衡紊乱

## 案例分析选择题（多选一）

1. 患者，男性，61 岁，患有肾功能衰竭；其血气指标检查结果显示：pH 为 7.28，$PaCO_2$ 为 30 mmHg，$[HCO_3^-]$ 为 14 mmol/L。

（1）该患者最可能出现下列哪项酸碱平衡紊乱？

    A. 代谢性酸中毒             B. 呼吸性酸中毒

    C. 代谢性碱中毒             D. 呼吸性碱中毒

    E. 以上都不是

（2）下列哪项是该患者体内最主要的代偿方式？

    A. 细胞外液缓冲             B. 骨骼代偿

    C. 细胞内外离子交换         D. 呼吸代偿

    E. 肾脏代偿

（3）下列哪项是该患者血液当中发挥缓冲作用的主要缓冲碱？

    A. $Na_2HPO_4$                 B. K-Hb

    C. $NaHCO_3$                 D. $HbO_2$

    E. $Pro^-$

（4）该患者体内血钾变化趋势是下列哪项？

    A. 降低                    B. 升高

    C. 不变                    D. 先降低后升高

    E. 先升高后降低

（5）关于该患者体内酸碱平衡指标变化趋势，下列哪项正确？

    A. AB 升高                B. SB 升高

    C. BB 升高                D. AB < SB

    E. AB > SB

（6）下列哪项不可能出现在该患者体内？

    A. 血 $K^+$ 升高             B. 血 $Ca^{2+}$ 升高

    C. 血肾上腺素浓度升高       D. 脑组织氧化磷酸化过程增强

    E. 脑内谷氨酸脱羧酶活性增强

（7）该患者不可能会出现下列哪种变化？

    A. 心律失常                    B. 心肌收缩力下降

    C. 肾上腺素分泌减少          D. 中枢神经系统代谢障碍

    E. 血管系统对儿茶酚胺的反应降低

（8）该患者治疗时的首选药物是下列哪项？

    A. 碳酸氢钠                    B. 枸橼酸钠

    C. 三羟甲基氨基甲烷          D. 乳酸钠

    E. 磷酸氢二钠

2. 患者，男性，6 岁，由于天气炎热，与小伙伴一起在河边玩耍时不幸溺水；送医院抢救后的血气分析结果为：pH 7.1，$PaCO_2$ 76 mmHg，[$HCO_3^-$] 28 mmol/L。

（1）该患者最有可能发生下列哪种酸碱平衡紊乱？

    A. 代谢性酸中毒              B. 急性呼吸性酸中毒

    C. 慢性呼吸性酸中毒        D. 代谢性酸中毒合并呼吸性酸中毒

    E. 以上都不是

（2）该患者体内最主要的代偿调节方式是下列哪项？

    A. 磷酸盐缓冲系统           B. 碳酸氢盐缓冲系统

    C. 非碳酸氢盐缓冲系统       D. 血浆蛋白质缓冲系统

    E. 肾脏调节

（3）下列哪项不可能是该患者的临床表现？

    A. 肾前性肾功能衰竭         B. 心律失常

    C. 高钾血症                    D. 血压降低

    E. 持续头痛

（4）下列哪项变化不可能出现在该患者体内？

    A. 血 $K^+$ 升高                  B. 血 $Ca^{2+}$ 升高

    C. 血 $Na^+$ 正常               D. 血 $Cl^-$ 升高

    E. 脑血管扩张

3. 某女性患者，68 岁，因气温骤降受凉入院。肺心病 25 年。查血气：pH 7.33，$PaCO_2$ 70 mmHg，[$HCO_3^-$] 36 mmol/L。

（1）该患者发生了下列哪种酸碱平衡紊乱？

    A. 代谢性酸中毒              B. 代谢性碱中毒

    C. 急性呼吸性酸中毒       D. 慢性呼吸性酸中毒

    E. 呼吸性碱中毒

（2）该患者酸碱紊乱发生的机制是下列哪项？

    A. 癔症                       B. 气道阻塞，$CO_2$ 潴留

    C. 内分泌失调               D. 肾功能不全

    E. 心力衰竭

（3）下列哪项是该患者体内最主要的代偿调节方式？

    A. 磷酸盐缓冲系统              B. 碳酸氢盐缓冲系统

    C. 非碳酸氢盐缓冲系统       D. 血浆蛋白质缓冲系统

    E. 肾脏调节

（4）关于该患者体内酸碱平衡指标变化趋势，下列哪项正确？

    A. AB 降低                    B. SB 降低

    C. BB 升高                   D. AB < SB

    E. ［BE］负值升高

（5）该酸碱失衡会引起何种水、电解质紊乱？

    A. 高钾血症                   B. 高钙血症

    C. 低磷血症                   D. 高氯血症

    E. 全身性水肿

（6）下列哪项酶变化可能发生于该患者中枢系统内？

    A. 碳酸酐酶活性↓           B. 谷氨酸脱羧酶活性↓

    C. 谷氨酰胺酶活性↓       D. γ-氨基丁酸转氨酶活性↓

    E. 生物氧化酶活性↑

（7）下列哪种治疗措施不恰当？

    A. 有效通气                  B. 抗生素控制感染

    C. 低浓度吸氧                D. 祛痰

    E. 口服补氯化钾

4. 男性患儿，12 岁，因发热、咳嗽、呼吸急促留发热门诊观察。BP 110/75 mmHg，R 28 次/min，肺部闻及湿啰音。实验室检查：［$K^+$］4.5 mmol/L，［$Na^+$］134 mmol/L，［$Cl^-$］106 mmol/L，pH 7.51，$PaCO_2$ 30 mmHg，［$HCO_3^-$］20.3 mmol/L。

（1）该患者发生了下列哪种酸碱平衡紊乱？

    A. 代谢性酸中毒          B. 呼吸性酸中毒

    C. 代谢性碱中毒          D. 呼吸性碱中毒

    E. 以上都不是

（2）下列哪项是该患者酸碱紊乱的发生机制？

    A. 体内挥发酸过多排出     B. 固定酸减少

    C. 胰岛素分泌减少        D. 脂肪酸减少

    E. 肺部感染

（3）下列哪项病因引起的酸碱平衡紊乱与该患者不同？

    A. 人工呼吸机流速过快    B. 大量输入库存血

    C. 甲状腺功能亢进       D. 癔症发作

    E. 铵盐类药物摄入过量

（4）该种酸碱平衡紊乱常见的并发症不包括下列哪项？

    A. 低钾血症                   B. 肌肉抽搐

    C. 高磷血症                   D. 缺氧

    E. 意识障碍

（5）下列哪项是该患者体内酸碱平衡指标的变化？

    A. AB 升高                    B. SB 升高

    C. BB 升高                    D. AB > SB

    E. AB < SB

（6）下列哪种治疗措施不恰当？

    A. 降温                       B. 吸入 $CO_2$

    C. 使用抗生素                  D. 高浓度氧疗

    E. 补液

5. 患者，女性，60 岁，反复呕吐后入院，诊断为幽门梗阻。血气检查结果显示：pH 7.5，$PaCO_2$ 48 mmHg，[$HCO_3^-$] 36 mmol/L。

（1）该患者最可能发生下列哪种酸碱平衡紊乱？

    A. 代谢性酸中毒             B. 呼吸性酸中毒

    C. 代谢性碱中毒             D. 呼吸性碱中毒

    E. 混合性酸碱紊乱

（2）下列哪项病因引起的紊乱与该患者不同？

    A. 肺炎                      B. 应用利尿剂（呋塞米）

    C. 肾上腺皮质增生          D. 低钾血症

    E. 肝功能衰竭

（3）该患者出现的酸碱紊乱与下列哪种机制无关？

    A. $H^+$ 丢失                  B. $Na^+$ 丢失

    C. $K^+$ 丢失                  D. 细胞外液大量丢失

    E. $Cl^-$ 丢失

（4）下列有关该患者体内代偿调节的论述哪项是不正确的？

    A. 肺的代偿较快            B. 血液缓冲能力有限

    C. 肾脏代偿发挥较早        D. 肾脏代偿发挥较晚

    E. 呼吸受抑制

（5）下列哪项是该患者体内起主要作用的缓冲系统？

    A. $HCO_3^-/H_2CO_3$           B. $Hb^-/HHb$

    C. $Pr/HPr$                 D. $HbO_2^-/HHbO_2$

    E. $HPO_4^{2-}/H_2PO_4^-$

（6）该患者中枢抑制介质减少与下列哪种酶活性的变化有关？

    A. 谷氨酸脱羧酶活性↓　　　　　　　B. γ-氨基丁酸转氨酶活性↓

    C. 碳酸酐酶活性↑　　　　　　　　　D. 谷氨酰胺酶活性↑

    E. 丙酮酸脱氢酶活性↓

（7）该患者体内可能出现下列哪种变化？

    A. $K^+$内流，近曲小管 $K^+$-$Na^+$ 交换↓　　B. $K^+$内流，近曲小管 $H^+$-$Na^+$ 交换↑

    C. $K^+$内流，近曲小管 $H^+$-$Na^+$ 交换↓　　D. $K^+$外流，近曲小管 $H^+$-$Na^+$ 交换↑

    E. $K^+$外流，近曲小管 $H^+$-$Na^+$ 交换↓

（8）该患者后期若出现手足抽搐，最有可能的原因是下列哪项？

    A. ［$K^+$］↓　　　　　　　　　　　　B. ［$Cl^-$］↓

    C. ［$Na^+$］↓　　　　　　　　　　　　D. ［$Ca^{2+}$］↓

    E. ［$Mg^{2+}$］↓

（9）下列哪种治疗措施不恰当？

    A. 噻嗪类利尿剂　　　　　　　　　　B. 口服生理盐水

    C. 氯化钾　　　　　　　　　　　　　D. 禁食、胃肠减压

    E. 补液

6. 患者，女性，46 岁，因发热就医。她患糖尿病 10 余年。体格检查：T 39 ℃，呼吸深大，28 次/min。实验室检查：血糖 10.1 mmol/L，［$Na^+$］160 mmol/L，［$Cl^-$］104 mmol/L；pH 7.38，$PaCO_2$ 24 mmHg，［$HCO_3^-$］13 mmol/L，尿糖(+++)。

（1）该患者发生了何种酸碱平衡紊乱？

    A. 代谢性酸中毒　　　　　　　　　　B. 代谢性碱中毒

    C. 呼吸性酸中毒　　　　　　　　　　D. 呼吸性碱中毒

    E. 代谢性酸中毒合并呼吸性碱中毒

（2）下列哪项变化不是该患者引发酸碱紊乱的原因？

    A. 挥发酸增多　　　　　　　　　　　B. 乳酸增多

    C. β-羟丁酸增多　　　　　　　　　　D. 乙酰乙酸增多

    E. 脂肪分解代谢增强

（3）下列哪项指标变化与该患者病症相符？

    A. 血氯增高　　　　　　　　　　　　B. 血氯降低

    C. AG 正常　　　　　　　　　　　　D. AG 增高

    E. AB > SB

7. 患者，老年男性，因近 2 日反复呕吐、尿少且无力而就医。他患有慢性阻塞性肺炎。体格检查：BP 118/68 mmHg，R 10 次/min，严重脱水貌。实验室检查：［$K^+$］2.8 mmol/L，［$Na^+$］147 mmol/L，［$Cl^-$］95 mmol/L；pH 7.48，$PaCO_2$ 52 mmHg，［$HCO_3^-$］38 mmol/L。

（1）该患者发生了下列哪种酸碱平衡紊乱？

  A. 代谢性酸中毒　　　　　　　　B. 代谢性碱中毒

  C. 呼吸性酸中毒　　　　　　　　D. 呼吸性碱中毒

  E. 呼吸性酸中毒合并代谢性碱中毒

（2）下列哪项是该患者酸碱紊乱的发生机制？

  A. 呕吐　　　　　　　　　　　　B. 低钾血症

  C. 低氯血症　　　　　　　　　　D. 慢性阻塞性肺炎

  E. 以上都是

（3）该患者目前没有以下哪种水、电解质紊乱？

  A. 低钾血症　　　　　　　　　　B. 高钠血症

  C. 低渗性脱水　　　　　　　　　D. 低氯血症

  E. 高渗性脱水

（4）如果治疗不及时，该患者不可能发生下列哪种并发症？

  A. 消化道出血　　　　　　　　　B. 肝性脑病

  C. 肺性脑病　　　　　　　　　　D. 心律失常

  E. 蛛网膜下腔出血

（5）下列哪种治疗措施不恰当？

  A. 葡萄糖输液　　　　　　　　　B. 生理盐水输液

  C. 氯化钾输液　　　　　　　　　D. 高速输氧

  E. 以上都是

## 案例分析问答题

[案例一]

某患者，男性，38 岁。因近 2 周反复呕吐并伴有间歇性腹泻，尿量明显减少而前往医院就诊。实验室检查：pH 7.54，$PaCO_2$ 6.8 kPa（52 mmHg），BB 65 mmol/L，$BE^+$12 mmol/L，SB 40 mmol/L，$[K^+]$3.1 mmol/L，$\triangle[HCO_3^-]$16 mmol/L。

问题：

（1）该患者发生了何种酸碱平衡紊乱？处于代偿还是失代偿阶段？为什么？

（2）患者体内的哪些酸碱指标发生了原发性改变，哪些发生了继发性改变？这些变化发生的原因是什么？

（3）患者为何会发生低钾血症？低血钾在该酸碱平衡紊乱中的作用是什么？

[案例二]

某患者，女性，55 岁。因右下腹及瘘口周围疼痛伴食欲下降、干呕和呼吸急促就诊。该患者患有Ⅰ型糖尿病、舒张性心力衰竭、慢性胰腺炎及胃排空障碍，曾做过阑尾与胆囊切除术、胰腺十二指肠切除术、小肠及结肠造瘘术。患者入院前几天回肠造口袋的清空次数增多，除入院当天外，每天按时注射胰岛素。体格检查显示：血压正常，HR 87 次/min，呼吸急促，血氧与体温正常，病容明显，恶病质。因为疼痛，患者并不舒服，黏膜干燥，腹部弥散性疼痛但无腹壁紧张及反跳痛。随后患者突然出现意识障碍。血液检查发现:血糖 594 mg/dL,[Na$^+$] 124 mmol/L,[K$^+$] 5.1 mmol/L,[Mg$^{2+}$] 0.9 mmol/L,[Ca$^{2+}$] 0.7 mmol/L,[Pi] 6.8 mg/dL(正常 3.0 ~ 4.5 mg/dL),[Cl$^-$] 68 mmol/L,pH 7.85,PaCO$_2$ 21 mmHg,PO$_2$ 99 mmHg,[HCO$_3^-$] 33 mmol/L,lactate 4.3 mmol/L(正常 0.5 ~ 1.7 mmol/L),BUN 44 mg/dL,creatinine 3.9 mg/dL,肝肾功能及凝血功能检查均未发现异常。

**问题:**

(1)该患者发生了哪种类型的酸碱平衡紊乱?

(2)该患者出现这种酸碱平衡紊乱的发病机制是什么?

(3)该患者还可能出现了哪些机能代谢变化? 这些变化的机制是什么?

**参考答案**

**案例分析选择题(多选一)**

**1**. ADCBDDCA;**2**. BCAD;**3**. DBECADE;**4**. DABCED;**5**. CABCAACDA;**6**. EAD;**7**. EECBE

**案例分析问答题**

[案例一]

(1)该患者发生了何种酸碱平衡紊乱? 处于代偿还是失代偿阶段? 为什么?

该患者发生了代谢性碱中毒:

① pH = 7.54 碱中毒。

② HCO$_3^-$↑/PaCO$_2$↑同向,单纯型或者混合型。

③ 病史有呕吐加腹泻,所以 HCO$_3^-$↑为原发。

④ 根据代碱代偿公式预测 PaCO$_2$ = 40 + (0.7△HCO$_3^-$ ± 5) = 40 + (0.7 × 16 ± 5) = 51.2 ± 5,实际 PaCO$_2$52 在此范围内,故为单纯型代谢性碱中毒。

该代谢性碱中毒处于失代偿阶段,原因是 pH = 7.54,偏离了正常范围 7.35 ~ 7.45。

(2)患者体内的哪些酸碱指标发生了原发性改变,哪些发生了继发性改变? 这些变化发生的原因是什么?

SB 和 BB 升高、BE 为正值属于原发性变化,原因是呕吐引起大量胃酸丢失,使体内未被中和的 HCO$_3^-$增多;PaCO$_2$ 增加属于继发性改变,原因是代碱发生后呼吸运动减弱,机体 CO$_2$ 排出减少。

(3)患者为何会发生低钾血症? 低血钾在该酸碱平衡紊乱中的作用是什么?

患者发生低钾的原因包括:

① 呕吐加腹泻导致消化道失钾。

② 消化液大量丢失可导致 RAAS 激活,释放醛固酮促肾排钾。

③ 碱中毒时细胞内外 H$^+$-K$^+$ 离子交换被启动,K$^+$ 流入细胞内。

④ 肾小管上皮细胞内 H$^+$ 减少,H$^+$-Na$^+$ 交换减弱,K$^+$-Na$^+$ 交换增强,K$^+$ 大量从尿中丢失。

低血钾促进代谢性碱中毒发生的机制包括:

① 细胞外液中 K$^+$ 减少,促进 H$^+$-K$^+$ 交换和 H$^+$ 流入细胞内。

② 肾小管上皮细胞内 K$^+$ 减少,K$^+$-Na$^+$ 交换减弱,H$^+$-Na$^+$ 交换增强。肾小管上皮细胞 H$^+$ 分泌增加,促进 HCO$_3^-$ 重吸收。

[案例二]

(1)该患者发生了哪种类型的酸碱平衡紊乱?

① 根据 Henderson 简化公式,评估血气分析结果的可靠性。

$[H^+] = 24 \times (PaCO_2)/[HCO_3^-] = 24 \times 21/33 = 15.3$，对应的 pH $7.81 \approx 7.85$，故血气结果可靠。

② pH $7.85 > 7.45$，故为失代偿碱中毒。患者有呼吸急促，结合 $PaCO_2$ 下降，判断为急性呼吸性碱中毒。$HCO_3^-$ 升高结合造口袋清空频率增加判定为代谢性碱中毒。$PaCO_2$ 与 $HCO_3^-$ 变化相反，无法相互代偿，所以该酸碱平衡紊乱为失代偿。

③ $AG = [Na^+] - ([Cl^-] + [HCO_3^-]) = 124 - (68 + 33) = 23$，由于 $AG > 16$，可判定还存在代谢性酸中毒。

所以该患者发生了呼碱合并代碱合并代酸的三重酸碱平衡紊乱。

（2）该患者出现这种酸碱平衡紊乱的发病机制是什么？

① 呼吸性碱中毒：患者呼吸急促引起肺通气过度，$CO_2$ 排出过多，导致原发性 $PaCO_2$ 的降低。

② 代谢性碱中毒：患者造口袋清空频率增加提示腹泻，可造成患者丢失大量消化液。消化液含钾量高，且失液所致有效循环血量的降低可激活 RAAS 并通过醛固酮促进肾排钾，导致严重的低钾血症。低钾血症通过细胞内外 $H^+$-$K^+$ 交换引起 $H^+$ 内流；而肾小管 $K^+$-$Na^+$ 交换减弱，$H^+$-$Na^+$ 交换增强促进 $H^+$ 排出。此外，低氯血症也会增加远端肾小管对 $H^+$ 的分泌但减少 $[HCO_3^-]$ 的分泌。而随后增加的 $HCO_3^-$ 重吸收导致了血浆 $[HCO_3^-]$ 的原发性升高。

③ 代谢性酸中毒：患者患有糖尿病，血糖异常升高提示糖代谢异常，乳酸升高提示体内乳酸堆积；同时患者体内碱中毒引发血红蛋白氧离曲线左移可致组织缺氧，无氧糖酵解增强而致乳酸堆积；进而导致了 AG 增高型代谢性酸中毒的发生。

（3）该患者还可能出现了哪些机能代谢变化？这些变化的机制是什么？

碱中毒引起中枢抑制性递质 GABA 分解增加可导致中枢神经系统兴奋。而碱中毒时血红蛋白氧离曲线左移还可导致脑缺氧。因此，患者可出现烦躁不安、精神错乱及意识障碍。碱中毒相关的组织缺氧还可引起胃黏膜缺血缺氧并导致消化道出血。此外，pH 升高会导致血浆钙离子浓度下降，神经-肌肉应激性增高，出现腱反射亢进与手足抽搐。

（郑　栋　赵　颖）

# 第四章　发　热

## 案例分析选择题（多选一）

1. 患者，女性，33 岁，妊娠晚期因大叶性肺炎住院。她有心肌炎病史。入院时体温 39 ℃且仍有升高的趋势，HR 120 次/min。

（1）该患者发热的病因最有可能是下列哪项？

    A. 感染　　　　　　　　　　　　B. 内分泌代谢障碍

    C. 变态反应　　　　　　　　　　D. 体温调节中枢障碍

    E. 结缔组织性疾病

（2）下列哪项体现了肺炎球菌在引起患者发热中的作用？

    A. 内生致热源                B. 肿瘤坏死因子

    C. 抗原抗体复合物        D. 外致热原

    E. 白细胞致热原

（3）该患者此时处于体温继续上升阶段，那么其热代谢特点是下列哪项？

    A. 散热 > 产热              B. 散热障碍

    C. 产热 = 散热              D. 产热障碍

    E. 产热 > 散热

（4）该患者的体温变化提示其发热类型为下列哪项？

    A. 不规则热                B. 弛张热

    C. 稽留热                  D. 间歇热

    E. 风湿热

（5）该患者要及时输液防止脱水，但需要防止输液造成下列哪种二度感染？

    A. 变态反应                B. 内毒素污染

    C. 外毒素污染             D. 支原体污染

    E. 病毒污染

2. 患者，男，2 岁，主要因为"咳嗽 3 天，发热 1 天伴抽搐 2 次"入院治疗；入院前最高体温 39.1 ℃，抽搐时双眼上吊，咬牙，颜面口唇发绀，四肢发硬抖动，呼之不应；父母口述患儿为足月顺产，生长发育无特殊之处，智力体力与正常同龄儿童一致。入院后经过一系列检查，诊断为小儿热惊厥。

（1）小儿热惊厥产生的机制是下列哪项？

    A. 大脑皮质处于兴奋，皮质下中枢兴奋性增强

    B. 先天性体温中枢疾病

    C. 体温调节机制障碍

    D. 中枢神经尚未发育成熟

    E. 大脑皮质处于抑制，皮质下中枢亦受抑制

（2）此患者若没有给予任何处理，首先容易发生下列哪种病症？

    A. 低渗性脱水              B. 呼吸性酸中毒

    C. 肾性水潴留              D. 高渗性脱水

    E. 等渗性脱水

（3）该患者体内并没有下列哪项物质代谢的变化？

    A. 维生素消耗减少         B. 糖原分解加强

    C. 脂肪分解加强          D. 负氮平衡

    E. 物质代谢率增高

（4）可以给该患儿用下述哪类药物进行解热？

    A. 去氧皮质酮              B. 苯海拉明

    C. 茶碱                    D. 环磷酸腺苷

    E. 布洛芬

3. 患者,男性,79 岁,因持续 1 个月不明原因的发热入院。他自述体温持续在 38 ℃左右,且服用解热药无效。入院后该患者由低热转为高热,体温达到 39.1 ℃,且抗炎治疗数日无效。后 PET/CT 结合骨髓穿刺活检结果给出的诊断为:非霍奇金淋巴瘤。

（1）该患者发热的内生致热原主要由下列哪种细胞产生?

    A. 单核细胞                 B. 巨噬细胞

    C. 肿瘤细胞                 D. 星状细胞

    E. 内皮细胞

（2）下列哪种物质属于内生致热原?

    A. PGE                      B. MIP-1

    C. LPS                      D. AVP

    E. MAN

（3）下列哪种处理方式能够有效为该患者降低体温?

    A. 水杨酸钠                 B. 糖皮质激素

    C. 尼克酸                   D. 冰毯

    E. 茶碱

## 案例分析问答题

[案例一]

患者,女性,70 岁,2 天前因受凉后出现头疼咳嗽并出现发热入院。患者食欲不佳,每餐只进食少量稀饭。入院体检:T 39 ℃,左下肺部有散在啰音。因身体虚弱,用轮椅送往住院部入院治疗。患者自述无其他既往病史。

问题:

（1）入院后在确诊与治疗前还需要进行哪些检查?

（2）该患者发热的可能原因是什么? 简述其机制。

（3）该患者食欲不佳的可能原因是什么?

[案例二]

患者,男性,68 岁,因咳嗽加剧及胸痛入院诊治。患者已婚,退休。发热伴咳嗽、咳痰 5 天,长期吸烟史,高血压病史 15 年;自服感冒药(布洛芬)后体温略减;次日体温又逐渐升高至 39 ℃。

入院体检:T 39.5 ℃,P 100 次/min,R 29 次/min,BP 160/82 mmHg。

实验室检查:白细胞(WBC) $12 \times 10^9$/L,中性粒细胞 75%。

胸部 X 线检查结果显示两侧肺纹理增多增粗,左侧胸腔积液。

因此,该患者初步诊断为上呼吸道感染引起的高热。

问题:

（1）该患者是否属于必须及时解热的患者? 为什么?

（2）该患者心血管系统会出现何种变化?

（3）该患者体内物质代谢会出现何种改变？

（4）该患者还可能出现哪些其他基本病理过程？

（5）该患者可采取的护理措施有哪些？

### 参考答案

**案例分析选择题（多选一）**

**1.** ADECB；**2.** DDAE；**3.** CBD

**案例分析问答题**

[案例一]

（1）入院后在确诊与治疗前还需要进行哪些检查？

血液检查（白细胞计数及分类，中性粒细胞计数），尿液检查，放射学检查（包括胸部 X 线摄片），痰培养。

（2）该患者发热的可能原因是什么？简述其机制。

患者上呼吸道感染引起病原体入侵，经过层层信息传递与整合，最终引起发热。其机制为：

① 发热激活物的作用阶段：发热激活物（包括外致热原和体内产物）作用于产 EP 细胞（包括单核细胞、巨噬细胞及淋巴细胞等），产生和释放 EP（IL-1、TNF、IFN、IL-6 和 MIP-1），通过血脑屏障或 OVLT 部位将信号传递进入体温调节中枢，即 POAH 区域。

② 调定点上移：正调节中枢产生正调节介质，如 $PGE_2$、cAMP、$Na^+/Ca^{2+}$、CRH 和 NO；负调节中枢产生负调节介质，如 AVP、α-MSH 和 LC-1；正负调节作用的结局是体温调定点上移。

③ 发热的效应阶段：机体一方面通过皮肤血管收缩方式减少散热，另一方面通过寒战和增加物质代谢的方式增加产热，最终导致发热。

（3）该患者食欲不佳的可能原因是什么？

发热导致患者消化液分泌减少，各种消化酶活性降低。

[案例二]

（1）该患者是否属于必须及时解热的患者？为什么？

患者体温已高达 39 ℃，且有高血压病史，因此属于必须及时解热的病例。一方面考虑高热本身的危害，另一方面考虑高血压患者心脏负荷过重引起心力衰竭。

（2）该患者心血管系统会出现何种变化？

该患者血温增高刺激窦房结致使心率加快，感染后血液中 LPS 及下丘脑中 $PGE_2$ 含量的增加都可激活交感-肾上腺髓质系统，导致心率增快，心输出量也增加。但心率大于 180 次/min 时，心输出量反而会降低。而且患者长期高血压及吸烟会极大地削弱其心血管系统代偿机能，在高热下心肌负担的加重更易诱发心力衰竭。

（3）该患者体内物质代谢会出现何种改变？

发热时体内物质消耗都升高，分别体现在：

① 糖代谢：糖原分解增高，血糖增高，糖原储备减少。

② 蛋白质代谢：蛋白质分解代谢加强，尿素氮明显增高，呈负氮平衡。

③ 脂肪代谢：患者食欲低下，糖类摄入不足导致脂肪分解加强，大量脂肪分解而氧化不全可使血中酮体增加。

④ 水、电解质与维生素代谢：高热引发水分大量丢失易引发脱水；患者食物摄入有限且消耗增加导致体内维生素不足。

（4）该患者还可能出现哪些其他基本病理过程？

① 该患者退热后皮肤、呼吸道大量蒸发水分，出汗增多及尿量增多，可引起高渗性脱水。

② 严重时因乳酸和酮体增多，可发生代谢性酸中毒。

③ 发热时，一方面组织分解代谢增强，细胞内钾释放入血；另一方面酸中毒也会引起钾离子的外移，都可能引起高钾血症。

（5）该患者可采取的护理措施有哪些？

① 控制原发病。

② 物理降温，包括头部冷敷、酒精擦拭或温水浴。

③ 遵医嘱采用药物降温，包括对乙酰氨基酚类的药物等。

④ 鼓励饮水，给高热量流质或半流质的饮食，必要时配合输液，纠正水、电解质代谢紊乱。

（孙丽娜）

# 第五章　应　激

## 案例分析选择题（多选一）

1. 患者，男性，32 岁，厨师，因接触高温油引发烧伤急诊入院。体格检查：意识不清，T 36.3 ℃，P 143 次/min，R 36 次/min，BP 82/68 mmHg。4 小时后患者意识清醒，生命体征平稳，2 天后患者出现水样腹泻，并柏油样便 3 次，伴有腹胀。大便潜血试验（＋＋＋＋）。患者否认有任何胃部疾病的病史。

（1）该患者最有可能发生下列哪种疾病？

　　A. 原发性高血压　　　　　　　　B. 动脉粥样硬化

　　C. 应激性溃疡　　　　　　　　　D. 支气管哮喘

　　E. 冠心病

（2）该患者体内不可能出现下列哪种反应？

　　A. 心率增快　　　　　　　　　　B. 心肌收缩力增强

　　C. 心输出量增加　　　　　　　　D. 骨骼肌血管扩张

　　E. 肾动脉扩张

（3）该患者体内减少的激素最有可能是下列哪种？

　　A. β-内啡肽　　　　　　　　　　B. 胰岛素

　　C. 胰高血糖素　　　　　　　　　D. ADH

　　E. 催乳素

（4）该患者临床表现的发病机制不包括以下哪个选项？

　　A. 胃黏膜缺血　　　　　　　　　B. 胆汁逆流

　　C. 胃黏液蛋白分泌增多　　　　　D. $H^+$ 向黏膜内反向弥散

　　E. 酸中毒

（5）该患者体内浓度迅速变化的蛋白不包括下列哪项？

    A. C-反应蛋白　　　　　　　　　　B. 血红素结合蛋白

    C. 热休克蛋白　　　　　　　　　　D. 铜蓝蛋白

    E. 纤维蛋白原

2. 患者,男性,60 岁,主诉胸闷、心悸 1 年,1 天前因情绪激动胸痛加重入当地医院。患者有高血压病史 10 年,入院后血压 160/100 mmHg;床边心电图结果:ST 段压低,该导联 T 波倒置,诊断结果为“急性非 ST 段抬高型心肌梗死”。

（1）该患者情绪激动与其发病相关的主要机制是下列哪项？

    A. 交感-肾上腺髓质系统兴奋　　　　B. 使心肌发生向心性肥大

    C. 血胆固醇升高,血液黏度增高　　　D. 激活肾素-血管紧张素-醛固酮系统

    E. 肾血管收缩,水钠潴留

（2）该患者体内下列哪一种内分泌腺最可能发生应答？

    A. 甲状腺　　　　　　　　　　　　B. 肾上腺

    C. 甲状旁腺　　　　　　　　　　　D. 性腺

    E. 胰腺

（3）该患者发病前心血管系统的基本变化为下列哪项？

    A. 心室纤颤的阈值升高　　　　　　B. 冠状动脉血流量减少

    C. 心率减慢,心输出量减少　　　　D. 心输出量增加, 血压升高

    E. 总外周阻力下降

（4）该患者体内最有可能出现下列哪种变化？

    A. 肾上腺素浓度降低　　　　　　　B. 胰高血糖素浓度降低

    C. 胰岛素浓度降低　　　　　　　　D. 内啡肽浓度降低

    E. 去甲肾上腺素浓度降低

（5）该患者若出现少尿,其可能的机制是下列哪项？

    A. 交感-肾上腺髓质系统兴奋　　　　B. 肾素-血管紧张素-醛固酮系统抑制

    C. 心房钠尿肽分泌增多　　　　　　D. 下丘脑-垂体-肾上腺皮质系统兴奋

    E. 抗利尿激素分泌减少

3. 患者,男性,17 岁,初三,主诉其近 1 年里总会有莫名的压抑感,很痛苦;对一切无兴趣,情绪极度低落,甚至有自杀未遂的经历,遂入院进行心理辅导。

（1）该患者身体可能会出现下列哪种病理生理变化？

    A. 多尿　　　　　　　　　　　　　B. 血糖降低

    C. 游离脂肪酸增多　　　　　　　　D. 血液凝固性降低

    E. 心率降低

（2）该患者血液系统的变化可能是下列哪项？

    A. 白细胞数量减少　　　　　　　　B. 凝血因子Ⅷ减少

    C. 补体成分 C3 减少　　　　　　　D. 纤维蛋白原浓度减少

    E. 红细胞数目减少

（3）该患者消化系统可能的变化是下列哪项？

    A. 胃酸分泌减少            B. 胃血流量增加

    C. 胃蛋白酶分泌减少     D. 胃黏膜糜烂

    E. 胃黏膜修复能力增加

（4）该患者泌尿系统可能的变化是下列哪项？

    A. 尿量增多               B. 尿比重降低

    C. 蛋白尿                 D. 肾小球滤过率降低

    E. 肾小管泌 $H^+$ 功能降低

## 案例分析问答题

[案例一]

患者，男性，50 岁，因吐血和柏油样大便入院。患者 3 天前发生了翻船事故，差点溺水身亡。之后 3 天，他持续激动得睡不着觉。患者否认有任何胃病史。入院时 T 37.5 ℃，HR 125 次/min，BP 135/80 mmHg。实验室检查显示：轻度贫血，WBC $1.5 \times 10^9$/L，胃泌素正常，血糖 10 mmol/L（正常 3.9~6.0 mmol/L）。食管胃十二指肠镜检查显示患者胃黏膜血管外漏，是胃溃疡。

问题：

（1）该患者为什么出现黑便？请简述其发病机制。

（2）该患者神经-内分泌系统可能发生哪些变化？

[案例二]

患者，女性，17 岁，高中生，由母亲陪同就诊。自述：精神紧张，睡不着觉，看到试卷就头脑一片空白等。母亲所述：患者从小学习成绩优良，性格开朗；但自从上了重点中学后，学习压力突然增大，加上自我要求又高，所以变得更加刻苦，希望考上重点大学。为了成绩进步，该患者放弃了其他业余爱好。即便如此，随着高考考期临近，患者逐渐出现了紧张、失眠、消瘦、易怒、喜欢独处等反常行为，学习成绩也一直在下降；并且每到考试前期就出现"肚子痛"的现象，检查后并未发现有异常。

心理医生和她沟通后，帮助她重新调整了学习目标，合理地调配学习和休息、娱乐时间。半年后症状逐渐消失。

问题：

（1）患者为何会出现上述表现？

（2）简述患者出现这些症状的神经内分泌变化机制。

（3）简单分析其"肚子痛"现象属于哪种病理过程。

参考答案

案例分析选择题（多选一）

1. CEBCC；2. ABDCA；3. CEDD

**案例分析问答题**

**[案例一]**

（1）该患者为什么出现黑便？请简述其发病机制。

患者发生应激性溃疡，在遭受各类重伤、重病和其他应激情况（如该患者大面积烫伤）下，会出现胃、十二指肠黏膜的急性病变，主要表现为胃、十二指肠黏膜的糜烂、浅溃疡、渗血等，少数可较深或穿孔。

发生机制如下：

① 胃肠黏膜缺血：蓝斑-交感-肾上腺髓质系统强烈兴奋，引起胃、十二指肠黏膜缺血缺氧，是造成应激时胃黏膜糜烂、溃疡和出血的基本原因。

② 黏膜屏障功能降低：ATP 生成减少，碳酸氢盐及黏液不足；缺血引发胃腔内 $H^+$ 向黏膜内的反向弥散增多，不能及时中和又无法及时运走，进一步造成损伤。

③ 胆汁反流和自由基等可能也参与黏膜缺血性损伤。

（2）该患者神经-内分泌系统可能发生哪些变化？

① 蓝斑-交感-肾上腺髓质系统兴奋，其中枢效应为：患者产生兴奋和警觉，并产生紧张、焦虑等情绪反应；其外周效应为：血浆肾上腺素和去甲肾上腺素浓度迅速升高。

② 下丘脑-垂体-肾上腺皮质系统兴奋，其中枢效应为：下丘脑室旁核分泌 CRH 增多，调控应激时的情绪行为反应，促进内啡肽释放；其外周效应为：CRH 刺激垂体分泌 ACTH，最终诱导糖皮质激素分泌增多。

③ RAAS 兴奋，血浆中醛固酮增多，血压升高，少尿，维持血容量。

**[案例二]**

（1）患者为何会出现上述表现？

心理性应激过度强烈带来的不良后果。

（2）简述患者出现这些症状的神经内分泌变化机制。

① 蓝斑-交感-肾上腺髓质系统兴奋：蓝斑 NE 神经元过度兴奋导致其上行投射脑区中（杏仁体、海马、边缘系统和新皮质）的 NE 水平过度增高→引发患者产生焦虑和害怕的不良情绪。

② 下丘脑-垂体-肾上腺皮质系统兴奋：PVN 释放大量 CRH→过量 CRH 引起患者的适应机制障碍，如焦虑、抑郁、学习与记忆能力下降、食欲减退等。

（3）简单分析其"肚子痛"现象属于哪种病理过程。

属于功能性胃肠病，不伴有形态学和生化方面的异常，与患者长期精神压力过大、过度焦虑和抑郁情绪有直接关系。机制：神经内分泌系统调节出现障碍。

（孙丽娜）

# 第六章　缺　氧

## 案例分析选择题（多选一）

1. 患者，女性，血氧指标检测如下：$PaO_2$ 为 98 mmHg，$CO_2max$ 为 13 mL/dL，$CaO_2$ 为 15 mL/dL，$C(a\text{-}v)O_2$ 为 3 mL/dL。

（1）该患者最可能患有下列哪种疾病？

    A. 哮喘                            B. 贫血

    C. 维生素 $B_1$ 缺乏             D. 一氧化碳中毒

    E. 心肌肥大

（2）下列哪项是该患者引起组织缺氧的机制？

    A. 毛细血管平均氧分压上升      B. 血氧含量减少

    C. 血氧容量上升               D. 血氧分压降低

    E. 组织血流减少

（3）下列哪项是该患者可能出现的代谢变化？

    A. 代谢性碱中毒              B. 细胞内 $Na^+$ 减少

    C. 有氧氧化增强              D. 糖酵解增强

    E. 机体耗氧增多

（4）该患者体内细胞可能出现下列哪种代偿性变化？

    A. 溶酶体膜通透性升高        B. 细胞内 $K^+$ 外流

    C. 细胞内 $Na^+$ 减少             D. 线粒体数目增多

    E. 毛细血管密度减少

2. 患者，男性，18 岁，高考后和同学相约去西藏旅游。因到达海拔 4 000 米处后较为兴奋而出现过度通气，逐渐全身麻木，四肢抽搐，继而昏厥。经当地医院抢救后恢复健康。

（1）该患者最可能发生了哪种类型的缺氧？

    A. 血液性缺氧              B. 缺血性缺氧

    C. 低张性缺氧              D. 组织性缺氧

    E. 淤血性缺氧

（2）该患者循环系统不可能出现下列哪种代偿反应？

    A. 心率加快                   B. 心肌收缩力加强

    C. 心、脑血管扩张           D. 静脉回流量增加

    E. 肺血管扩张

（3）下列哪项不可能是该患者出现昏厥的机制？

    A. 脑细胞 ATP 生成不足      B. 脑细胞脱水

    C. 脑微血管通透性增高      D. 神经细胞膜电位降低

    E. 神经细胞结构破坏

（4）该患者体内可能会出现下列哪一种变化？

    A. 交感神经兴奋，心输出量减少

    B. 脑细胞脱水，出现精神症状

    C. 心肌收缩加强，腺苷产生增多，冠状动脉收缩

    D. 肺小动脉收缩，肺动脉压升高

    E. 促红细胞生成素合成增多，红细胞数量及血红蛋白含量明显增加

3. 一位住院患者李某的血气检测结果如下：$PaO_2$ 85 mmHg，$PvO_2$ 60 mmHg，血氧容量 10.8 mL/dL，动脉血氧饱和度 97%，动-静脉血氧含量差 2.8 mL/dL。

（1）下列有关血氧指标的叙述哪一项不正确？

　　A. 血氧容量决定于血液中 Hb 的浓度及 Hb 和 $O_2$ 的结合力

　　B. 血氧饱和度的高低与血液中血红蛋白的量无关

　　C. 动脉血氧分压取决于吸入气中氧分压的高低

　　D. 血氧含量是指 100 mL 血液中实际含有 $O_2$ 的毫升数

　　E. 正常动-静脉血氧含量差约为 5 mL/dL

（2）该患者有哪种类型的缺氧？

　　A. 乏氧性缺氧　　　　　　　　　　B. 血液性缺氧

　　C. 循环性缺氧　　　　　　　　　　D. 组织性缺氧

　　E. 混合性缺氧

（3）如果缺氧未及时纠正，该患者会出现下列哪种细胞膜内、外的离子变化？

　　A. 细胞内 $Na^+$ 增多　　　　　　　B. 细胞外 $K^+$ 减少

　　C. 细胞内 $Ca^{2+}$ 减少　　　　　　D. 细胞外 $H^+$ 减少

　　E. 细胞内 $H^+$ 减少

（4）下列关于该患者的说法哪一项是正确的？

　　A. 呼吸运动和肺通气量显著增加　　B. 脑血管收缩

　　C. 应及时给患者输血　　　　　　　D. 皮肤黏膜呈樱桃红色

　　E. 高压氧治疗后患者症状明显缓解

4. 患儿，6 个月，因哭闹后呼吸急促并伴有青紫而入院。最终诊断为先天性心脏病（法洛四联症）。

（1）下列哪种变化导致患儿发绀？

　　A. 血红蛋白的增多　　　　　　　　B. 碳氧血红蛋白的增多

　　C. 高铁血红蛋白的增多　　　　　　D. 脱氧血红蛋白的增多

　　E. 氰化血红蛋白的增多

（2）该患儿发绀是由下列哪类缺氧引发？

　　A. 低张性缺氧　　　　　　　　　　B. 血液性缺氧

　　C. 循环性缺氧　　　　　　　　　　D. 组织性缺氧

　　E. 混合性缺氧

（3）下列哪项是该患儿发生缺氧的原因？

　　A. 吸入气氧分压降低　　　　　　　B. 血红蛋白含量减少

　　C. 全身循环功能障碍　　　　　　　D. 线粒体损伤

　　E. 静脉血分流入动脉血

（4）该患儿不会出现下列哪项血氧变化？

    A. 动脉血氧分压降低           B. 动脉血氧饱和度降低

    C. 动脉血氧容量降低           D. 动脉血氧含量降低

    E. 动-静脉血氧含量差降低

（5）有关该患儿的治疗下列哪项不正确？

    A. 镇静                       B. 让婴儿平躺

    C. 吸氧                       D. 姑息性手术

    E. 前列腺素治疗

5. 22 岁女性，在一起交通事故后因严重的左上腹疼痛被送入急诊室。入院体检发现：面色惨白，BP 80/40 mmHg，P 125 次/min，R 26 次/min。腹部 CT 发现脾破裂及腹腔大量出血。诊断为脾破裂和失血性休克。

（1）该患者最可能发生下列哪种类型的缺氧？

    A. 乏氧性缺氧             B. 血液性缺氧

    C. 循环性缺氧             D. 组织性缺氧

    E. 以上都有可能

（2）该患者可能出现下列哪种血气变化？

    A. 动脉血氧分压降低           B. 动脉血氧饱和度降低

    C. 动脉血氧容量降低           D. 动脉血氧含量降低

    E. 动-静脉血氧含量差增高

（3）有关该患者发生缺氧的描述下列哪项不正确？

    A. 患者外呼吸功能正常，血氧分压及饱和度并不降低

    B. 患者外周组织缺血缺氧

    C. 由于细胞从血液中摄取的氧减少，所以不易出现发绀

    D. 组织缺氧后血红蛋白的氧离曲线右移

    E. 患者血红蛋白的数量与质量变化不大

（4）如果患者大量输液后导致血液过度稀释，可能发生下列哪种类型的缺氧？

    A. 低张性缺氧 + 血液性缺氧       B. 血液性缺氧 + 循环性缺氧

    C. 循环性缺氧 + 低张性缺氧       D. 组织性缺氧 + 低张性缺氧

    E. 组织性缺氧 + 血液性缺氧

6. 患儿 6 岁，晚餐进食一锅酸菜炖肉后，出现头疼无力，由父母送入急诊。病人面色青紫，发绀明显。经血检等检查诊断为亚硝酸盐中毒。

（1）该患者最可能发生下列哪种类型的缺氧？

    A. 乏氧性缺氧             B. 血液性缺氧

    C. 循环性缺氧             D. 组织性缺氧

    E. 以上都有可能

（2）下列哪项改变导致患儿发绀？

  A. 血红蛋白增多       B. 碳氧血红蛋白增多

  C. 高铁血红蛋白增多      D. 脱氧血红蛋白增多

  E. 亚铁血红蛋白增多

（3）下列哪项血气变化并不可能出现在该患儿体内？

  A. 动脉血氧分压降低      B. 动脉血氧饱和度降低

  C. 动脉血氧容量降低      D. 动脉血氧含量降低

  E. 动-静脉血氧含量差降低

（4）该患儿一定要进行下列哪项治疗？

  A. 催吐、洗胃去除毒素     B. 吸氧增加动脉血氧分压

  C. 治疗高铁血红蛋白血症    D. 饮水、输液促毒素排出

  E. 以上都不对

## 案例分析问答题

**[案例一]**

  患者，女性，67 岁，咳嗽、痰多、喘憋加重伴发热 3 天来院就诊。患者 15 年前开始咳嗽、咳痰反复发作，上述症状逐年加重，并逐渐伴有喘憋。本次于入院前 2 天受凉后出现发热、畏寒、咳嗽、咳脓痰、喘憋加重并且夜间不能平卧。

  体格检查：口唇和指尖部皮肤发绀。T 39.0 ℃，P 120 次/min，R 28 次/min。胸廓略呈桶状，肋间隙增宽，双肺呼吸音粗，可闻及大量痰鸣音，右下肺呼吸音低。

  动脉血气分析结果：pH 7.14，$PaO_2$ 50 mmHg，$PaCO_2$ 80 mmHg，患者 AB、SB 和 BB 均降低，AG 18 mmol/L，$[K^+]$ 6.6 mmol/L，$[Na^+]$ 140 mmol/L，$[Cl^-]$ 92 mmol/L。

  病人的初步诊断为慢性阻塞性肺疾病，给予吸氧治疗后患者症状得以缓解。

  问题：

  （1）该患者体内出现了何种类型的缺氧？出现了哪些典型表现？其血氧变化特点是什么？

  （2）患者入院后输氧的意义和原则是什么？

  （3）患者入院时发生了何种类型的酸碱平衡紊乱？其原因和发病机制是什么？

**[案例二]**

  患者男性，张某，12 岁，入院前 1 小时被家人发现卧倒在浴室，患者意识不清，呈昏迷状态。送至医院后患者开始出现四肢抽搐及大小便失禁的症状，予导尿、输液和输氧等对症处理。

  诊断：重度一氧化碳中毒。

  神志清醒后体检发现：T 36.5 ℃，P 110 次/min，BP 110/62 mmHg，$SaO_2$ 100%，每日行高压氧仓治疗，注意防治脑水肿，且给予营养疗法帮助恢复。

  问题：

  （1）该患者属于哪种类型的缺氧？其血气指标变化特点是什么？患者会有何种特征性的表现？

（2）该患者进行高压氧仓治疗的目的是什么？

（3）请分析为什么该患者易出现脑水肿。

**参考答案**

**案例分析选择题（多选一）**

**1.** BBDD；**2.** CEBD；**3.** CEAC；**4.** DAECB；**5.** CECB；**6.** BCAC

**案例分析问答题**

**［案例一］**

（1）该患者体内出现了何种类型的缺氧？出现了哪些典型表现？其血氧变化特点是什么？

慢性阻塞性肺疾病患者由于呼吸道阻塞导致肺泡通气不足，因此缺氧的原始病因是肺泡气的氧分压过低，属于低张性缺氧。该患者出现了典型的发绀，是毛细血管血液中脱氧血红蛋白浓度超过 5 g/dL 时导致皮肤与黏膜呈青紫色的症状。血氧变化特点：$PaO_2$ 下降（50 mmHg < 100 mmHg），$CaO_2$ 和 $SaO_2$ 下降，$CO_2max$ 上升，$C(a\text{-}v)O_2$ 变化应不大。

（2）患者入院后输氧的意义和原则是什么？

氧疗能提高肺泡内氧分压，进而提高 $PaO_2$ 和 $SaO_2$，减轻组织损伤，恢复脏器功能，降低缺氧性肺动脉高压进而减轻右心负荷。

临床上根据患者病情和靶向血氧水平选取不同的给氧浓度和给氧方法。原则是保证迅速提高 $PaO_2$ 到 60 mmHg 或脉搏容积血氧饱和度（$SpO_2$）达 90% 以上的前提下，尽量降低吸氧浓度。

（3）患者入院时发生了何种类型的酸碱平衡紊乱？其原因和发病机制是什么？

根据原发病为慢性阻塞性肺疾病（COPD）及 $PaO_2$ 降低，$PaCO_2$ 升高，AB、SB 和 BB 均降低，且 pH 也大幅度降低可初步断定该患者存在呼吸性酸中毒合并代谢性酸中毒。尽管 AG > 16，但是 AB、SB、BB 均减小且血氯正常，表明并不存在代谢性碱中毒，不是三重性的酸碱平衡紊乱。COPD 引起长期低张性缺氧导致 $PaO_2$ 持续较低水平，细胞无氧酵解增加，酸性物质产生增多，致使 AG 升高及 AB、SB 和 BB 的降低。而 COPD 导致通气障碍及 $CO_2$ 排出受阻，致使 $PaCO_2$ 远高于正常水平。

**［案例二］**

（1）该患者属于哪种类型的缺氧？其血气指标变化特点是什么？患者会有何种特征性的表现？

该患者属于血液性缺氧，其血液中血红蛋白变成碳氧血红蛋白，失去携氧能力。血气指标变化特点为：体内 $CO_2max$ 降低以致 $CaO_2$ 降低，$PaO_2$ 和 $SaO_2$ 可正常，$C(a\text{-}v)O_2$ 减少。CO 与血红蛋白结合形成的碳氧血红蛋白会令患者的皮肤与黏膜呈现樱桃红色。

（2）该患者进行高压氧仓治疗的目的是什么？

该患者属于血液性缺氧，高压氧仓治疗并不能明显改善患者呼吸系统功能，但是高压氧的治疗能够快速提高患者的血液储氧能力及脑组织的氧含量，改善脑组织和其他组织的缺氧情况，减少细胞损伤，尤其是脑细胞的损伤；另外，高压氧的治疗能够加速机体的代谢，加速患者体内一氧化碳的清除。

（3）请分析为什么该患者易出现脑水肿。

① 缺氧会引起脑血管扩张，脑血流量增大而液体外漏，引起脑水肿。

② 脑细胞由于能量代谢紊乱，ATP 生成降低，钠泵功能障碍，细胞内出现钠、水潴留而引起脑细胞水肿。

③ 缺氧引起脑组织血管内皮损伤，通透性增大，引起脑水肿。

（孙丽娜）

# 第七章 休 克

## 案例分析选择题（多选一）

1. 患儿,男,8 岁,接种疫苗 1 小时后出现皮疹,奇痒,伴心慌、头晕、皮肤发绀及呼吸困难。

（1）该患儿可能出现了何种病理过程？
    A. 感染性休克　　　　　　　　　　B. 低血容量性休克
    C. 心源性休克　　　　　　　　　　D. 神经源性休克
    E. 过敏性休克

（2）这种类型的休克发生时,应立即给予该患儿下列哪种药物？
    A. 缩血管药　　　　　　　　　　　B. 肾上腺皮质激素
    C. 扩血管药,并输液　　　　　　　D. 纠正酸中毒的药物
    E. 抗生素

（3）该患儿的血压可能发生何种变化？
    A. 收缩压升高　　　　　　　　　　B. 舒张压升高
    C. 显著降低　　　　　　　　　　　D. 变化不明显
    E. 脉压差减小

（4）下列哪项是该患儿发生休克的始动环节？
    A. 血容量减少　　　　　　　　　　B. 心脏泵功能障碍
    C. 血管床容积增大　　　　　　　　D. 血管床容积增大 + 血容量减少
    E. 心脏泵功能障碍 + 血管床容积增大

2. 患者,男,65 岁,患冠心病 15 年,凌晨睡眠中突然出现胸痛、胸闷及呼吸急促,同时伴有乏力、全身大汗、心悸及四肢厥冷,血压 60/40 mmHg。

（1）该患者可能出现了哪种类型的休克？
    A. 感染性休克　　　　　　　　　　B. 失血性休克
    C. 创伤性休克　　　　　　　　　　D. 心源性休克
    E. 过敏性休克

（2）患者可能出现下列哪种酸碱平衡紊乱？
    A. 代谢性酸中毒合并呼吸性碱中毒　　B. 呼吸性酸中毒
    C. 代谢性碱中毒　　　　　　　　　　D. 代谢性碱中毒合并呼吸性酸中毒
    E. 代谢性碱中毒合并呼吸性碱中毒

（3）此类型休克的始动环节是什么？

    A. 血容量减少          B. 心脏泵功能障碍

    C. 血管床容积增大      D. 血容量增加

    E. 外周血管收缩

（4）下列哪项是该患者血压下降的原因？

    A. 血容量减少          B. 血管床容积增大

    C. 心输出量减少       D. 肺循环淤血

    E. 外周血管收缩

3. 患者，女，31 岁，产后大出血，神志淡漠，皮肤出现发绀、花斑，24 小时尿量280 mL，血压 80/55 mmHg，使用缩血管药物血压略回升。

（1）该患者处于休克哪一期？

    A. 微循环缺血缺氧期      B. 微循环淤血缺氧期

    C. 微循环衰竭期        D. 代偿期

    E. 难治期

（2）该患者微循环最可能发生的变化是什么？

    A. 少灌多流、灌少于流，组织细胞缺血性缺氧

    B. 少灌少流、灌少于流，组织细胞缺血性缺氧

    C. 灌而少流、灌大于流，组织细胞淤血性缺氧

    D. 不灌不流、血液高凝，组织细胞无血供

    E. 弥漫性血管内凝血

（3）该患者血管阻力可能发生何种变化？

    A. 毛细血管前后阻力均升高    B. 毛细血管前后阻力均降低

    C. 毛细血管前阻力大于后阻力  D. 毛细血管后阻力大于前阻力

    E. 毛细血管前阻力增大，后阻力降低

（4）下列哪项是患者皮肤出现发绀和花斑的原因？

    A. 皮肤血管收缩        B. 皮肤血液淤滞，脱氧血红蛋白增多

    C. 脱氧血红蛋白减少    D. 毛细血管血浆外渗

    E. 血压显著降低

## 案例分析问答题

[案例一]

患者，女，45 岁，夜间由家人送至急诊科。当天早上，患者发现便中带血，颜色鲜红，她以为是痔疮，并未在意，继续日常活动。然而出血持续了一整天，到了晚上，患者脸色苍白，出冷汗，四肢湿冷，神情焦虑，呼吸加深加快，尿量减少，急诊入院。急诊科检查显示，患者血压 105/85 mmHg，心率 100 次/min。

患者于急诊科输注生理盐水，并抽取血液样本进行交叉配型，为输血做准备。结肠镜检查显示，该患者出血来自结肠壁的疝气，检查时出血已自发停止。由于失血量大，输血 400

mL,留院观察。第二天早上,患者皮肤颜色恢复,不再出冷汗,呼吸、血压和心率恢复正常。

**问题:**

(1)该患者是否发生了休克?请分析该患者出现休克的病因和类型。

(2)休克病程分为哪几期?该患者入院时处于哪一期?此期患者微循环血液灌流特点是什么?

(3)患者出血一整天,为何动脉血压降低不明显?

(4)为什么患者皮肤苍白,出冷汗,且尿量减少?

**[案例二]**

患者,男,18 岁,因发热、四肢皮疹入院。入院后检查 T 39.5 ℃,HR 120 次/min,BP 90/40 mmHg;动脉血气分析显示 pH 7.30,$HCO_3^-$浓度 16 mmol/L,$PaCO_2$ 26 mmHg,乳酸升高(3.5 mmol/L);胸片显示双侧肺间质-肺泡浸润;脑脊液染色提示革兰氏阴性球菌阳性,后期血液和脑脊液培养出脑膜炎奈瑟菌。入院后给予补液、广谱抗生素及多巴胺治疗,因患者持续低血压和少尿,增大多巴胺剂量和生理盐水输注量,并给予肾上腺素,患者的平均动脉压和尿量有所增加。12 小时后,患者动脉乳酸水平下降,病情好转。

**问题:**

(1)该患者是否发生了休克?请分析该患者出现休克的病因、类型及始动环节。

(2)该患者的脉压差为何增大?

(3)根据患者的血气分析结果,请分析该患者出现了何种酸碱平衡紊乱。

(4)患者乳酸升高的原因是什么?

**参考答案**

**案例分析选择题(多选一)**

**1.** EACD;**2.** DABC;**3.** BCDB

**案例分析问答题**

**[案例一]**

(1)该患者是否发生了休克?请分析该患者出现休克的病因和类型。

该患者因失血出现休克早期的表现:脸色苍白,出冷汗,四肢湿冷,神情焦虑,呼吸加深加快,血压稍降低,脉压差减少,心率加快,尿量减少,且患者入院后经过输血输液治疗症状消失,可判断该患者发生了休克。患者的病因是结肠壁疝气出血导致的血容量减少。按病因进行分类,患者发生的是失血性休克;按休克的始动环节进行分类,该患者发生的是低血容量性休克。

(2)休克病程分为哪几期?该患者入院时处于哪一期?此期患者微循环血液灌流特点是什么?

休克病程分为三期:微循环缺血缺氧期(代偿期)、微循环淤血缺氧期(失代偿期)及微循环衰竭期(难治期)。该患者症状体征符合休克代偿期的临床表现,如皮肤无花斑和发绀,血压降低不明显,神志清醒,故尚处于休克代偿期。休克代偿期血液灌流特点为:少灌少流,灌少于流,组织细胞缺血性缺氧。

(3)患者出血一整天,为何动脉血压降低不明显?

该患者处于休克代偿期,出血后血量减少导致交感神经系统兴奋,缩血管体液因子释放增加,可引起:

① 容量血管和肝脾等储血器官收缩,通过"自身输血"增加回心血量。

② 毛细血管前阻力血管收缩强度大于微静脉,毛细血管中流体静压下降,通过"自身输液"增加回心血量。

③ 阻力血管收缩,外周阻力升高。

④ 心肌细胞 β 受体兴奋,心率加快,心肌收缩力增强,增加心输出量。回心血量增加,外周阻力增加,心输出量增加有助于动脉血压的维持。

(4)为什么患者皮肤苍白、出冷汗,且尿量减少?

失血导致交感-肾上腺髓质系统和肾素-血管紧张素-醛固酮系统激活,引起外周血管收缩,其中皮肤、肾脏血管收缩更明显。皮肤缺血导致肤色苍白、四肢冰冷;肾脏血流减少引起尿量减少;交感神经兴奋刺激汗腺分泌,患者出冷汗。

[案例二]

(1)该患者是否发生了休克? 请分析该患者出现休克的病因、类型及始动环节。

该患者有低血压、少尿和酸中毒等有效循环血量减少、组织血液低灌注的表现,表明他发生了休克。根据患者发热以及血液和脑脊液培养出脑膜炎奈瑟菌的感染证据,按病因分类,他发生了因脑膜炎奈瑟菌感染所致的感染性休克(脓毒性休克)。其始动环节涉及休克发生的 3 个始动环节:

① 细胞因子和血管活性物质可增加毛细血管通透性,使血浆外渗,血容量减少。

② 血管活性物质引起血管扩张,血管床容积增大。

③ 细菌毒素及炎症介质可直接损伤心肌细胞,造成心脏功能障碍。

(2)该患者的脉压差为何增大?

感染性休克(脓毒性休克)引起交感-肾上腺髓质系统兴奋,激活心肌 β 受体,增强心肌收缩力,有助于维持收缩压;同时机体产生大量炎症介质和扩张血管的活性物质,使外周阻力降低,因此舒张压降低更明显,脉压差增大。

(3)根据患者的血气分析结果,请分析该患者出现了何种酸碱平衡紊乱。

pH 7.30,且 $HCO_3^-$ 浓度降低,乳酸升高,提示该患者出现了代谢性酸中毒。根据代谢性酸中毒预计代偿公式,$PaCO_2 = 1.5 \times [HCO_3^-] + 8 \pm 2$,预测 $PaCO_2$ 为 $32 \pm 2$,该患者实际 $PaCO_2$ 26 mmHg,说明该患者发生的酸碱平衡紊乱为代谢性酸中毒合并呼吸性碱中毒。

(4)患者乳酸升高的原因是什么?

休克组织细胞缺血缺氧,细胞发生无氧糖酵解,乳酸生成增多;肝功能受损,乳酸代谢障碍;肾缺血,乳酸排出减少。

(赵丽梅)

# 第八章 凝血与抗凝血平衡紊乱

## 案例分析选择题（多选一）

1. 患者,男性,56 岁,咳嗽、胸痛 5 天,咳黄色脓痰 3 天。体格检查发现:T 39 ℃,HR 96 次/min,R 24 次/min,BP 129/85 mmHg,肺呼吸音粗,右下肺有明显湿啰音,双下肢大片瘀斑。实验室检查:血常规 WBC $22 \times 10^9$/L,血红蛋白(Hb)94 g/L(正常 120~160 g/L),血小板(PLT)$100 \times 10^9$/L;凝血功能活化部分凝血活酶时间(APTT)48.2 s(对照30.2 s),血浆凝血酶原时间(PT)19.5 s(对照 14.2 s),凝血酶时间(TT)35.6 s(对照 12.8 s),纤维蛋白原(Fg)1.6 g/L(正常 1.8~4.5 g/L)。X 线显示双肺纹理增粗,右下肺可见片状阴影。

（1）医生高度怀疑病人发生了 DIC，下列哪项指标可以帮助医生确诊？

    A. 白细胞计数                    B. 血小板功能

    C. D-二聚体检查                D. 血小板数

    E. APTT

（2）如果病人确诊发生了 DIC，在发病过程中血液凝固性的变化为？

    A. 凝固性增高                    B. 凝固性降低

    C. 凝固性先增高后降低          D. 凝固性先降低后增高

    E. 凝固性无明显变化

（3）如果病人确诊发生 DIC，下列哪项描述不正确？

    A. 肺部感染是 DIC 发生的原因

    B. 双下肢瘀斑提示局部出现出血

    C. PLT 减少参与了病人双下肢瘀斑的形成

    D. 患者凝血功能检查结果提示其体内凝血因子减少

    E. Fg 的减少与病人双下肢瘀斑的形成无关

（4）患者确诊 DIC 后，需立即进行的治疗不包括下列哪项？

    A. 抗休克                      B. 抗感染

    C. 输入新鲜冰冻血浆            D. 应用低分子肝素

    E. 补充凝血因子

2. 患者，女性，49 岁，高热、寒战 1 周，少尿 3 天，意识模糊 1 天。体格检查：T 39.6 ℃，HR 129 次/min，R 28 次/min，BP 79/55 mmHg，皮肤有散在出血点和瘀斑。实验室检查：WBC 27 ×10$^9$/L，Hb 88 g/L，PT 21 s（对照 13.5 s），Fg 1.4 g/L（正常 1.8 ~4.5 g/L），D-二聚体（DD）>1.0 mg/L（对照 <0.5 mg/L）；外周血涂片可见裂体细胞；血培养提示大肠埃希菌生长。核磁共振提示蛛网膜下腔出血。患者诊断为大肠埃希菌败血症合并 DIC。

（1）引发该患者发生 DIC 的原因为下列哪项？

    A. 恶性肿瘤                    B. 产科意外

    C. 代谢性疾病                  D. 大手术创伤

    E. 感染性疾病

（2）以下哪项不是患者发生 DIC 的临床表现？

    A. 寒战、高热                    B. 少尿

    C. 贫血                        D. 皮肤瘀斑

    E. 意识模糊

（3）患者出血的机制不包括以下哪项？

    A. 凝血功能障碍                B. 纤溶系统激活

    C. 纤维蛋白降解产物形成      D. 骨髓功能抑制

    E. 微血管损伤

（4）以下哪项是与 DIC 中裂体细胞生成相关的变化？

    A. 贫血                        B. 出血

    C. 休克                        D. 肾衰竭

    E. 希恩综合征

（5）有关患者外周血涂片中的裂体细胞，下列哪项描述不正确？

    A. 裂体细胞是红细胞碎片

    B. 裂体细胞形态相似

    C. 裂体细胞脆性高

    D. 微血管中纤维蛋白丝的形成导致了裂体细胞的形成

    E. 裂体细胞提示患者的溶血性贫血

3. 女，37 岁，孕 39 周时因不规律宫缩 1 小时入院。患者 5 年前已顺利产下一位健康女婴。入院时，患者 HR 70 次/min，BP 110/80 mmHg，R 18 次/min，氧饱和度 98%。实验室检查未见任何异常。胎心 150 次/min。入院 4 小时内，患者自动破水，羊水清澈，宫颈已开至 10 cm。10 分钟后，病人出现呼吸困难、烦躁不安及嘴唇发绀，BP 98/60 mmHg，HR 120 次/min，胎心降至 70 次/min。在产钳的帮助下，一个重 3 150 g 的女婴出生并转入新生儿 ICU。大约 20 分钟后患者胎盘排出，随后大量未凝固的血液从她的阴道流出。她在 1 小时内失血 2 100 mL，BP 降至 40/20 mmHg，HR 156 次/min。随后她失去意识，嘴唇发白，呼吸变得极度困难。她被转入 ICU，给予红细胞悬液、新鲜冷冻血浆、止血剂及大量胶体/晶体溶液。呼吸机、血液透析和各种支持措施都先后实施。实验室检查：Hb 54 g/L，PLT $67 \times 10^9$/L，凝血功能 APTT > 180 s（对照 30.2 s），PT 40 s（对照 14.2 s），DD > 20 μg/mL，纤维蛋白降解产物（FDP）> 120 μg/mL。诊断结果为羊水栓塞并发 DIC。

（1）该患者 DIC 是下列哪一型？

    A. 急性代偿型　　　　　　　　　B. 急性失代偿型

    C. 急性过度代偿型　　　　　　　D. 急性消耗低凝型

    E. 急性纤溶亢进型

（2）患者发生 DIC 的关键机制可能是下列哪项？

    A. 组织因子入血，外源性凝血系统激活，启动凝血过程

    B. 内毒素损伤内皮细胞

    C. 白细胞的破坏

    D. 血小板的原发性激活

    E. 原发性急性溶血

（3）影响该患者发生 DIC 的因素是下列哪项？

    A. 单核-巨噬细胞系统功能的受损　　B. 肝功能严重障碍

    C. 血液高凝状态　　　　　　　　　　D. 微循环障碍

    E. 以上都不是

（4）下列哪项是该患者出现呼吸困难的机制？

    A. 肺栓塞导致限制性通气不足　　　B. 肺栓塞导致阻塞性通气不足

    C. 肺梗死导致的肺泡通气障碍　　　D. 妊娠时心脏前负荷升高

    E. 妊娠时心脏后负荷升高

（5）下列关于该患者发生休克的机制分析,哪项不正确?

    A. DIC 中微血栓的形成阻塞微血管导致回心血量降低

    B. 患者大出血导致血容量减少

    C. 患者发生 DIC 中产生的血管活性物质舒张血管,降低外周阻力

    D. 患者 DIC 时贫血的发生并不影响休克的发生

    E. 患者 DIC 发生中微血管的损伤是休克进展的重要机制

### 案例分析问答题

**[案例]**

男性,36 岁,转诊入院。患者咽痛 3 周,1 周前加重,发热 39 ℃,伴鼻出血和皮肤点状出血,咳嗽,痰中带血丝。外院实验室检查:Hb 94 g/L,WBC $2.4 \times 10^9$/L,PLT $38 \times 10^9$/L。患者患病后无尿血及便血,进食少,睡眠差。既往健康,无肝肾疾病和结核病史。入院查体:T 37.8 ℃,R 20 次/min,HR 88 次/min,BP 120/80 mmHg,皮肤出现散在出血点和瘀斑,浅表淋巴结不大,巩膜无黄染,咽充血(+),扁桃体Ⅰ度肿大,无分泌物,甲状腺不大,胸骨有轻压痛,心界不大,心律齐,无杂音,右下肺可闻及少量湿啰音,腹平软,肝脾未触及。实验室检查:Hb 90 g/L(正常 120 ~ 160 g/L),WBC $2.8 \times 10^9$/L,分类见原始粒细胞 12%,早幼粒细胞 28%,中幼粒细胞 8%,分叶核粒细胞 8%,淋巴细胞 40%,单核细胞 4%,PLT $30 \times 10^9$/L(正常 $100 \times 10^9$ ~ $300 \times 10^9$/L),骨髓增生明显,极度活跃,早幼粒细胞 91%,红系细胞 1.5%,全片见一个巨核细胞,过氧化酶染色强阳性。凝血检查:PT 19.9 s(对照 15.3 s),Fg 1.5 g/L(正常 1.8 ~4.5 g/L),FDP 180 μg/mL(对照 5 μg/mL),3P 试验阳性。大便隐血(−),尿蛋白微量,红细胞(−),胸片显示右下肺云雾状阴影。患者诊断为急性早幼粒细胞白血病、肺部感染合并 DIC。

**问题:**

（1）请问医生诊断患者发生 DIC 的依据是什么?

（2）DIC 的分期与分型有哪些? 案例中患者 DIC 的分期与分型分别是什么?

（3）请结合 DIC 的发生发展机制,说明该患者后续可能出现的临床表现及其发生的原因。

（4）请分析本案例中患者发生 DIC 的机制。

（5）3P 试验检测的是什么? 在患者确诊 DIC 中有何作用?

### 参考答案

**案例分析选择题(多选一)**

**1.** CCED; **2.** EADAB; **3.** BACCD

**案例分析问答题**

（1）请问医生诊断患者发生 DIC 的依据是什么?

该患者罹患早幼粒细胞白血病和肺部感染,这两类疾病都是 DIC 发生的主要病因之一,且患者体格检查示全身多部位出血——DIC 典型的临床症状。实验室检查发现 PT 延长,Fg 降低,FDP 增高,3P 试验阳性,展现了 DIC 中同时存在凝血功能障碍与纤溶系统的激活。

（2）DIC 的分期与分型有哪些？案例中患者 DIC 的分期与分型分别是什么？

典型的 DIC 病程可分为三期：高凝期、消耗性低凝期、继发性纤溶亢进期。按病情进展速度，DIC 可分为急性型、亚急性型及慢性型；根据 DIC 发生后的代偿情况，可将 DIC 分为代偿型、失代偿型和过度代偿型。案例中病人的 DIC 在数天内形成，所以属于亚急性型，而 FDP 的大量形成表明为继发性纤溶亢进期，血小板减少考虑该患者处于 DIC 失代偿期。

（3）请结合 DIC 的发生发展机制，说明该患者后续可能出现的临床表现及其发生的原因。

患者病情有迅速恶化的可能，出现大出血、休克、多器官功能障碍等临床表现。

① 大出血主要是由于 DIC 的凝血机制障碍及继发性纤溶亢进所致。

② 休克：大量微血栓形成，阻塞微血管，减少回心血量；广泛的出血可使血容量减少；心肌损伤减少心输出量；激肽、补体和纤溶系统的激活产生血管活性物质，如激肽、组胺、补体成分等，增加血管通透性，促进血管舒张并降低外周阻力，减少回心血量；FDP 的某些成分可增强组胺、激肽的作用，进一步促进微血管扩张。

③ MODS：微血栓阻塞局部微循环，造成器官缺血及局部性坏死，促进休克的发展，以及肾、胃肠道和心功能障碍的发生。

（4）请分析本案例中患者发生 DIC 的机制。

该患者发生 DIC 的主要机制：恶性肿瘤及感染会造成组织损伤，组织因子释放，启动凝血系统；恶性肿瘤及感染会损伤血管内皮，凝血、抗凝调控失调；白血病患者的血细胞大量破坏，血小板激活。

（5）3P 试验检测的是什么？在患者确诊 DIC 中有何作用？

3P 试验用来检测 FDP 的存在。DIC 时，继发性纤溶亢进，纤维蛋白在纤溶酶的作用下分解为 FDP，这些碎片可与纤维蛋白单体形成可溶性复合物。如果受检血浆中存在这些可溶性复合物，将鱼精蛋白加入患者的血浆后，鱼精蛋白可使复合物中的纤维蛋白单体和 FDP 分离，分离的纤维蛋白单体在血浆中自行聚集而形成可见的白色沉淀，3P 试验呈阳性反应。3P 试验在确诊 DIC 中的意义：DIC 存在时，3P 试验呈阳性反应。

（刘立民　赵丽梅）

# 第九章　缺血-再灌注损伤

## 案例分析选择题（多选一）

1. 患者，女性，74 岁，因突然出现左侧肢体无力、言语不清 1 小时入院。头颅 MRI 提示右侧额叶、颞叶片状新鲜梗死灶，确诊为"脑梗死"，行保守溶栓治疗后情况好转。不久患者家属发现患者呼之不应、枕头上有中等量呕吐物，左侧肢体完全不能动。急诊头颅 CT 显示右侧额叶、颞叶大量高密度出血灶，量约 40 mL。

（1）下列哪项是患者在行保守溶栓治疗情况好转后却出现严重脑出血的可能原因？

  A. 脑缺血　　　　　　　　　　　B. 脑血栓

  C. 再灌注　　　　　　　　　　　D. 脑血栓-再灌注

  E. 脑缺血-再灌注损伤

（2）下列哪项机制与该患者溶栓后损伤加重无直接联系？

    A. 兴奋性氨基酸增多　　　　　　B. 自由基增多

    C. 炎症反应过度激活　　　　　　D. 钙超载

    E. 星形胶质细胞增生

（3）下列哪项是该患者损伤加重时脑细胞的变化？

    A. cAMP↑和cGMP↑　　　　　　B. cAMP↓和cGMP↓

    C. cAMP↑和cGMP↓　　　　　　D. cAMP↓和cGMP↑

    E. cAMP和cGMP均正常

2. 患者，男性，53岁，因胸部剧烈疼痛半小时入院。心电图检查等确诊为 ST 段抬高的心肌梗死。行经皮冠脉介入治疗，患者症状缓解。10 分钟后，心电监护显示心动过速。

（1）下列哪项是患者在介入治疗后反而出现心动过速的原因？

    A. 心输出量降低　　　　　　　　B. 心室舒张末期压力增高

    C. 心肌收缩力降低　　　　　　　D. 心脏缺血-再灌注损伤

    E. 心肌顿抑

（2）下列哪种心律失常是该患者最可能出现的类型？

    A. 房性心律失常　　　　　　　　B. 房室传导阻滞

    C. 房室交界部阻滞　　　　　　　D. 室性心律失常

    E. 房颤

（3）患者治疗后出现可逆性心肌收缩和舒张功能障碍的变化是下列哪项？

    A. 心输出量降低　　　　　　　　B. 心室舒张末期压力降低

    C. 心室收缩峰压降低　　　　　　D. 心室内最大变化速率降低

    E. 心肌顿抑

3. 患者，71 岁，于护理院出现轻微腹痛、便秘与四肢苍白冰冷，并于 12 小时后死亡。患者有高血压病史，无腹部疾病史及手术史。出现上述不适后并未接受任何药物治疗。死亡 4 小时前，患者四肢极度苍白冰冷，收缩压 76 mmHg。在接受生理盐水输注后，出现心跳骤停，经抢救无效死亡。尸检发现：死者腹腔内有约 1 000 mL 的血液，肠系膜血肿且血肿的动脉周围分支破裂，乙状结肠扭转并已松解。推测患者死因：肠缺血-再灌注损伤引发的失血性休克。

（1）有关患者缺血-再灌注损伤的分析，下列哪项是正确的？

    A. 缺血-再灌注损伤主要是由于缺血引发

    B. 缺血-再灌注损伤反而加重了缺血性损伤

    C. 缺血-再灌注损伤为不可逆损伤

    D. 肠道发生再灌注损伤前缺血的时间与心脑相近

    E. 再灌注损伤的发生与再灌注液中电解质浓度无关

（2）下列哪种因素会影响患者发生肠缺血-再灌注损伤？

    A. 缺血时间                      B. 再灌注时血液的压力

    C. 再灌注血液的 pH            D. 上面三种因素都可以

    E. 上述答案都不正确

（3）下列哪项是患者死亡前四肢苍白冰冷的主要原因？

    A. 疼痛应激导致交感系统的激活

    B. 疼痛应激导致糖皮质激素释放增加

    C. 腹腔出血后 RAAS 的激活

    D. 失血性休克后心输出量下降与交感系统的激活

    E. 以上都不正确

（4）患者发生失血性休克后，下列哪种代谢变化可能是心脏骤停的原因？

    A. 高钾血症                      B. 低钾血症

    C. 呼吸性碱中毒             D. 分解代谢减弱

    E. 以上都不正确

## 案例分析问答题

［案例一］

患者，男性，50 岁，因持续剧烈胸痛 5 小时入院，疼痛为深压痛，向左臂放射，伴有出汗和恶心。体检：窦性心律，HR 110 次/min，BP 75/50 mmHg。患者精神错乱，呼吸困难。实验室检查：血清酶显示肌酸磷酸激酶（CK）1 660 U/L（正常 <198 U/L），肌酸磷酸激酶同工酶 35 U/L（正常 <16 U/L），血清丙二醛水平升高。心电图显示前胸导联 $V_1 - V_6$ 的 ST 段抬高，左室射血分数为 31%，胸部 X 线检查显示严重肺水肿。患者确诊为心肌梗死，给予静脉注射速尿（利尿剂）和组织纤溶酶原激活剂（溶栓剂）治疗，然而血压仍然是 80/50 mmHg。冠脉造影检查发现左冠状动脉主干完全闭塞，通过球囊血管成形术打开后，患者呼吸困难明显改善，疼痛消失。术后血压恢复到 100/70 mmHg，左室射血分数恢复到 38%，但很快观察到暂时性室性心动过速。

问题：

（1）该患者发生的休克为哪种类型？请结合病例简述其发生机制。

（2）请简述该患者发生呼吸困难及肺水肿的机制。

（3）该患者冠脉再通后血压及左室射血分数明显回升，但出现暂时性室性心动过速，考虑为何种原因？请分析该现象的病理生理学机制。

（4）如何预防心肌梗死冠脉再通后的缺血-再灌注损伤？

［案例二］

患者，男性，25 岁，因一氧化碳中毒入 ICU。入院前患者发生过两次心脏骤停，经心肺复苏后心跳恢复。入院时，患者无意识，低效自主呼吸并出现低血压。立即给予机械通气及输注肌力性儿茶酚胺。实验室检查发现 CO-Hb 48.7%，给予纯氧 1 小时，CO-Hb 降至 12.1%，并在 5 小时后降为 1.2%。患者尿量 >250 mL/h，在给予抗利尿激素（ADH）后缓解。血清肌酐低于1.0 mg/dL。患者40小时后神经状态无改善,判定为脑死亡,其肾脏用于肾移植。

接受肾移植的患者,男性,46岁,慢性肾小球肾炎引发终末期肾病,已连续腹膜透析20个月。该患者由于髂外动脉广泛动脉粥样硬化斑块,动脉吻合术时不得不添加人造血管,导致移植供体肾脏缺血时间长达100分钟。但是令人惊讶的是,移植后的肾脏并未出现明显的缺血-再灌注损伤。尽管未使用透析与利尿剂,患者的血清肌酐稳定回落,患者于手术后10天出院。

**问题:**

(1)影响肾移植后缺血-再灌注损伤的因素有哪些?

(2)肾移植后患者发生缺血-再灌注损伤的机制是什么?

(3)请分析患者未出现缺血-再灌注损伤的可能原因。

**参考答案**

**案例分析选择题(多选一)**

**1.** EEC;**2.** DDE;**3.** BDDA

**案例分析问答题**

[案例一]

(1)该患者发生的休克为哪种类型?请结合病例简述其发生机制。

该患者发生了心源性休克。其机制为:心肌梗死→心功能障碍→输出量下降→血压及脉压差降低→心源性休克。

(2)请简述该患者发生呼吸困难及肺水肿的机制。

左心衰竭→左心室舒张末期容积增大、压力上升→左心房压力上升→肺静脉回流障碍→肺循环淤血→毛细血管压升高、毛细血管通透性增加→肺水肿→呼吸困难。

(3)该患者冠脉再通后血压及左室射血分数明显回升,但出现暂时性室性心动过速,考虑为何种原因?请分析该现象的病理生理学机制。

该患者心肌功能未完全恢复,并很快出现暂时性室性心动过速,此为再灌注性心律失常,与心肌缺血-再灌注损伤有关。再灌注心律失常的发生机制与心肌动作电位时程不均一、心肌的延迟后除极、心肌电生理特性改变等有关。

(4)如何预防心肌梗死冠脉再通后的缺血-再灌注损伤?

再灌注损伤的发生与心肌缺血的程度、时间长短、缺血心肌数量、电解质紊乱、再灌注血流速度等因素有关。防治措施包括控制再灌注条件、改善心肌的代谢、清除自由基、减轻钙负荷、拮抗白细胞等。

[案例二]

(1)影响肾移植后缺血-再灌注损伤的因素有哪些?

肾脏移植手术本身就是缺血-再灌注损伤发病的原因。移植肾的缺血时间以及再灌注液体的压力、温度、pH和电解质浓度都会影响缺血-再灌注损伤的发生。本案例中供体肾缺血时间长于60分钟,但并未出现器质性的坏死,因此本身发生损伤的概率是升高的。而通常移植中为了降低再灌注损伤,会降低再灌注液的灌注速度、压力、温度、pH及钠钙离子的含量,而增加灌注液中钾镁离子含量也有利于减轻再灌注损伤。

(2)肾移植后患者发生缺血-再灌注损伤的机制是什么?

目前认为,自由基增多、钙超载和炎症反应过度激活是发生缺血-再灌注损伤的关键机制。自由基增多通过促进膜脂质过氧化,抑制细胞结构蛋白与酶的功能,破坏核酸引发DNA断裂导致机体损伤。钙超载引发的能量代谢障碍,细胞膜及结构蛋白分解以及酸中毒加重也是损伤发生的重要机制。炎症反应对微血管及细胞的损伤也参与了缺血-再灌注损伤的发生。

（3）请分析患者未出现缺血-再灌注损伤的可能原因。

首先,本案例患者肾脏供体因为 CO 中毒已经历过缺血缺氧,这种预适应可能激活了内源性保护机制。其次,也是最可能的原因是 CO 对肾脏缺血-再灌注损伤的保护作用。实验研究发现,CO 的少量吸入或者局部释放可有效对抗实验动物主要器官(心、肝、肾、肺与肠)的缺血-再灌注损伤,微量的 CO 不仅增强细胞的抗损伤能力,减少缺血性细胞凋亡,还可抑制炎症反应。

（刘立民　赵丽梅）

# 第十章　心功能不全

## 案例分析选择题（多选一）

1. 患者,男,59 岁,夜间于睡梦中突感憋闷,惊醒后被迫坐起,剧烈咳嗽,咳粉红色泡沫痰。

（1）该患者可能出现了何种病理过程?
    A. 左心衰竭                 B. 右心衰竭
    C. 心功能不全代偿期       D. 感染性休克
    E. 过敏性休克

（2）患者出现的呼吸困难的机制不包括下列哪项?
    A. 平卧时下肢水肿液回吸收入血增多
    B. 平卧时下半身血液回流增加,加重肺淤血
    C. 平卧时膈肌上移,肺泡通气减少
    D. 入睡后迷走神经抑制,小支气管扩张
    E. 入睡后中枢神经敏感性减低,只有严重的低氧血症、通气费力才能将患者唤醒

（3）下列哪一项指标与该患者相符合?
    A. HR 50 次/min             B. pH 7.59
    C. BP 120/80 mmHg      D. 口唇发绀
    E. $PaO_2$ 100 mmHg

（4）下列哪项不是该患者发病的病因?
    A. 高血压                  B. 冠心病
    C. 肺动脉瓣关闭不全      D. 主动脉瓣狭窄
    E. 二尖瓣狭窄

2. 患者,女,62 岁,患主动脉瓣狭窄 12 年。近半年出现上楼梯或做家务后心慌、气喘。肝脾未见肿大,下肢无水肿。超声心动图检查可见左心室肥厚,左室射血分数 53%。

（1）该患者出现心力衰竭的主要病因是下列哪项？

    A. 左心容量负荷过度　　　　　B. 右心容量负荷过度

    C. 左心压力负荷过度　　　　　D. 右心压力负荷过度

    E. 心肌收缩成分减少

（2）关于该患者劳累后出现呼吸困难的机制，下列哪项描述正确？

    A. 体力活动时，机体需氧量减少　　B. 体力活动时，左心室充盈增加

    C. 体力活动时，回心血量减少　　　D. 体力活动时，肺淤血水肿加重

    E. 劳累导致呼吸肌麻痹

（3）该患者可能出现的变化不包括下列哪项？

    A. 血容量增加　　　　　　　　B. 肾血流减少

    C. 红细胞减少　　　　　　　　D. 心率加快

    E. 心室重塑

（4）按左室射血分数分类，该患者的心力衰竭类型为下列哪种？

    A. 射血分数升高的心力衰竭　　B. 射血分数保留的心力衰竭

    C. 射血分数中间范围的心力衰竭　D. 射血分数降低的心力衰竭

    E. 低输出量性心力衰竭

（5）患者出现左心室肥厚，对机体的代偿意义不包括下列哪项？

    A. 单位重量心肌收缩性增强　　B. 心室壁增厚，降低心室壁张力

    C. 减少心肌耗氧量　　　　　　D. 减轻心脏负担

    E. 有助于维持心输出量

3. 患者，男，56岁，前列腺切除术后卧床5天，突然出现气短和晕厥，急诊入院。超声心动图显示左室射血分数正常，右心室收缩压升高，右心室中度扩张，右心室功能下降。胸部CT显示广泛的双侧肺栓塞，静脉扫描显示急性左下肢深静脉血栓。

（1）该患者出现心力衰竭的主要病因是下列哪项？

    A. 左心容量负荷过度　　　　　B. 右心容量负荷过度

    C. 左心压力负荷过度　　　　　D. 右心压力负荷过度

    E. 心肌收缩成分减少

（2）该患者不会出现下列哪种症状或体征？

    A. 血压降低　　　　　　　　　B. 呼吸频率加快

    C. 咳粉红色泡沫痰　　　　　　D. 氧饱和度降低

    E. 中心静脉压升高

（3）该患者可能出现的变化不包括下列哪项？

    A. 下肢压陷性水肿　　　　　　B. 颈静脉充盈

    C. 肝颈静脉回流征阳性　　　　D. 肝脾肿大

    E. 肺动脉楔压降低

**案例分析问答题**

**[案例一]**

患者,68 岁,男,因近 3 日呼吸急促加重就诊。患者自述体力活动时呼吸困难加重,乏力,休息时有所缓解,夜间平卧入睡后常惊醒并剧烈咳嗽,咳粉红色的痰液,被迫坐起。患者有 20 年高血压史,15 年冠心病史,近期因遭遇电信诈骗情绪低落,其父亲 20 年前因心肌梗死去世。

入院检查显示:身高 170 cm,体重 90 kg,R 24 次/min,HR 112 次/min,脉搏细弱,BP 150/90 mmHg,T 37 ℃,双脚踝肿胀,按压后出现凹陷,颈静脉压力升高,听诊心尖向左下移位,可闻及第四心音及肺底部湿啰音,肝脏边缘在肋缘下 10 cm 处可触及。

问题:

(1)什么是心力衰竭?患者发生的心力衰竭的类型是什么?

(2)该患者出现静脉淤血的表现有哪些?

(3)该患者存在哪些可导致心力衰竭的因素?

(4)该患者出现咳粉红色泡沫痰的原因是什么?

**[案例二]**

患者,63 岁,女,因呼吸急促急诊就医。自述 2 天前感冒后出现休息时呼吸困难,健忘,轻度疲劳,双侧下肢肿胀,后因感到虚弱、疲倦和呼吸急促,卧床 2 天。患者有 30 年的吸烟史,因呼吸急促,2 年前戒烟。自述 1 年前出现类似症状,并伴慢性阻塞性肺疾病(COPD)急性加重,住院治疗。

入院检查显示:T 38.6 ℃,HR 120 次/min,R 24 次/min,BP 104/54 mmHg,$SaO_2$ 90% ,心指数 1.4 L/(min·m²),左室射血分数 40% ,颈静脉怒张,双侧下肢出现压陷性水肿。动脉血气分析:pH 为 7.49,$PaCO_2$ 27.6 mmHg,$PaO_2$ 53.6 mmHg,$[HCO_3^-]$ 20.6 mmol/L,氧饱和度为 90% 。胸部 X 线检查提示肺泡水肿,心包积液,心脏肥大,双侧胸腔少量积液,左肺部分不张。

问题:

(1)请分析该患者心脏功能是否发生改变及改变的原因。

(2)试述感冒在该患者心功能变化中的作用及机制。

(3)该患者为何出现心率加快?心率加快对心功能有何影响?

(4)该患者出现脚踝肿胀和颈静脉压力升高的机制是什么?

**参考答案**

<u>案例分析选择题(多选一)</u>

**1.** ADDC; **2.** CDCBA; **3.** DCE

<u>案例分析问答题</u>

[案例一]

(1)什么是心力衰竭?患者发生的心力衰竭的类型是什么?

心力衰竭是在机体有足够循环血量的前提下,因心脏结构和功能的改变,导致心室射血能力和/或充盈功能受损,心输出量明显减少到已不能满足日常代谢需要,出现全身组织器官灌流不足,肺循环和/或体循环静脉淤血等一系列临床综合征。该患者出现的呼吸困难是左心衰竭的表现,下肢压陷性水肿、肝脏扩大及颈静脉压力升高是右心衰竭的表现,因此该患者发生的是急性全心衰竭。

(2)该患者出现静脉淤血的表现有哪些?

患者出现劳力性呼吸困难、夜间阵发性呼吸困难及咳粉红色泡沫痰是肺循环淤血的表现;患者下肢压陷性水肿、肝脏扩大及颈静脉压力升高是体循环淤血的表现。

(3)该患者存在哪些可导致心力衰竭的因素?

家族遗传史、高血压、冠心病、肥胖、情绪波动。

(4)该患者出现咳粉红色泡沫痰的原因是什么?

咳粉红色泡沫痰提示患者出现肺水肿。左心衰竭引起心输出量减少,舒张期肺循环血液回流阻力增大,导致肺循环淤血。肺静脉和肺毛细血管压力升高,毛细血管通透性增大,血浆渗出到肺间质与肺泡引起肺水肿。

[案例二]

(1)请分析该患者心脏功能是否发生改变及改变的原因。

该患者心指数 < 2.2 L/(min·m²),左室射血分数 < 50%,提示心功能降低。该患者心功能降低的根本原因是 COPD 引起右心室后负荷增加,机体缺氧,导致右心衰竭并累及左心,感冒诱发并加重了心功能降低。

(2)试述感冒在该患者心功能变化中的作用及机制。

上呼吸道感染引起发热,一方面基础代谢率升高,增加心脏负荷,另一方面心率加快,增加心肌耗氧量,舒张期缩短也影响冠脉血液灌注;上呼吸道感染引起肺血管阻力升高,增加右心后负荷;炎症介质及细菌毒素可直接抑制心肌功能。

(3)该患者为何出现心率加快?心率加快对心功能有何影响?

心输出量减少引起交感-肾上腺髓质系统兴奋,进而激活心肌 β 受体,使心率加快。在一定范围内,心率加快可提高心输出量,并可提高舒张压,有利于冠脉的血液灌流,对维持动脉血压、保障重要器官的血流供应有积极意义。但心率加快可增加心肌耗氧量,且心率超过 180 次/min 可明显缩短舒张期,使心室血液充盈及冠脉血液灌注减少,导致心输出量减少和心肌缺血缺氧加重。

(4)该患者出现脚踝肿胀和颈静脉压力升高的机制是什么?

右心衰竭引起右心输出量减少,右心室舒张期压力增高,因此上下腔静脉回流受阻,导致下肢淤血、颈静脉怒张。

(赵丽梅)

# 第十一章 肺功能不全

## 案例分析选择题(多选一)

1. 某高中男生,17 岁,因体育课后突发右侧胸痛伴呼吸困难 1 小时而被送入医院。查体:HR 145 次/min,BP 92/60 mmHg,口唇青紫,右侧胸廓膨隆,叩诊呈鼓音,以闭合性气胸收治入院。

（1）病人可能发生下列哪种病理过程？

    A. 阻塞性通气不足            B. 限制性通气不足

    C. 弥散障碍                     D. 死腔气量增加

    E. 肺表面活性物质减少

（2）下列哪个血气指标可以帮助确定患者发生呼吸衰竭的类型？

    A. $PaO_2$ 和 $SO_2$           B. $PaCO_2$ 和 $[HCO_3^-]$

    C. $PaO_2$ 和 $PaCO_2$        D. $CO_2$ 和 $[H^+]$

    E. $CO_2max$ 和 $[HCO_3^-]$

（3）有关患者呼吸循环系统的变化，下列解释哪项不正确？

    A. 缺氧可兴奋心血管运动中枢，提高心率及心肌收缩力

    B. 气胸影响静脉回流，减少心输出量，导致收缩压降低

    C. 心血管运动中枢兴奋有利于外周阻力的维持与血流重分布

    D. 患者的呼吸困难表现在呼吸运动变浅变快

    E. 肺缺氧与二氧化碳潴留所致血液 $H^+$ 浓度过高，导致肺血管扩张

（4）此类患者常发生下列哪种酸碱平衡紊乱？

    A. 代谢性酸中毒             B. 代谢性碱中毒

    C. 呼吸性酸中毒             D. 呼吸性碱中毒

    E. 混合型酸碱平衡紊乱

（5）下列有关该患者的诊治哪项不正确？

    A. X 线胸片检查可明确诊断闭合性气胸

    B. 本案例患者可因闭合性气胸发生急性呼吸衰竭

    C. 心包穿刺排气可缓解患者的呼吸困难

    D. 胸腔穿刺排气可缓解患者的呼吸困难

    E. 吸氧有利于缓解患者的缺氧症状

2. 男，65 岁，患慢性支气管炎 10 余年，近 1 个月症状加重，呼吸困难明显。血气分析结果：pH 7.2，$PaO_2$ 50 mmHg，$SaO_2$ 80%，$PaCO_2$ 82 mmHg，$[HCO_3^-]$ 36.2 mmol/L。

（1）该患者诊断为慢性呼吸衰竭的最重要依据是下列哪项？

    A. 有呼吸困难症状         B. 有慢性支气管炎病史

    C. $SaO_2 < 90\%$           D. $PaO_2 < 60$ mmHg，$PaCO_2 > 50$ mmHg

    E. pH < 7.35

（2）该患者主要的呼吸困难是下列哪种？

    A. 吸气困难                B. 呼气困难

    C. 呼吸减慢                D. 呼吸变浅

    E. 以上都不是

（3）该患者发生慢性呼吸衰竭的主要机制是下列哪项？

    A. 弥散障碍                B. 部分肺泡通气不足

    C. 阻塞性通气不足         D. 部分肺泡血流不足

    E. 静脉血分流入动脉血

（4）下列哪项患者呼吸系统的病理变化可能不参与慢性呼吸衰竭的发生？

  A. 气道管壁增厚狭窄       B. 支气管痉挛

  C. 表面物质减少,表面张力减少

  D. 黏液腺及杯状细胞分泌黏液增多,堵塞小气道

  E. 肺组织增生与纤维化压迫小气道

（5）下列哪个指标可以有效地反映患者的气道阻力？

  A. 用力肺活量（FVC）

  B. 一秒钟用力呼气容积（FEV1）

  C. 一秒率（FEV1% : FEV1/FVC×100%）

  D. 每分通气量（VE）

  E. 每分钟肺泡通气量（VA）

（6）下列哪项变化反映了该患者肺部发生了功能性分流？

  A. 全肺 $V_A/Q=0.8$       B. 全肺 $V_A/Q<0.8$

  C. 全肺 $V_A/Q>0.8$       D. $CaO_2$ 升高

  E. $CaCO_2$ 降低

（7）通过血气分析,可以判断该患者发生了下列哪种酸碱平衡紊乱？

  A. 代谢性酸中毒       B. 呼吸性酸中毒

  C. 代谢性碱中毒       D. 呼吸性碱中毒

  E. 混合型酸碱平衡紊乱

（8）下列哪项治疗措施不应该用于该患者？

  A. 预防和治疗呼吸道感染    B. 给予吸氧,尽快提高 $PaO_2$ 至 60 mmHg 以上

  C. 增加肺通气,降低 $PaCO_2$    D. 纠正酸碱平衡和电解质紊乱

  E. 改善内环境,保护心、脑等重要脏器功能

3. 女,25 岁,因左腿股骨段开放性骨折和胫腓骨骨折进行伤口清创手术。手术结束时在伤口上覆盖了含去甲肾上腺素的纱布。患者在到达康复室时苏醒。BP 165/115 mmHg, HR 110 次/min,R 20 次/min。1 小时后,其血压突然下降至 106/74 mmHg, 心率加快（HR 135 次/min）。血气及血液检测发现:pH 7.35, $PaO_2$ 64 mmHg, $SaO_2$ 91.6%, $PaCO_2$ 34 mmHg,[$HCO_3^-$]19 mmol/L, Hb 8.9 mg/dL, [$Na^+$] 131 mmol/L, [$K^+$] 2.26 mmol/L。病人被缓慢输注 500 mL 红细胞及含 20 mEq KCl 的 800 mL Ringer's 乳酸盐溶液。患者的心率却升高到 145 次/min。胸腔听诊发现双侧湿啰音。患者中心静脉压27 $cmH_2O$（正常 3~10 $cmH_2O$）且少尿。速尿治疗 50 分钟后通过胸片确诊为肺水肿。1 小时后,患者血压降低（BP 82/59 mmHg）并出现缺氧（$SpO_2$ <85%）,咳粉红色泡沫痰。行气管插管后血气检测发现: pH 7.09, $PaO_2$ 45 mmHg, $SaO_2$ 63.7%, $PaCO_2$ 52 mmHg, [ $HCO_3^-$] 15.6 mmol/L, Hb 12.5 mg/dL, [$Na^+$] 131 mmol/L, [$K^+$] 8.0 mmol/L。

（1）根据患者确诊肺水肿前的动脉血检测结果判断,下列描述哪项正确？

  A. 患者有 I 型呼吸衰竭       B. 患者有 II 型呼吸衰竭

  C. 患者有急性呼吸衰竭       D. 患者有慢性呼吸衰竭

  E. 以上都不对

（2）根据患者行气管插管后的血气分析判断当时患者发生了下列哪种呼吸衰竭。

    A. Ⅰ型呼吸衰竭　　　　　　　　B. Ⅱ型呼吸衰竭

    C. 急性Ⅰ型呼吸衰竭　　　　　　D. 急性Ⅱ型呼吸衰竭

    E. 慢性Ⅱ型呼吸衰竭

（3）下列哪项是该患者发生呼吸衰竭的病理生理学机制？

    A. 限制性通气不足　　　　　　　B. 阻塞性通气不足

    C. 弥散障碍　　　　　　　　　　D. 肺泡通气/血流比失调

    E. 以上都是

（4）下列有关患者行气管插管前的呼吸变化哪项是正确的？

    A. 吸气、呼气都困难　　　　　　B. 仅吸气困难

    C. 仅呼气困难　　　　　　　　　D. 呼吸变浅

    E. 呼吸减慢

（5）患者发生肺水肿后，可能出现下列哪项循环系统的变化？

    A. 血压升高　　　　　　　　　　B. 心脏骤停

    C. 左心后负荷增大　　　　　　　D. 右心后负荷降低

    E. 以上都不对

（6）患者在行气管插管后出现了下列哪种酸碱平衡紊乱？

    A. 代谢性酸中毒　　　　　　　　B. 呼吸性酸中毒

    C. 代谢性碱中毒　　　　　　　　D. 呼吸性碱中毒

    E. 代酸合并呼酸

（7）在救治中，患者可能出现下列哪个并发症？

    A. 急性肾功能衰竭　　　　　　　B. 胃肠黏膜出血

    C. 脑疝　　　　　　　　　　　　D. 多器官功能衰竭

    E. 以上都有可能

4. 女，20岁，因轻微呼吸困难和弥散性右上腹部疼痛急诊入院。体格检查发现 T 38.6 ℃，P 72 次/min，R 15 次/min，BP 98/70 mmHg，心、肺检测无明显异常。腹部柔软但右上腹有压痛，肠鸣音减弱。无远端深度静脉血栓的征兆。2 小时后患者右上腹部紧张且有反跳痛。电解质、血糖、血肌酐、血尿素氮浓度均无异常。血细胞计数、β-人绒毛膜促性腺激素与甲状腺激素含量也正常。血气分析发现 pH 7.42，$PaO_2$ 65 mmHg，$PaCO_2$ 31 mmHg，肺泡动脉氧梯度[$P_{(A-a)}O_2$] 46 mmHg。胸片未发现异常而腹部 B 超也排除了肠梗阻。肺部通气灌流扫描结合肺血管造影诊断为肺栓塞。

（1）下列哪项有关该患者呼吸功能障碍的描述是正确的？

    A. 患者有Ⅰ型呼吸衰竭　　　　　B. 患者有Ⅱ型呼吸衰竭

    C. 患者有肺通气功能障碍　　　　D. 患者有肺换气功能障碍

    E. 以上都不对

（2）根据患者的血气分析结果判断下列哪项是其呼吸功能发生改变的原因。

  A．弥散障碍       B．功能性分流

  C．死腔样通气      D．解剖分流

  E．真性分流

（3）下列有关该患者的肺通气/血流比值及血气变化的描述哪项是正确的？

  A．全肺 $V_A/Q = 0.8$     B．全肺 $V_A/Q < 0.8$

  C．全肺 $V_A/Q > 0.8$     D．$CaO_2$ 升高

  E．$CaCO_2$ 升高

（4）下列哪项是患者肺栓塞对心脏功能的影响？

  A．心输出量增加     B．外周阻力降低

  C．左心前负荷增大    D．右心前负荷增大

  E．右心后负荷增大

（5）下列哪项是对患者最关键的治疗措施？

  A．溶栓治疗，预防呼吸衰竭  B．吸纯氧，提高 $PaO_2$

  C．增加肺通气，降低 $PaCO_2$  D．纠正酸碱平衡紊乱和电解质紊乱

  E．改善内环境，保护心、脑等重要脏器功能

## 案例分析问答题

[案例一]

患者，男，68 岁，因近日咳喘加重、呼吸困难和嗜睡而入院。患者有吸烟史 30 年，15 年前开始出现咳嗽、咳痰，量不多，白色痰，冬季好发。后发作频繁，症状加重，痰液呈黄色，治疗后好转。近 3 年来出现劳累后心悸、气促伴双下肢水肿，休息后气促可缓解。10 天前出现咳喘并不断加重至呼吸困难。近 2 日出现嗜睡。

查体：T 36.5 ℃，BP 120/80 mmHg，HR 118 次/min，R 25 次/min，意识模糊，口唇发绀，呼吸稍促，颈静脉怒张。肺部叩诊呈过清音，双肺可闻及干湿啰音。心音弱，心界无明显扩大，心脏听诊无杂音。腹平软，右上腹有压痛，肝肋下可触及，移动性浊音（+）。双下肢凹陷性水肿。

入院后，该患者经吸氧后呼吸困难进一步加重。血气分析：pH 7.10，$PaO_2$ 70 mmHg，$PaCO_2$ 90 mmHg，$[HCO_3^-]$ 27.3 mmol/L。

诊断结果：COPD、肺心病、肺性脑病。

**问题：**

（1）COPD、肺心病与肺性脑病的发病机制是什么？

（2）该患者出现腹水与双下肢水肿的机制是什么？

（3）该患者出现意识障碍的机制是什么？

（4）该患者发生了何种酸碱平衡紊乱？

（5）该患者为何经吸氧后呼吸困难进一步加重？此时应首选什么治疗措施？

[案例二]

患者，男，48 岁，因发热、咳嗽及呼吸困难 8 天入院诊治。患者有高血压病史并接受治

疗。入院检测发现：BP 131/78 mmHg，HR 88 次/min，R 30 次/min，T 37.7 ℃，$SpO_2$ 77%，双侧肺有干啰音。胸部 CT 扫描显示磨玻璃样混浊和双肺外周的多灶碎路石征象。实验室检查发现淋巴细胞减少、中性粒细胞增多、红细胞沉降率增加与 D-二聚体升高。入院前血气分析显示：pH 7.5，$PaO_2$ 57 mmHg，$PaCO_2$ 29 mmHg，$[HCO_3^-]$ 22.4 mmol/L，$SpO_2$ 92.2%。新冠病毒核酸检测呈阳性。随后患者被诊断为新冠肺炎引发的 I 型呼吸衰竭与 ARDS。

患者转入 ICU 后高流速鼻导管给氧后血氧饱和度回升至正常并应用多种药物进行抗病毒治疗。住院第 4 天，患者病情出现恶化，血氧分析发现：pH 7.45，$PaO_2$ 69.9 mmHg，$PaCO_2$ 31.9 mmHg，$[HCO_3^-]$ 22.1 mmol/L，$SpO_2$ 95.5%。随后给予患者插管并用机械通气支持。实验室检测发现 D-二聚体 4.49（N<0.05）。次日开始给予了 4 天的肝素治疗。在住院的第 14 天，X 线胸片显示右侧肺出现液气胸和肺不张。随即给予患者水封排水管。支气管镜检查发现左右主支气管内出现黏液堵塞。支气管灌洗液培养发现鲍曼不动杆菌。治疗 4 天后 X 线胸片显示液气胸和肺不张有所改善，血氧饱和度上升；但血液检测发现明显的 DIC，遂给予患者新鲜冰冻血浆救治。随后患者慢慢恢复，在第 36 天移除了插管并于第 41 天出院。出院前最后一次 X 线胸片检查发现右肺广泛纤维化以及右胸膜增厚。这些病理变化在出院 2 周后仍有残留但已有所改善。

**问题：**

（1）该患者入院诊断为 I 型呼吸衰竭及 ARDS 的依据是什么？

（2）该患者新冠肺炎与 I 型呼吸衰竭和 ARDS 间有何关系？

（3）该患者发生 ARDS 的发病机制是什么？

（4）患者血液里的什么指标能帮助患者确诊 DIC？

（5）为什么患者发生 DIC 与 ARDS 有关？

（6）患者出院时胸片检测结果提示其可能有哪些呼吸功能障碍？

**参考答案**

**案例分析选择题（多选一）**

**1．** BCEEC；**2．** DBBCCBBB；**3．** EDEABEE；**4．** DCCEA

**案例分析问答题**

[案例一]

（1）COPD、肺心病与肺性脑病的发病机制是什么？

COPD 是指慢性支气管炎和肺气肿引起的慢性气道阻塞。可从患者的慢性病史（咳喘、呼吸困难）和肺部检查结果（肺部叩诊呈过清音，双肺可闻及干湿啰音）来确诊。其发病机制主要包括：

① 阻塞性通气障碍（炎症引发的支气管壁肿胀、气道高反应性、支气管痉挛、支气管堵塞）。

② 限制性通气障碍（呼吸肌衰竭）。

③ 弥散功能障碍（肺泡损伤和肺泡膜增厚）。

④ 肺泡通气/血流比例失调（部分肺泡的低通气和低灌注或者肺血管收缩与改建）。

肺心病：COPD 患者出现右心衰竭所致的体循环淤血（颈静脉怒张、腹水及上下肢凹陷性水肿）。其发病机制主要包括：

① COPD 患者肺泡缺氧和 $CO_2$ 潴留导致 $H^+$ 升高使肺小动脉血管收缩，长期作用后引发血管壁重建，

形成持久性肺动脉高压,加重右心后负荷。

②缺氧和酸中毒降低心肌的舒、缩功能。

③长期缺氧促进促红细胞生成素(EPO)生成,红细胞增多导致血液黏度升高,加重心脏负荷。

④肺部病变引起的胸内压的异常波动影响心脏的舒、缩活动。

肺性脑病:COPD 中的肺性脑病是由呼吸衰竭引起的脑功能障碍。嗜睡是本案例中患者神经认知障碍的表现。其发病机制与高碳酸血症、酸中毒和缺氧引发的脑水肿及神经功能障碍有关。

①酸中毒和缺氧促进脑血管扩张与脑血流量增加,而脑血管内皮的损伤不仅增加了血管的通透性,导致脑间质水肿,还可引发血管内凝血。

②缺氧导致的 ATP 生成减少影响钠钾泵,继而导致脑细胞水肿。

③酸中毒使抑制性递质 GABA 生成增多导致中枢抑制。

④酸中毒增强磷脂酶活性,促进溶酶体水解酶释放引发神经组织损伤。

(2)该患者出现腹水与双下肢水肿的机制是什么?

腹水与双下肢水肿是患者体循环淤血的表现,这是呼吸衰竭引发右心衰竭的结果。患者肺部病变通过引起肺动脉高压增加右心的后负荷而引发右心衰竭,外周血无法有效回心又进一步导致了体循环淤血。毛细血管静水压的增高是水肿发生的主要机制。

(3)该患者出现意识障碍的机制是什么?

患者发生了肺性脑病,其意识障碍是由缺氧、高碳酸血症和酸中毒引发脑血管和脑细胞损伤所致的脑水肿和中枢神经系统功能障碍的表现。

(4)该患者发生了何种酸碱平衡紊乱?

通过患者吸氧后的血气 pH 7.10 可知患者出现了失代偿酸中毒。结合患者的原发病 COPD 及 $PaCO_2$ 升高可以判定其发生了呼吸性酸中毒。由于 COPD 为慢性病,其 $\Delta[HCO_3^-] = 0.35 \times \Delta PaCO_2 \pm 3 = 0.35 \times (90 - 40) \pm 3 = 17.5 \pm 3$,但实际 $\Delta[HCO_3^-]$ 只为 27.3 − 24 = 3.3,不在代偿范围,表明其还发生了缺氧引发的代谢性酸中毒。

(5)该患者为何经吸氧后呼吸困难进一步加重?此时应首选什么治疗措施?

患者为 Ⅱ 型呼吸衰竭,在 $PaCO_2$ 未得到纠正时给予高浓度高流量吸氧,在缺氧纠正后,反而会由高碳酸血症引起呼吸抑制,进而使病情更加恶化。因此,该患者首先要改善通气,降低 $PaCO_2$。

[案例二]

(1)该患者入院诊断为 Ⅰ 型呼吸衰竭及 ARDS 的依据是什么?

Ⅰ 型呼吸衰竭的诊断依据是 $PaO_2$(57 mmHg)低于 60 mmHg 而 $PaCO_2$(29 mmHg)并未高于 50 mmHg。ARDS 是急性肺损伤引起的一种急性呼吸衰竭,本案例中患者为新冠肺炎引发的弥漫性肺泡损伤,诊断依据是胸部 CT 扫描显示磨玻璃样混浊和双肺外周的多灶碎路石征象。

(2)该患者新冠肺炎与 Ⅰ 型呼吸衰竭和 ARDS 间有何关系?

本案例中患者 ARDS 是由新冠病毒引发急性肺损伤,肺泡-毛细血管膜的损伤及炎症介质导致肺泡上皮和毛细血管内皮通透性增高,引起渗透性肺水肿及透明膜形成,引发弥散功能障碍。弥散功能障碍、肺内功能性分流增多和死腔样通气均使 $PaO_2$ 降低,进而引发 Ⅰ 型呼吸衰竭。

(3)该患者发生 ARDS 的发病机制是什么?

①病毒作用于肺毛细血管、肺泡上皮细胞及肺泡膜,进而引起广泛性肺损伤。

②病毒激活白细胞、巨噬细胞和血小板,间接引起肺损伤。

③病毒引发大量中性粒细胞粘附于肺泡毛细血管内皮并浸润入肺,中性粒细胞活化促进释放细胞因子、氧自由基、蛋白酶和其他炎症介质,进而损伤肺泡上皮细胞及毛细血管内皮细胞。

④血管内膜与肺组织损伤、中性粒细胞浸润刺激及肺组织释放的促凝物质,导致血管内凝血,形成微血栓;进而阻断血流进一步加重肺损伤,并通过形成纤维蛋白降解产物及释放 $TXA_2$ 等血管活性物质增加

肺血管通透性。

（4）患者血液里的什么指标能帮助患者确诊 DIC？

DIC 是弥散性血管内凝血，血管系统中同时存在广泛凝血与出血的病理学过程。在致病因子作用下大量促凝物质入血，凝血因子和血小板激活，使凝血酶增多引起微循环中形成广泛的微血栓，继而因凝血因子和血小板的大量消耗，引起继发性纤维蛋白溶解功能增强。D-二聚体是纤溶酶分解纤维蛋白多聚体的产物。因原发性的纤溶亢进不存在纤维蛋白多聚体的生成，故无 D-二聚体的升高，所以 D-二聚体升高反映了继发性的纤溶亢进。临床根据 ISTH 评分系统来诊断 DIC，评分所需的参数包括：血小板计数（减少:0~2）、D-二聚体（增加:0、2、3）、凝血酶原时间（延长:0~2）和纤维蛋白原（ >1.0 g/L =0，<1.0 g/L =1）。当这些参数的评分相加大于或等于 5 时可诊断为明显的 DIC。

（5）为什么患者发生 DIC 与 ARDS 有关？

患者发生 ARDS 是 DIC 发生的重要病因。新冠病毒引发的急性肺损伤可通过以下机制促进 DIC 的发生：

① 急性肺组织损伤导致组织因子释放增多，激活外源性凝血系统，启动凝血。

② 血管内皮细胞损伤，不仅促进组织因子启动凝血，其自身抗凝血功能也减弱。

③ 白细胞的破坏可释放组织因子启动凝血。

④ 急性肺损伤中血管基底膜胶原暴露也可激活血小板。

（6）患者出院时胸片检测结果提示其可能有哪些呼吸功能障碍？

患者出院时发现肺部广泛的纤维化及胸膜增厚，这可能会通过引起限制性通气不足、弥散障碍、功能性分流和死腔样通气等病理过程而导致呼吸功能不全。

（孙晓东　赵　颖）

# 第十二章　肝功能不全

## 案例分析选择题（多选一）

1. 患者，男，56 岁，嗜睡、神智欠清 2 天入院。患者患肝硬化 10 余年。查体:P 95 次/min，R 32 次/min。肝肋下 2 指，质硬，腹水征(+)。初步诊断:肝性脑病。

（1）该患者处于肝性脑病的哪期？

　　A. 一期　　　　　　　　　　　B. 二期

　　C. 三期　　　　　　　　　　　D. 四期

　　E. 五期

（2）有关患者病情的分析，下列哪项不正确？

　　A. 患者的神经精神综合征继发于肝硬化

　　B. 患者已处于肝性脑病的晚期

　　C. 患者应该有明显的扑翼样震颤

　　D. 患者会存在门静脉高压

　　E. 患者血浆白蛋白合成不足

（3）患者发生肝性脑病的机制中,下列哪项不正确?

  A. 肝硬化可导致鸟氨酸循环障碍

  B. 肝脏 ATP 生成减少也影响着氨代谢

  C. 患者消化吸收功能减弱

  D. 患者肠道产氨增多

  E. 肾小管泌氨增多

（4）肝性腹水的形成机制中,下列哪项不正确?

  A. 门脉高压          B. 血浆胶体渗透压降低

  C. 淋巴循环障碍        D. 肾小球滤过率下降

  E. 醛固酮减少

（5）该患者有可能发生下列哪种酸碱平衡紊乱?

  A. 代谢性酸中毒        B. 呼吸性酸中毒

  C. 代谢性碱中毒        D. 呼吸性碱中毒

  E. 以上都不是

（6）该患者有可能发生下列哪种水、电解质紊乱?

  A. 低钾血症          B. 高渗性脱水

  C. 低渗性脱水         D. 盐中毒

  E. 以上都不是

（7）下列对该患者的治疗措施中哪一项是不妥当的?

  A. 硫酸镁导泻         B. 口服乳果糖

  C. 给予碱性药物        D. 给予左旋多巴

  E. 口服或静脉输注以支链氨基酸为主的氨基酸混合液

2. **患者,男,55 岁,突然呕血 500 mL 就诊。乙型肝炎肝硬化史 10 年。查体:贫血貌, BP 90/60 mmHg,HR 90 次/min,腹软,肝肋下 3 cm,质硬。血液检测发现:Hb 70 g/L, WBC 5.5×10⁹/L,PLT 100×10⁹/L。初步诊断:上消化道出血;慢性乙型肝炎、肝硬化。**

（1）患者呕血的原因可能是下列哪项?

  A. 胃出血           B. 胆道出血

  C. 应激性溃疡出血       D. 出血性溃疡病

  E. 食管下端静脉曲张破裂出血

（2）患者若有门静脉高压,其机制不包括下列哪项?

  A. 脾肿大           B. 肝内纤维组织增生

  C. 肝细胞结节状再生      D. 肝动脉-门静脉肝内吻合支形成

  E. 肝门静脉受压

（3）如果上消化道出血诱发了肝性脑病,其主要机制是下列哪项?

  A. 血脑屏障破坏        B. 肠道产氨增加

  C. 脑组织缺血、缺氧      D. 脑内假性神经递质增加

  E. 大量失血导致休克

（4）如果上消化道出血诱发了肝性脑病，其诱因是下列哪项？

    A. 缺氧所致脑敏感性增加

    B. 肠腔内血红蛋白分解所致氮负荷增加

    C. 肝肾综合征所致内源性氮负荷增加

    D. 能量代谢异常所致血脑屏障通透性增加

    E. 以上都是

（5）如果患者出现肝性脑病，其发病机制不包括下列哪项？

    A. 血氨升高后造成脑毒性作用

    B. 血氨升高后减弱 GABA 能神经元抑制功能

    C. 血氨升高后促进芳香族氨基酸产生

    D. 脑内芳香族氨基酸增加促进假性神经递质形成

    E. 脑内支链氨基酸减少不利于脑内氨的解毒

（6）如果患者发生肝肾综合征，该患者不会出现下列哪项变化？

    A. 血尿素氮升高　　　　　　　　B. 器质性肾衰竭

    C. 交感-肾上腺髓质系统被激活　　D. RAAS 被激活

    E. ADH 水平会升高

## 案例分析问答题

**[案例一]**

患者，男，50 岁，农药厂工人，因吃饭时呕吐鲜血由救护车送急诊。吐出血量约 1 200 mL，伴头晕、心悸、出冷汗。患者有肝硬化史 5 年。经输血与止血治疗病情稳定后收住院。1 天后出现睡眠障碍和幻听，语无伦次；继而转为意识不清，进入昏迷状态。血生化检查：血氨 140 μg/dL，血糖 3.5 mmol/L，BUN 7.3 mmol/L。诊断为肝性脑病。

问题：

（1）什么是肝性脑病？该患者的哪些临床表现提示其患有肝性脑病？

（2）该患者发生肝性脑病的诱因是什么？肝性脑病还有哪些诱因？

（3）请简述该患者血氨增高的机制及血氨增高对中枢神经系统的毒性作用。

（4）肝性脑病有哪些治疗措施？

**[案例二]**

患者，男，35 岁，因发现肝硬化腹水而转至我院处理。前期因黑便 2 天，当地医院以"胃肠出血"给予了输血与止血治疗。患者有 5 年酒精性肝病史。体检可见黄疸、胸部蜘蛛痣和腹部移动性浊音。实验室检测结果：血清白蛋白 17 g/L（正常 34 ~ 47 g/L），总胆红素 350.6 μmol/L（正常 1.7 ~ 21 μmol/L），凝血酶原时间 14.9 s（正常 8.9 ~ 10.7 s），血尿素氮 17.5 mmol/L（正常 2.9 ~ 7.1 mmol/L），血肌酐 185.6 μmol/L（正常 61.9 ~ 106.1 μmol/L）；肝炎病毒学指标未见异常。腹部 B 超显示腹腔积液、肝结节与脾肿大，未见肾实质性与堵塞性病变。诊断结果：酒精性肝病、肝硬化；肝肾综合征。经过 8 个月治疗后，血尿素氮和血肌酐分别降至 5.4 mmol/L 和 79.6 μmol/L。

**问题:**

（1）有哪些体征与实验室检测结果反映该患者肝功能异常？

（2）什么是肝肾综合征？该患者的哪些变化表明其患有肝肾综合征？

（3）该患者腹水形成的主要机制是什么？

（4）该患者发生肝肾综合征的机制是什么？

（5）该患者是否容易发生肝性脑病？为什么？

## 参考答案

**案例分析选择题（多选一）**

**1**．BBEEDAC；**2**．EABEBB

**案例分析问答题**

**［案例一］**

（1）什么是肝性脑病？该患者的哪些临床表现提示其患有肝性脑病？

肝性脑病是指在排除其他已知脑疾病的前提下,继发于肝功能障碍或门体分流的一系列严重的神经精神综合征。上消化道出血可能是患者肝硬化门静脉高压的结果。患者还出现了睡眠障碍、幻听、语无伦次、意识不清和昏迷等一系列的中枢神经系统障碍的征状。

（2）该患者发生肝性脑病的诱因是什么？肝性脑病还有哪些诱因？

患者上消化道出血是其发生肝性脑病的诱因。

肝性脑病的诱因涉及:引起氮负荷增加的各种内外源性因素;引起血脑屏障通透性增强的各种因素;引起神经元对毒性物质敏感性增高的各种因素。

（3）请简述该患者血氨增高的机制及血氨增高对中枢神经系统的毒性作用。

本案例中的患者有由肝硬化、门静脉高压引发的上消化道出血,导致肠道产氨过多;而肝脏鸟氨酸循环障碍也大大降低了其对氨的清除力。因此,氨生成增加且清除减少共同致使血氨水平显著升高。

血氨增加对中枢神经系统的毒性作用包括:干扰脑细胞能量代谢;使脑内神经递质发生改变;氨对神经细胞膜功能的抑制作用。

（4）肝性脑病有哪些治疗措施？

① 防止诱因:减少氮负荷;防止上消化道出血;防止便秘;纠正水、电解质紊乱;慎用镇静剂、麻醉剂。

② 降低血氨:清洁灌肠或口服硫酸镁导泻;口服新霉素,抑制肠道细菌;口服乳果糖,"酸透析";应用谷氨酸、精氨酸降低血氨。

③ 其他治疗措施:口服或静脉输注以支链氨基酸为主的氨基酸混合液,纠正氨基酸失衡;应用左旋多巴,促使患者清醒。

④ 肝移植恢复肝脏代谢功能。

**［案例二］**

（1）有哪些体征与实验室检测结果反映该患者肝功能异常？

① 黄疸与总胆红素水平升高提示患者肝脏摄取、运载、酯化和排泄胆红素障碍。

② 蜘蛛痣反映患者肝脏灭活雌激素能力减弱。

③ 血清白蛋白降低与凝血酶原时间延长反映该患者肝脏合成能力下降。

（2）什么是肝肾综合征？该患者的哪些变化表明其患有肝肾综合征？

肝肾综合征是肝硬化失代偿期或急性重症肝炎时,继发于肝功能衰竭的可逆性肾衰竭。患者体内的下列变化表明了肝肾综合征的发生:

① 黄疸、蜘蛛痣与总胆红素升高表明患者出现了肝功能不全,腹部移动性腹水是肝硬化失代偿期的

表现。

② 血浆尿素氮、血浆肌酐水平异常增高反映肾功能降低。

③ 腹部 B 超检查未见肾实质性与堵塞性病变,提示肾功能下降是慢性肝病性腹水引起有效循环血量减少、肾脏供血不足所致。

④ 患者治疗后血尿素氮与血肌酐的下降表明该肾衰竭具有可逆性。

（3）该患者腹水形成的主要机制是什么?

① 血清白蛋白显著降低,引起血浆胶体渗透压下降。

② 脾肿大提示门静脉高压,可能与肝结节状再生压迫门静脉分支有关。

③ 水钠潴留:肝肾综合征时有效循环血量降低,引起交感神经系统、RAAS 激活及 ADH 分泌增多。

④ 淋巴回流不足:可能是肝静脉与淋巴管受压所致。

（4）该患者发生肝肾综合征的机制是什么?

患者慢性肝病性腹水的形成,造成血容量与有效循环血量明显减少,通过下列途径加重肾脏供血不足,促进肾衰竭:

① 激活交感-肾上腺髓质系统,血儿茶酚胺增加,促使肾动脉收缩,肾血流量与肾小球滤过率降低。

② 激活 RAAS,血管紧张素 II 水平升高,促使肾动脉收缩,肾血流量与肾小球滤过率降低。

③ ADH 分泌增加,促进肾脏水潴留,同时肾血管阻力明显增加,肾血流量与肾小球滤过率降低。

（5）该患者是否容易发生肝性脑病? 为什么?

该患者易发生肝性脑病。由于肝肾综合征时肾衰竭引起尿素排出减少,尿素会弥散至肠腔并被大肠杆菌释放的尿素酶分解而释放出氨,后者再经肠道吸收;因肝功能下降,不能通过鸟氨酸循环清除氨,会促使血氨浓度增高,诱发肝性脑病。

（孙晓东　赵　颖）

# 第十三章　肾功能不全

## 案例分析选择题（多选一）

1. 患者,女,36 岁,因黄疸、少尿 2 日入院。她 6 日前自服 10 余斤重鲤鱼鱼胆 1 枚后出现恶心、呕吐、腹痛、腹泻,并伴腰痛。查体:皮肤、巩膜黄染,心、肺无异常,腹软,肝肋下 2 cm 压触痛,BP 120/80 mmHg。实验室检查:血钾 5.6 mmol/L,血糖 6.7 mmol/L,血尿素氮（BUN）18.4 mmol/L,血肌酐（SCr）158.6 μmol/L。谷丙、谷草转氨酶正常。

（1）病人并未发生以下哪种病症?

    A. ARF                 B. 乙型肝炎

    C. 急性胃肠炎        D. 急性胆囊炎

    E. 高钾血症

（2）下列哪项是患者出现少尿的原因？

  A. 肾小管中毒      B. 原发性肾小球肾炎

  C. 肾盂肾炎       D. 腰肌劳损

  E. 尿路结石

（3）患者不会出现下列哪种疾病状态？

  A. 血尿        B. 蛋白尿

  C. 酸中毒       D. 水肿

  E. 碱中毒

（4）下列哪项不会是患者的尿检结果？

  A. 低尿钠       B. 低渗尿

  C. 低比重尿      D. 蛋白尿

  E. 管型尿

（5）患者出现泌尿系统问题的主要发病机制不包括以下哪个因素？

  A. 肾小管上皮细胞损伤   B. 肾灌注压降低

  C. GFR 下降      D. 肾小管离子转运体受损

  E. 肾小管刷状缘受损

2. 患者，女，37 岁，因血肌酐反复升高入院治疗。患者于 2 年前无明显诱因出现头晕的症状，血液检查发现血肌酐 475 μmol/L，BP 182/104 mmHg。她前后在多家医院治疗，但病情一直反复，血肌酐也持续上升。最近患者饮食差，反酸，怕冷，夜尿 3～4 次。入院检查发现血肌酐 1 021 μmol/L，腱反射消失。

（1）患者目前的主要诊断可能是下列哪项？

  A. 慢性肾功能不全代偿期  B. 慢性肾功能不全期

  C. 急性肾功能不全代偿期  D. 尿毒症期

  E. 急性肾功能不全

（2）下列哪项是患者腱反射消失的原因？

  A. 周围神经病变     B. 高磷血症

  C. 生长激素分泌增多   D. 蛋白质合成增强

  E. 高脂血症

（3）下列哪项是患者反酸的原因？

  A. 尿素减少      B. 胰岛素减少

  C. PTH 减少      D. 产氨减少

  E. 胃泌素增多

（4）下列哪项是患者体内可能出现的毒素物质？

  A. 尿素        B. 胍类化合物

  C. PTH        D. 多胺

  E. 上述所有

（5）以下哪种治疗措施不应该用于该患者？

    A. 营养支持

    B. 富含碳水化合物和脂肪的高卡路里食物

    C. 高蛋白质饮食

    D. 抗感染治疗

    E. 纠正水、电解质紊乱

3. 患者，男，30 岁，半小时前突发车祸致股骨骨折入院，入院检查测 BP 90/64 mmHg。实验室检测发现血肌酐 132 μmol/L，尿比重 1.021，尿钠 <20 mmol/L，血尿素氮/肌酐为 40:1，尿蛋白微量。

（1）该患者目前的主要诊断是下列哪项？

    A. 功能性肾衰竭            B. 慢性肾功能不全期

    C. 器质性肾衰竭            D. 尿毒症期

    E. 慢性肾功能衰竭期

（2）该患者出现肾功能异常的机制是下列哪项？

    A. 有效循环血量减少        B. 骨折

    C. 高血糖                D. 蛋白质合成增强

    E. 高脂血症

（3）下列哪项可能出现在该患者的尿沉渣镜检中？

    A. 变形上皮细胞         B. 大量红细胞

    C. 白细胞管型           D. 颗粒管型

    E. 以上都不是

（4）如果患者在扩容后血肌酐持续上升至 300 μmol/L，此时尿渗透压可能是下列哪项？

    A. 550 mM              B. 700 mM

    C. 330 mM              D. 500 mM

    E. 600 mM

（5）下列哪项是该患者目前的首要治疗方法？

    A. 外在固定股骨         B. 补充血容量

    C. 营养支持              D. 抗感染治疗

    E. 纠正水、电解质紊乱

## 案例分析问答题

[案例]

患者，女，32 岁，尿闭 1 天急诊入院。21 年前患"肾小球肾炎"，在此之前没有长期服用的药物。此后患者出现反复眼睑浮肿（不受重力影响）。7 年来排尿次数增多，每天 10 余次，夜尿 4~5 次，尿量 2 000 mL/d。其间她的 BP 145/100 mmHg。血液检查发现 Hb 40~70 g/L，红细胞（RBC）$1.3 \times 10^{12}$~$1.76 \times 10^{12}$/L。尿检结果：蛋白（+）（蛋白尿），RBC（-），

WBC（－），上皮细胞 0 ~ 2/HP（高倍镜下）。3 年来夜尿更明显，尿量达 2 500 ~ 3 500 mL/d，比重固定在 1.010 左右（1.015 ~ 1.025）。全身骨痛并逐渐加重，经"抗风湿"及针灸治疗无效。近 15 天来尿少、浮肿加重、食欲锐减、恶心呕吐、腹痛、全身瘙痒，四肢麻木并有轻微抽搐。体检发现：T 37 ℃，R 20 次/min，HR 120 次/min，BP 150/98 mmHg，RBC 1.49 × 10$^{12}$/L，Hb 47 g/L，WBC 9.6 × 10$^9$/L（正常 4 × 10$^9$ ~ 10 × 10$^9$/L），血磷 1.9 mmol/L（正常 0.74 ~ 1.39 mmol/L），血钙 1.3 mmol/L（正常 2.25 ~ 2.75 mmol/L）。血肌酐 320 μmol/L，尿检见蛋白（＋），RBC 10 ~ 15/HP，WBC 0 ~ 2/HP，上皮细胞 0 ~ 2/HP，颗粒管型 2 ~ 3/HP。X 线检查：双肺正常，心界略扩大，手骨质普遍性稀疏、骨质变薄。诊断结果：慢性肾衰竭。

**问题：**

（1）患者发生慢性肾衰竭的机制是什么？患者出现了哪些典型的临床表现？

（2）患者为何会有夜尿、多尿、等渗尿？

（3）患者存在哪些并发症？发生机制如何？

**参考答案**

**案例分析选择题（多选一）**

**1.** BAEAB；**2.** DAEEC；**3.** AAECB

**案例分析问答题**

（1）患者发生慢性肾衰竭的机制是什么？患者出现了哪些典型的临床表现？

患者患"肾小球肾炎"、反复浮肿 20 年，即慢性肾小球肾炎，可造成肾单位慢性进行性破坏。一方面，健存肾单位血流动力学代偿性改变（高灌注、高压力、高滤过），其中包括系膜细胞增殖和细胞外基质增多和聚集，反过来又造成另一部分肾小球损伤，功能性肾单位进一步减少以及残存功能性肾单位的进一步代偿，形成恶性循环，最终导致继发性肾小球硬化；另一方面，多种因素导致的慢性炎症、慢性缺氧、肾小管高代谢使得肾小管-间质损伤，功能性肾单位进行性减少。另外，还有许多因素如高血压、蛋白尿、尿毒症毒素等也与慢性肾衰竭的进展相关。综上，患者逐渐出现肾功能不全、肾衰竭的临床表现：早、中期的夜尿（夜间尿量＞白天尿量）、多尿（＞2 000 mL/d）、低渗尿发展为晚期的少尿/无尿、等渗尿、血尿和管型尿。患者还有氮质血症（血肌酐 320 μmol/L）、高磷血症（1.9 μmol/L ＞1.39 μmol/L）、低钙血症（1.3 mmol/L ＜ 2.25 mmol/L）并出现严重贫血（Hb 47 g/L ＜120 g/L）、高血压（150/98 mmHg ＞140/90 mmHg）和骨营养不良（手骨质普遍性稀疏、骨质变薄）等症状。

（2）患者为何会有夜尿、多尿、等渗尿？

夜尿：慢性肾衰竭早期即有夜尿出现，即夜间尿量和白天尿量相近，甚至超过白天尿量的情况，发生的机制可能是肾的浓缩功能减退，而夜间平卧时回心血量增加、肾血流量相对增多，肾小球滤过也相应增多。

多尿机制：大量肾单位被破坏，残存肾单位代偿性血流增多，肾小球滤过率增加，导致强迫性利尿；原尿中溶质含量增加，导致渗透性利尿；髓袢受损，髓质高渗环境不能形成，导致尿液浓缩功能减低，使尿液增多；肾远曲小管和集合管上皮细胞受损，对抗利尿激素反应性下降，导致重吸收水减少。

等渗尿：慢性肾衰竭晚期，肾浓缩功能和稀释功能均丧失，使得尿比重固定在 1.008 ~ 1.012 之间，尿渗透压接近血浆渗透压。

（3）患者存在哪些并发症？发生机制如何？

患者存在肾性高血压，肾性贫血，肾性骨营养不良。发病机制如下：

① 肾性高血压：水钠潴留，血容量增加，引起容量依赖性高血压。肾实质缺血刺激肾素、血管紧张素分

泌增加,小动脉收缩和外周阻力增加,引起肾素依赖性高血压。肾实质损伤以后,肾内降压物质肾内激肽释放酶、激肽和前列腺素生成减少,也是肾性高血压的原因之一。肾小球疾病所导致的高血压多数为容量依赖性,少数为肾素依赖性,但两种高血压常混合存在,有时难以截然分开。近年发现肾脏局部交感神经过度兴奋也可以引起难治性高血压。

② 肾性贫血:促红细胞生成素生成减少。体内蓄积的毒性物质,如甲基胍等直接抑制骨髓造血功能并破坏红细胞。它们对血小板功能的抑制可导致出血。有些毒物还可引起肠道对铁和叶酸等造血原料的吸收减少或利用障碍。铝中毒(或铝负荷过多)可抑制血红蛋白合成时某些酶的作用而影响红细胞功能。

③ 骨性营养不良:由于慢性肾衰竭,体内钙、磷代谢异常而出现高血磷、低血钙,会刺激甲状旁腺激素大量分泌从而使骨钙大量释放,骨质会出现变软、脱钙的现象。肾脏疾病也会造成身体内活性维生素 $D_3$ 减少而不利于骨的钙化,并加重继发性甲状旁腺激素亢进从而出现骨的大量脱钙、骨质变软、关节疼痛、关节周围肌腱炎等一系列症状。另外,酸中毒、铝积聚也会促使骨性营养不良的发生。

(郑　栋　赵　颖)

# 第十四章　脑功能不全

## 案例分析选择题（多选一）

1. 男,55 岁,突发头晕、右侧肢体活动不利、不能言语 2 小时。有代谢综合征及房颤史,诊断为缺血性脑卒中。

(1) 该患者可能的病变部位在哪?

  A. 大脑左半球　　　　　　　　　　B. 大脑右半球

  C. 枕叶　　　　　　　　　　　　　　D. 额叶

  E. 颞叶

(2) 下列哪项检测结果最不可能是该患者的?

  A. Glucose 8.98 mmol/L　　　　　　B. LDL-C 2.7 mmol/L

  C. BP 150/95 mmHg　　　　　　　　D. BMI 30

  E. TG 2.7 mmol/L

(3) 该患者出现的下列临床表现,哪种属于认知障碍?

  A. 头晕　　　　　　　　　　　　　　B. 肢体活动不利

  C. 不能言语　　　　　　　　　　　　D. 高血压

  E. 房颤

(4) 有关患者认知障碍的发生机制,下列哪项不正确?

  A. 脑缺血导致神经元能量代谢异常　　B. 脑缺血导致神经细胞钙超载

  C. 脑缺血导致 GABA 能神经元兴奋　　D. 脑缺血引发炎症机制损伤神经元

  E. 脑缺血时氧自由基生成增多

（5）有关患者的治疗方法，下列哪项最重要？

    A. 尽快实现血管再通，减少神经元的损伤

    B. 调节患者情绪，进行心理治疗

    C. 调节神经递质，提升神经元功能

    D. 改善机体微环境，对症治疗

    E. 药物保守治疗

2. 女性，63 岁。患者半小时前在家突然躺倒在地，呼之不应，当时未发现患者出现肢体抽搐、双眼上翻、口吐白沫、大小便失禁。既往患者有高血压和糖尿病。查体：BP 140/85 mmHg，血糖 25 mmol/L，心、肺、腹无明显异常。患者呼之不应，双瞳等大等圆，双侧病理征阴性，疼痛刺激后肢体有回缩活动。

（1）该患者出现的脑功能不全属于哪一类？

    A. 认知障碍                B. 意识障碍

    C. 心理障碍                D. 情绪障碍

    E. 记忆障碍

（2）该患者的觉醒度状态为下列哪项？

    A. 嗜睡                   B. 昏睡

    C. 昏迷                   D. 意识模糊

    E. 谵妄

（3）该患者晕倒的最可能原因是下列哪项？

    A. 血压异常                B. 血糖代谢异常

    C. 电解质紊乱             D. 脑内神经递质代谢紊乱

    E. 脑卒中

（4）该患者脑功能不全的发生机制，并不包括下列哪项？

    A. ARAS 受损

    B. 大脑皮质的广泛损伤及功能抑制

    C. 中脑网状结构-丘脑-大脑皮质-中脑网状结构之间构成的正反馈环路的破坏

    D. 丘脑功能障碍

    E. 突触功能异常

（5）有关患者的治疗方法，下列哪项不正确？

    A. 调节神经递质          B. 保持患者呼吸道畅通

    C. 尽快明确病因，给予针对性治疗    D. 实时监测生命指征和意识状态

    E. 减少原发性与继发性脑损伤

3. 患者，女，68 岁，因无法找到回家的路前往医院就医。患者既往无高血压、心脏病、脑出血及缺血性病史。但近几年来，她记忆力逐渐减退，总是丢三落四，忘记一些事情。当天她一早出去买菜，但到中午也没回家。她的丈夫最后在菜场附近的小巷子里找到了患者，问她为什么不回家，她答说："不记得来时的路了，找不到家了。"到医院就诊查体：BP 130/85 mmHg，神清，但对上午走丢一事毫无印象。CT 显示脑广泛性萎缩。诊断为老年痴呆。

（1）该患者出现了哪种脑功能不全的表现？

    A. 认知障碍　　　　　　　　　　　　B. 意识障碍

    C. 学习障碍　　　　　　　　　　　　D. 痴呆

    E. 辨认障碍

（2）该患者为什么会出现失忆？

    A. 颅脑外伤　　　　　　　　　　　　B. 脑老化与神经元减少

    C. 脑缺血　　　　　　　　　　　　　D. 慢性全身性疾病

    E. 精神活动异常

（3）下列哪种机制不可能引发老人的痴呆？

    A. 脑内蛋白质异常聚集　　　　　　　B. 脑内蛋白质异常修饰

    C. 自由基损伤　　　　　　　　　　　D. 谷氨酸的兴奋毒性

    E. 基因变异

（4）除了脑萎缩，下列哪些异常还可导致患者学习记忆障碍？

    A. 神经调节因子与受体异常　　　　　B. 突触功能异常

    C. 神经回路功能异常　　　　　　　　D. 蛋白质合成受阻与磷酸化失衡

    E. 以上全部都是

## 案例分析问答题

**[案例]**

男性，70岁，因行动迟缓与手颤抖来院就诊。8年前无明显诱因下开始出现行动缓慢，当时伴有左上肢颤抖，幅度较小，后幅度逐渐增大，鼻子也没有以前灵敏了。家人没有太重视。5年前逐渐累及右上肢出现震颤，静止时明显，紧张时加重，并出现运动迟缓加重。曾用过美多芭0.125 g，bid。近1年来出现行走时身体向前、向右倾斜，动作缓慢加重明显，日常活动不能自理。饮食尚可，偶有呛咳。查体：BP 135/85 mmHg，神清，面具脸，双上肢静止性震颤，四肢肌张力增高，四肢肌力5级，双侧轮替试验执行缓慢。诊断结果：帕金森病。

**问题：**

（1）该患者诊断为帕金森病的依据有哪些？

（2）该患者发生脑功能不全的可能机制有哪些？

（3）该患者出现了哪些脑功能障碍？

### 参考答案

**案例分析选择题（多选一）**

**1.** ABCCA；**2.** BCBEA；**3.** ABDE

**案例分析问答题**

（1）该患者诊断为帕金森病的依据有哪些？

① 静止性震颤渐进性加重，由单侧发展为双侧（8年前出现行动缓慢，伴有左上肢颤抖，5年前震颤逐渐累及右上肢，静止时明显，紧张时加重，并出现运动迟缓加重）。

② 查体有帕金森病的典型表现，即面具脸，静止性震颤，行动缓慢。

③ 嗅觉功能障碍(鼻子没有以前灵敏)。

（2）该患者发生脑功能不全的可能机制有哪些?

① 脑内多巴胺递质代谢异常。

② 可能与其家族遗传基因有关。

③ 可能与其生活或以往的工作环境有关,如长期接触重金属、杀虫剂等。

④ 线粒体功能障碍、氧化应激、谷氨酸的毒性作用、免疫炎性机制、细胞凋亡、转运体失调等。

（3）该患者出现了哪些脑功能障碍?

① 运动障碍:上肢静止性震颤,肌张力增高,双侧轮替试验执行缓慢,运动迟缓。

② 感觉障碍:鼻子没有以前灵敏。

(单立冬)

# 第十五章　多器官功能障碍

## 案例分析选择题（多选一）

1. 患者,男,78 岁,因咳嗽 2 周就诊。CT 检查和肺穿刺诊断为肺癌,化疗后出院休息。3 周后患者先出现发热、呼吸急促,后又出现黄疸、少尿,再次入院。入院检查:T 38.6 ℃,R 30 次/min,BP 140/95 mmHg,HR 125 次/min。

（1）下列哪项是导致该患者化疗出院后再次入院最可能的原因?

　　A. 感染性休克　　　　　　　　　　B. 慢性肾功能障碍

　　C. 心功能不全　　　　　　　　　　D. MODS

　　E. 肝性脑病

（2）下列哪项是患者化疗出院后出现异常的原因?

　　A. 肺癌导致呼吸急促　　　　　　　B. 肺癌导致低氧血症

　　C. 肿瘤转移至各器官　　　　　　　D. 化疗药物副作用

　　E. 免疫功能低下和严重感染

（3）该患者体内可能存在的应答反应不包括下列哪项?

　　A. SIRS 引起全身炎症反应失控　　　B. 促炎反应大于抗炎反应

　　C. 抗炎反应大于促炎反应　　　　　D. 肠道内细菌移位

　　E. 炎症介质表达增多

（4）该患者肝脏受累的主要原因不包括下列哪项?

　　A. 肝脏血流增加,导致肝淤血水肿

　　B. 肝组织富含黄嘌呤氧化酶,易发生缺血-再灌注损伤

　　C. 肠道细菌和毒素入血后进入肝脏,损伤肝细胞

　　D. 肝脏富含 Kupffer 细胞,导致炎症介质产生和泛滥

　　E. 毒素损伤肝内血管内皮细胞,促进微血栓形成

2. 患者,女,58 岁,因急性右上腹疼痛入院,入院后诊断为急性坏死性胰腺炎。入院后症状持续加重,且出现急性呼吸窘迫综合征。经抗感染、补液、吸氧等综合治疗后病情有所缓解。3 天后体温再次升高,伴呼吸困难,之后又出现了少尿、心悸及腿部肌肉萎缩,诊断为 MODS。

(1) 该患者出现 MODS 的主要原因是下列哪项?

    A. 肺部感染                B. 急性坏死性胰腺炎导致的组织坏死

    C. 心功能不全             D. 肾功能障碍

    E. 免疫功能低下

(2) 该患者所患 MODS 属于哪一种类型?

    A. 单项速发型             B. 原发型

    C. 一次打击型             D. 双相迟发型

    E. 以上都不是

(3) 该患者出现腿部肌肉萎缩,反映了患者的代谢状态符合下列哪项?

    A. 高代谢                B. 耗氧量减少

    C. 高动力循环             D. 低动力循环

    E. 基础代谢率降低

(4) 下列哪项是 MODS 易发生急性肺功能障碍的原因?

    A. 肺循环接受来自全身的静脉血,其中的有害物质在肺内聚集

    B. 肺组织富含巨噬细胞,易被激活

    C. 肺血管内,活化的炎症细胞易损伤并激活内皮细胞

    D. 肺内易产生活性氧、溶酶体酶和炎症介质

    E. 以上都是

3. 患者,女,35 岁,因自然分娩后大出血入院。入院给予抗休克治疗,但患者血压持续降低。入院 4 天后患者 T 39 ℃,WBC $2.0 \times 10^{10}$/L,未发现感染病灶且血细菌培养阴性,HR 120 次/min,脉搏细弱,血清肌酐升高,并出现血小板减少、凝血时间延长、皮肤花斑及点状出血点。

(1) 该患者有感染症状,但未发现感染病灶且血细菌培养阴性,原因可能是下列哪项?

    A. 肠源性内毒素血症          B. 泌尿系统感染

    C. 生殖系统感染           D. 神经系统感染

    E. 呼吸系统感染

(2) 该患者血清肌酐升高可能还伴有下列哪项机体变化?

    A. 少尿或无尿             B. 高钾血症

    C. 血尿素氮增高           D. 水肿

    E. 以上都是

(3) 该患者早期出现血清肌酐升高的原因是下列哪项?

    A. 醛固酮和抗利尿激素分泌减少    B. 肾小管坏死

    C. 肾血流减少            D. 交感神经系统抑制

    E. 器质性损伤

（4）该患者出现的病理过程是下列哪项？

    A. 失血性休克

    C. 肾功能障碍

    E. 以上都是

    B. 全身炎症反应

    D. DIC

（5）该患者的治疗原则不包括下列哪项？

    A. 阻断炎症反应

    C. 抗凝血治疗

    E. 改善内脏器官血液灌流状态

    B. 改善氧代谢，纠正组织细胞的缺氧状态

    D. 防治缺血-再灌注损伤

**参考答案**

**案例分析选择题（多选一）**

**1.** DECA；**2.** BDAE；**3.** AECEC

（赵丽梅）

# 第十六章　"基于问题式学习"案例分析

## 案例一：小感冒引发的大麻烦

**第一幕**

王先生今年 40 岁，是一家广告公司的老总。他白手起家闯荡了十几年，从一无所有的外来打工者独自创业拼搏，到终于成立自己的公司。用王先生的话来说：天南地北，哪里没有留下他的脚印？他常常奔波于各地，吃饭睡觉都没个准点，经常连夜工作，需要大量吸烟提神来熬夜构思。平时免不了各种饭局，王先生酒量大、口味也偏重。不过王先生从来没担心过身体吃不消，他认为自己身体健壮得很，很少去医院，有时有点头疼脑热的挺一挺就过去了。由于工作忙碌，他连每年的体检也一拖再拖。3 年前他被发现血压有点升高，但是他并没有进行血压监测及任何治疗。半年前开始，他自己感觉比以往更容易疲乏，吃饭也没有以前香了，有时忙碌劳累后会感觉胸闷、气急，偶尔觉得胸口疼痛，但休息一会儿就很快可以缓解，以前喜欢的羽毛球运动也变得心有余而力不足了，但他并没有放在心上。3 天前他"感冒"了，开始流较多清鼻涕，自己到药店买了些感冒药吃，吃药以后鼻涕明显减少，但又出现咳嗽，而且晚上尤其明显，小便量减少，脚也有点肿起来了。今天晚上公司聚餐，他作为老总少不得大喝一顿，回家后感觉到胸口憋闷得很厉害，有"缺氧"的感觉，休息了很长时间，却没有明显减轻，于是他来到医院就诊。

**第二幕**

接诊医生在询问了简单病史后，立即进行了体格检查：T 36.5 ℃，HR 115 次/min，

R 30 次/min,BP 160/105 mmHg。患者呈强迫体位,端坐呼吸状态,卧位时气急加重。颈静脉怒张,肝颈静脉回流征阳性。下肢和脚踝凹陷性水肿。肺部听诊:双肺肺底细湿啰音。心脏听诊:心界向左扩大,心尖搏动点位于左侧第六肋间锁骨中线外约 1 cm 处,第一心音减弱,可闻及舒张期奔马律(第三心音),心尖区可闻及 2/6 级吹风样收缩期杂音。

**第三幕**

血常规:RBC $6.4 \times 10^{12}$/L($4.3 \times 10^{12} \sim 5.8 \times 10^{12}$/L),WBC $12 \times 10^9$/L($3.5 \times 10^9 \sim 9.5 \times 10^9$/L),N 81%(40% ~ 75%),PLT $230 \times 10^9$/L($125 \times 10^9 \sim 350 \times 10^9$/L),Hb 185 g/L(130 ~ 175 g/L)。

血生化:TB 28.7 μmol/L(3.5 ~ 20.5 μmol/L),ALT 80 U/L(4 ~ 43 U/L),Cr 79 μmol/L(59 ~ 104 μmol/L),GLU 6.6 mmol/L(3.89 ~ 6.11 mmol/L),TC 4.5 mmol/L(0 ~ 5.69 mmol/L),TG 1.2 mmol/L(0.3 ~ 1.7 mmol/L),LDL-C 3.62 mmol/L(2.07 ~ 3.36 mmol/L),CK 46 U/L(38 ~ 172 U/L),肌钙蛋白(TRO)(−)。

尿常规:Pro(−)。

特殊标志物检测:NT-proBNP 5 600 pg/mL( <300 pg/mL)。

心电图:窦性心动过速,HR 110 次/min,ST-T 改变(图 1)。

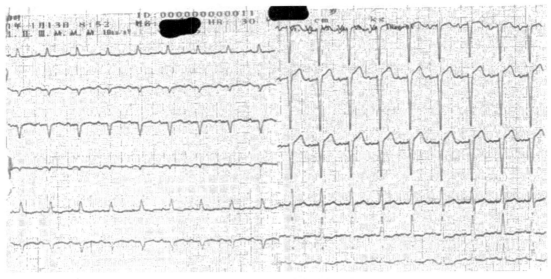

**图 1 心电图检查结果**

X线胸片:普大型心脏,心胸比为0.66,肺水肿(图2)。

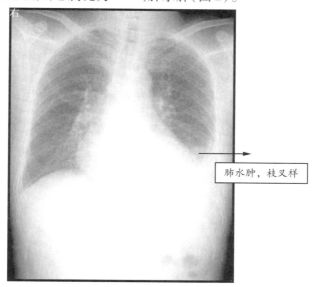

**图2 X线胸片检查结果**

冠状动脉造影:右冠状动脉大致正常(图3A),左前降支近段40%狭窄(图3B),左回旋支40%狭窄(图3C)。

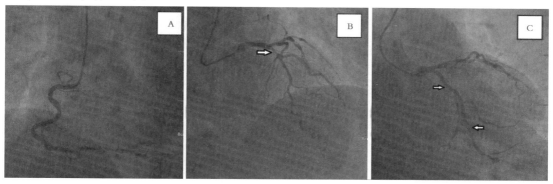

**图3 冠状动脉造影结果**

超声心动图:全心扩大,左室收缩功能明显降低(左室射血分数23.67%),二尖瓣、三尖瓣中度反流,中度肺动脉高压,主动脉瓣硬化伴轻微关闭不全。

## 第四幕

诊断:扩张型心肌病;全心衰竭,NYHA Ⅳ级;高血压2级;冠状动脉粥样硬化。

药物治疗:

| | | |
|---|---|---|
| 呋塞米注射液 | 20~40 mg | 每日分3次静推,急症缓解后改口服 |
| 地高辛 | 0.125 mg | qd |
| 培哚普利 | 4 mg | qd |
| 螺内酯 | 20 mg | qd |

冠脉造影后加用：

| | | |
|---|---|---|
| 阿托伐他汀 | 20 mg | qn |
| 阿司匹林 | 0.1 g | qd |

水肿消退、体重稳定 4 天后加用：

| | | |
|---|---|---|
| 美托洛尔缓释片 | 11.875 mg | qd |

患者住院共 10 天，经治疗后明显好转，自觉休息和平躺后不再有呼吸气促的现象，肺部啰音、下肢水肿消失，各项血检及尿检指标都正常。

出院后服用的药物：

| | | |
|---|---|---|
| 呋塞米 | 20 mg | qd |
| 地高辛 | 0.125 mg | qd |
| 培哚普利 | 4 mg | qd |
| 美托洛尔缓释片 | 11.875 mg | qd |
| 螺内酯 | 20 mg | qd |
| 阿托伐他汀 | 20 mg | qn |
| 阿司匹林 | 0.1 g | qd |

医嘱：戒烟戒酒，低钠、限水饮食，避免重体力活动及受凉感冒，保持心情舒畅。

## 第五幕

出院后患者改善生活方式并依嘱用药，身体状态持续好转，下肢没有水肿，在家中适当做些家务也完全没有气喘的症状。

第 10 天晨起后，患者自觉厌食、恶心，并未在意。下午在看报纸时突然出现视物模糊，告诉其妻子他所看到的东西都是黄色的，并感觉心悸。

患者即赴医院，接诊医生进行了相关检查。

心电图：HR 120 次/min，频发室性早搏，二联律。

## 第六幕

医生追问病史，患者误服过量的地高辛（因为每片含 0.25 mg 地高辛）。

检测地高辛血药浓度：4.0 ng/mL（0~2 ng/mL）。

诊断：地高辛中毒。

医生立即停用地高辛，并给予氯化钾 1.5 g 加入 500 mL 生理盐水缓慢静滴，同时口服补钾（氯化钾缓释片 1.0 g，tid），予苯妥英钠 0.1 g，bid 口服。同时监测血钾和患者尿量。当天晚上患者上述症状消失。

在接下来的几周，医生将医嘱中的地高辛停药，继用余药，并逐渐增加培哚普利及美托洛尔剂量，患者症状继续好转，病情未有反复。

3 个月后，王先生休息和轻微运动时无症状，医院复诊示：HR 80 次/min，BP 110/70 mmHg，左室射血分数增加到 40%。

### 核心学习问题

（1）结合心血管的组织解剖学特点及泵血功能分析本案例心脏 ECG 结果。

（2）结合心血管的组织解剖学特点及泵血功能分析本案例心脏听诊结果。

（3）结合心血管的组织解剖学特点及泵血功能分析本案例心脏超声结果。

（4）结合案例分析病人全心衰竭临床表现的发生机制，并解释为什么正性肌力药物不再是心力衰竭治疗的首选药。

（5）结合案例分析病人发生心力衰竭的病因及发病机制。

（6）冠状动脉粥样硬化性心脏病发生、发展的病理基础是什么？与心力衰竭有何关系？

（7）高血压、扩张型心肌病的病理变化是什么？有何临床表现和体征？

（8）结合病例分析本病案使用药物的药理作用，分析降脂药和利尿剂的作用机制。

（9）地高辛有哪些不良反应，如何防治？在本病例中为什么要给予患者氯化钾和苯妥英钠？

（10）抗心力衰竭药物的种类和代表药物有哪些？地高辛、血管紧张素转换酶（ACE）抑制剂和 β 受体阻断药治疗心力衰竭的药理作用和作用机制分别是什么？

（盛 瑞 李 晖）

## 案例二：闵大叔，请听医生的话！

**第一幕**

闵大叔，今年 56 岁，退休在家。40 岁离异后一直单身。自己不爱做饭，几乎都是在外面饭店解决吃饭问题。他抽烟已超过 30 年，每天 1 ~ 2 包香烟。退休后喜欢打麻将，而且经常通宵不停。闵大叔一直认为自己身体不错，单位组织的体检多因为打麻将而忘记或错过。2015 年 7 月开始，闵大叔发现自己的尿中有大量泡沫，下肢有点浮肿，因为讳疾忌医，并未前往医院检查。3 个月后间断性地出现身体乏力，时有头晕不适，在给 82 岁母亲过生日时，姐姐们发现他的腿很肿，让他赶紧去医院检查。闵大叔也感觉越来越不好，于是就来到医院就诊。

**第二幕**

闵大叔告诉医生自己并未患过传染病，也没有药物过敏、外伤及手术史。父母都很健康。

体格检查：BW 75 kg，身高 175 cm，T 36.8 ℃，P 75 次/min，R 16 次/min，BP 145/95 mmHg，面部浮肿，无颈静脉怒张，心肺无异常，腹软，肝脾未触及，肾区无叩痛，下肢凹陷性浮肿，指压痕（+++）。

血检报告：血细胞正常，[K$^+$] 3.76 mmol/L（3.5 ~ 5.5 mmol/L），[Na$^+$] 143.5 mmol/L（135 ~ 145 mmol/L），[Cl$^-$] 107.9 mmol/L（97 ~ 107 mmol/L），[Ca] 2.38 mmol/L（2.3 ~ 2.7 mmol/L），TP（总蛋白）42.5 g/L（65 ~ 80 g/L），Alb（白蛋白）19.2 g/L（35 ~ 55 g/L），Glob（球蛋白）23.3 g/L（20 ~ 35 g/L），Alb/Glob = 0.8（1 ~ 2），ALT 15 U/L（0 ~ 40 U/L），AST 20 U/L（0 ~ 40 U/L），AST/ALT = 1.33（1 ~ 2），T-Bil（总胆红素）12.8 μmol/L（3.42 ~ 20.5 μmol/L），D-Bil（直接胆红素）2.1 μmol/L（0 ~ 6.8 μmol/L），

I-Bil(间接胆红素)10.7 μmol/L（0 ~ 17 μmol/L），TC(总胆固醇)8.51 mmol/L（0 ~ 5.17 mmol/L），TG(甘油三酯)1.7 mmol/L（0.5 ~ 1.7 mmol/L），HDL-C 1.8 mmol/L（1.04 ~ 1.66 mmol/L），LDL-C 4.74 mmol/L（0 ~ 3.12 mmol/L），BUN(尿素氮)4.5 mmol/L（1.7 ~ 8.3 mmol/L），SCr(血肌酐)76.5 μmol/L（60 ~ 115 μmol/L），BUN/SCr = 58.82（20 ~ 100），UA(尿酸)399 μmol/L（202 ~ 417 μmol/L），HBsAg(−)，梅毒(−)，艾滋病毒(−)。

尿检：比重 1.010（1.003 ~ 1.02），pH 6.0（6.0 ~ 8.0），RBC（++, 80/μL），WBC（−），蛋白（+++，≥3.0 g/L），葡萄糖（−），维生素 C 0.6 mmol/L，胆红素（−），酮体（−），URO（尿胆原）（−），亚硝酸盐（−）。闵大叔住院后 24 小时的尿量为 1.2 L，含蛋白 6.88 g。

### 第三幕

特殊检查：血清 anti-PLA2R IgG4（+++）。
肾活检结果（图 4）：

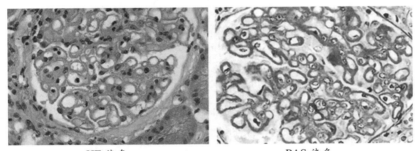

HE 染色　　　　　　　　　　　　PAS 染色

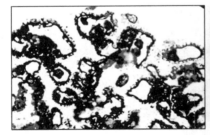　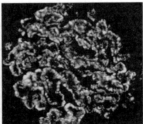　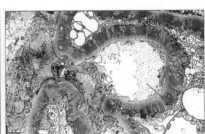

PASM 染色　　　　　　免疫荧光染色　　　　　　电镜

**图 4　肾活检结果**

光镜：全片见 2 条肾皮质组织，共见 21 个肾小球，未见小球硬化及新月体形成。肾小球体积稍大，细胞数 80 ~ 100 个/小球。系膜细胞 1 ~ 2 个/系膜区，系膜基质无增生。毛细血管袢开放，基底膜可见明显弥漫性增厚，外观僵硬感。PAS 染色：基底膜明显增厚，上皮侧可见嗜复红物质沉积。PASM 染色：基底膜可见"钉突"形成。

免疫荧光检查：基底膜团块状沉积，IgG（+++），C3（+++）。

电镜：上皮侧电子致密物（免疫复合物）沉积及"钉突"形成。

诊断结果：肾病综合征、膜性肾病Ⅱ期。

### 第四幕

医生的治疗方案:强的松 60 mg/(kg·d),口服(早晨 6 点至 8 点),环磷酰胺 0.6 g/m²,静脉注射。

建议患者定期复查,好好睡觉休息,戒烟戒酒,控制饮食(控制蛋白质、脂肪、钠、钾的摄入,适当增加碳水化合物,避免过度)与饮水。

### 第五幕

闵大叔回家后,开始按时按量服用强的松。闵大叔烟瘾较大,所以戒烟一直不是很顺利;麻将打得少了,但是有时兴致高起来还是会熬夜玩。由于常常感到饥饿,所以他的饮食量不断增大,一次可以吃 3 个苹果,一顿吃 2 碗饭,排骨等肉类也可以吃一大碗。由于口味一向偏重,所以他白天不停地喝水,医生的饮食嘱咐已全部遗忘。1 个月后,闵大叔发现自己的尿量明显减少,而且还感到没力气,运动后出现明显的气喘。这两天闵大叔发现自己几乎不怎么上厕所,下肢的浮肿又出现,最严重的是呼吸越来越困难,于是他来到医院就诊。

### 第六幕

体检:BW 80 kg,T 37 ℃,R 25 次/min,HR 110 次/min,BP 160/100 mmHg,面部浮肿,无结膜充血、水肿;向心性肥胖,双肺呼吸音低,未闻及干湿啰音,叩诊有浊音;心律齐,未闻及杂音;腹部隆起,移动性浊音阳性,双下肢重度凹陷性浮肿。

血细胞计数:WBC $6.31 \times 10^9$/L ($3.5 \times 10^9 \sim 9.5 \times 10^9$/L),Neu 71.9%,Lym 21.9%,HGB 98 g/L (130 ~ 175 g/L),RBC $4.35 \times 10^{12}$/L ($4.3 \times 10^{12} \sim 5.8 \times 10^{12}$/L),HCT 43.9 (40 ~ 50),PLT $275 \times 10^9$/L ($125 \times 10^9 \sim 350 \times 10^9$/L)。

血生化检查:$[K^+]$ 3.2 mmol/L (3.5 ~ 5.5 mmol/L),$[Na^+]$ 139 mmol/L (135 ~ 145 mmol/L),$[Ca]$ 1.8 mmol/L (2.3 ~ 2.7 mmol/L),$[HCO_3^-]$ 25 mmol/L (22 ~ 29 mmol/L),葡萄糖 7.2 mmol/L,TP 47 g/L (65 ~ 80 g/L),Alb 20 g/L (35 ~ 55 g/L),ALT 25 U/L (0 ~ 40 U/L),AST 20 U/L (0 ~ 40 U/L),TC 7.13 mmol/L (0 ~ 5.17 mmol/L),TG 1.37 mmol/L (0.5 ~ 1.7 mmol/L),HDL-C 1.8 mmol/L (1.04 ~ 1.66 mmol/L),LDL-C 4.8 mmol/L (0 ~ 3.12 mmol/L),BUN 33 mmol/L (1.7 ~ 8.3 mmol/L),SCr 552 μmol/L (60 ~ 115 μmol/L),UA 652 μmol/L (202 ~ 417 μmol/L),凝血酶原时间 13.30 s (9 ~ 14 s),凝血时间 14 s (4 ~ 14 s),纤维蛋白原 3.8 g/L (2 ~ 4 g/L),FDP 2.07 μg/mL (<5.0 μg/mL)。

尿检:比重 1.020,pH 6.0,隐血(−),WBC(−),蛋白(++),葡萄糖(−),维生素 C(+),胆红素(−),酮体(−),尿胆原(−),亚硝酸盐(−),24 小时尿蛋白定量 7.42 g/L × 0.5 L = 3.71 g。

心电图:窦性心动过速。

胸部 CT:双侧胸腔积液伴右肺不张。

腹部 B 超:右肾 118 mm × 68 mm × 55 mm,左肾 120 mm × 70 mm × 52 mm,皮质回声增强,皮质厚度及肾窦未见异常,皮髓质界限清晰;胆囊和肝脏未见异常,腹部现液性暗区。

诊断结果:膜性肾病、急性肾损伤。

## 第七幕

医生给出的住院治疗方案:

① 补钾,定时监测电解质和血气水平。

② 透析 2 周。

③ 强的松 60 mg/(kg·d),环磷酰胺 0.6 g/m²。

④ 螺内酯 60 mg/d,络活喜 5 mg/d,立普妥 10 mg/d。

⑤ 补钙。

治疗期间,闵大叔的尿量不断增加,血压被有效控制,且水肿和呼吸困难都有所缓解。

出院后,医生让病人继续膜性肾病维持治疗:强的松 60 mg/d,环磷酰胺 0.6 g/m²;并在激素服用 3 个月后开始逐渐减量(每周减 5 mg 到 30 mg/d)。他需要继续补钙和服用螺内酯 20 mg/d,络活喜 5 mg/d,立普妥 10 mg/d。医生再次强调要戒烟酒,好好休息,控制饮食和饮水。

经过这次突发事件后,闵大叔谨遵医嘱,按时休息、服药。3 个月后的检查发现他的膜性肾病得到明显控制。

### 核心学习问题

(1)正常肾单位的结构特点是什么?分析本案例中病人肾活检的病理变化及这些变化与膜性肾病间的关系。

(2)正常肾脏的生理功能有哪些?分析急性肾损伤患者出现了哪些功能异常。

(3)分析膜性肾病病人出现水肿的机制。

(4)分析膜性肾病病人出现高血脂的机制。

(5)分析膜性肾病选用强的松和环磷酰胺治疗的理论基础,以及治疗期间需要注意控制饮食和饮水的原因。

(6)分析糖皮质激素的生理功能和服用糖皮质激素的副作用。

(7)分析案例中膜性肾病患者发生急性肾损伤的机制。

(8)分析案例中病人发生急性肾损伤时出现的电解质紊乱的类型及发生机制。

(9)分析案例中患者急性肾损伤治疗方案的合理性。

(10)哪类降压药和利尿剂适用于肾病患者?

(赵　颖　李　明)

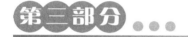

# 实验拓展与思考

## 第二章　水、电解质代谢紊乱

### ◇ 水、钠代谢紊乱

[课程实验]：过量肾上腺素引发的肺水肿

（选自：谢可鸣，王国卿，蒋星红，等.机能学实验[M].北京：高等教育出版社，2014.）

**1. 早期临床前发病机制的研究及综述分析**

➤ AUER J，GATES F L. Experiments on the causation and amelioration of adrenalin pulmonary edema[J]. J Exp Med，1917，26（2）：201－220.

➤ HURLEY J V. Current views on the mechanisms of pulmonary oedema[J]. J Pathol，1978，125（2）：59－79.

**2. 临床案例**

➤ ERSOZ N，FINESTONE S C. Adrenaline-induced pulmonary oedema and its treatment：a report of two cases[J]. Br J Anaesth，1971，43（7）：709－712.

➤ CHANG Y J，MIN S K，YOO J Y，et al. Acute pulmonary edema after local infiltration of epinephrine during mastoidectomy：a case report[J]. Korean J Anesthesiol，2009，56（4）：462－465.

**思考题：**

（1）除了上面文献报道的家兔，还有哪种小型实验动物可以用于诱导肺水肿？

（2）实验中可通过哪些实验指标来确定动物肺水肿的发生？

（3）肾上腺素引发的肺水肿液是漏出液还是渗出液？

（4）过量肾上腺素注射如何诱导小鼠肺水肿的发生？涉及组织局部中哪些系数（毛细血管静水压/胶体渗透压、组织液的静水压/胶体渗透压）的改变？

（5）实验动物肺水肿发生对机体代谢的影响及机制分别是什么？

[拓展实验]

1. 炎性水肿模型

➤ HORAKOVA Z, BEAVEN M A. Time course of histamine release and edema formation in the rat paw after thermal injury[J]. Eur J Pharmacol, 1974,27(3):305 – 312.

➤ PIETRA G G, SZIDON J P, LEVENTHAL M M, et al. Histamine and interstitial pulmonary edema in the dog[J]. Circ Res, 1971,29(4):323 – 337.

➤ MORRIS C J. Carrageenan-induced paw edema in the rat and mouse[J]. Methods Mol Biol, 2003,225:115 – 121.

2. 淋巴性水肿模型

➤ FRUEH F S, GOUSOPOULOS E, REZAEIAN F, et al. Animal models in surgical lymphedema research—a systematic review[J]. J Surg Res, 2016,200(1):208 – 220.

➤ SAARISTO A, KARKKAINEN M J, ALITALO K. Insights into the molecular pathogenesis and targeted treatment of lymphedema[J]. Ann N Y Acad Sci, 2002,979:94 – 110.

3. 低钠血症与脑水肿

➤ OVERGAARD-STEENSEN C, STØDKILDE-JØRGENSEN H, LARSSON A, et al. The frequently used intraperitoneal hyponatraemia model induces hypovolaemic hyponatraemia with possible model-dependent brain sodium loss[J]. Exp Physiol, 2016, 101(7):932 – 945.

4. 水中毒与脑细胞水肿

➤ KOZLER P, MARESOVA D, POKORNY J. Cellular brain edema induced by water intoxication in rat experimental model[J]. Neuro Endocrinol Lett, 2018, 39(3):209 – 218.

思考题：

（1）不同水肿模型是如何打破体液交换平衡的？
（2）水肿与细胞水肿间的区别是什么？
（3）各类水肿模型通过什么指标明确水肿的发生？
（4）器官水肿的表现有哪些？

## ◇ 钾代谢紊乱

[课程实验]：高血钾引发的家兔心脏功能障碍及其治疗

（选自：王建枝,钱睿哲.病理生理学实验指导[M].北京:人民卫生出版社,2017.）

1. 早期临床前发病机制的研究及综述分析

➤ PATERSON D J, BLAKE G J, LEITCH S P, et al. Effects of catecholamines and po-

tassium on cardiovascular performance in the rabbit[J]. J Appl Physiol, 1992,73(4):
1413 – 1418.

➤ GREENBERG A. Hyperkalemia:treatment options[J]. Semin Nephrol, 1998,18(1):
46 – 57.

## 2. 临床案例

➤ LAMBREW C T, CARVER S T, PETERSON R E, et al. Hypoaldosteronism as a
cause of hyperkalemia and syncopal attacks in a patient with complete heart block[J].
Am J Med, 1961,31:81 – 85.

➤ SAAD S M, YASIN S, JAIN N, et al. Cardiac manifestations in a case of severe hyperkalemia[J]. Cureus, 2021,13(3):e13641.

思考题:

(1)通过哪些实验指标可以明确心功能的改变?

(2)实验动物体内高血钾引发心肌功能改变的机制是什么?

(3)实验动物体内高血钾还引发哪些机能代谢改变?这些改变可通过什么检查明确?

## [拓展实验]

## 1. Ⅱ型假性低醛固酮症与高钾血症

➤ LÓPEZ-CAYUQUEO K I, CHAVEZ-CANALES M, PILLOT A, et al. A mouse model
of pseudohypoaldosteronism type Ⅱ reveals a novel mechanism of renal tubular acidosis
[J]. Kidney Int, 2018,94(3):514 – 523.

## 2. 挤压综合征与高钾血症

➤ CLEMENS M S, STULL M C, RALL J M, et al. Extracorporeal filtration of potassium
in a swine model of bilateral hindlimb ischemia-reperfusion injury with severe acute hyperkalemia[J]. Mil Med, 2018,183(11 – 12):e335 – e340.

➤ MURATA I, OOI K, SASAKI H, et al. Characterization of systemic and histologic injury after crush syndrome and intervals of reperfusion in a small animal model[J]. J
Trauma, 2011,70(6):1453 – 1463.

## 3. 地高辛中毒与高钾血症

➤ HACK J B, WOODY J H, LEWIS D E, et al. The effect of calcium chloride in treating
hyperkalemia due to acute digoxin toxicity in a porcine model[J]. J Toxicol Clin Toxicol, 2004,42(4):337 – 342.

## 4. 糖尿病相关的高钾血症

➤ KIM H J. Mechanisms of hyperkalemia associated with hyporeninemic hypoaldosteronism in streptozotocin-induced diabetic rats[J]. J Korean Med Sci, 1994,9(2):
107 – 115.

5. 醛固酮诱导的高钾血症

➤ ORENA S, MAURER T S, SHE L, et al. PF-03882845, a non-steroidal mineralocorticoid receptor antagonist, prevents renal injury with reduced risk of hyperkalemia in an animal model of nephropathy[J]. Front Pharmacol, 2013,4:115.

➤ BARRERA-CHIMAL J, GIRERD S, JAISSER F. Mineralocorticoid receptor antagonists and kidney diseases: pathophysiological basis[J]. Kidney Int, 2019,96(2):302 – 319.

思考题:

(1) 上述拓展实验模型中引发高血钾的机制各是什么?

(2) 上述拓展实验模型的发病机制还有哪些尚不清楚?

## ◇ 镁代谢紊乱

### [拓展实验]:噻嗪类利尿剂引发小鼠的低镁血症

1. 早期临床前发病机制的研究及综述分析

➤ NIJENHUIS T, VALLON V, VAN DER KEMP A W, et al. Enhanced passive $Ca^{2+}$ reabsorption and reduced $Mg^{2+}$ channel abundance explains thiazide-induced hypocalciuria and hypomagnesemia[J]. J Clin Invest, 2005,115(6):1651 – 1658.

➤ WHANG R. Magnesium deficiency: pathogenesis, prevalence, and clinical implications [J]. Am J Med, 1987,82(3A):24 – 29.

2. 临床案例

➤ BARNES J N, DREW P J, SKEHAN J D. Diuretic associated hypomagnesaemia[J]. Br Med J (Clin Res Ed), 1983,286(6359):146 – 147.

➤ SAAD S M, YASIN S, JAIN N, et al. Cardiac manifestations in a case of severe hyperkalemia[J]. Cureus, 2021,13(3):e13641.

思考题:

(1) 除了利尿剂可以诱发低镁血症,还有哪些方法可以诱导实验动物出现低镁血症?

(2) 实验动物体内低镁血症引发心功能变化的机制是什么?

(3) 实验性低镁血症可引发哪些机能代谢改变? 这些改变可通过什么检查明确?

## ◇ 钙磷代谢紊乱

### [拓展实验]:肾上腺切除引发家兔的高钙血症

1. 早期临床前发病机制的研究及综述分析

➤ GILDERSLEEVE D L, PEARSON T A, BAGHDIANTZ A, et al. Effect of ACTH, alpha-MSH, and beta-Lipotropin on calcium and phosphorus metabolism in the rabbit [J]. Endocrinology, 1975,97(6):1593 – 1596.

➢ WALSER M, ROBINSON B H, DUCKETT J W Jr. The hypercalcemia of adrenal insufficiency[J]. J Clin Invest, 1963,42(4):456 – 465.

## 2. 临床案例

➢ PEDERSEN K O. Hypercalcaemia in Addison's disease: report on two cases and review of the literature[J]. Acta Med Scand, 1967,181(6):691 – 698.

➢ AGRAWAL S, GOYAL A, AGARWAL S, et al. Hypercalcaemia, adrenal insufficiency and bilateral adrenal histoplasmosis in a middle-aged man: a diagnostic dilemma[J]. BMJ Case Rep, 2019,12(8):e231142.

**思考题:**

(1) 除了肾上腺切除术,还有哪些方法可以诱导实验动物出现高钙血症?

(2) 实验动物体内高钙血症引发心功能变化的机制是什么?

(3) 实验动物体内高血钙还引发哪些机能代谢改变? 这些改变可通过什么检查明确?

(赵丽梅  赵  颖)

# 第三章  酸碱平衡紊乱

## [课程实验]:实验性家兔代谢性酸碱平衡紊乱

(选自:刘健翔. 生理学与病理生理学实验[M]. 杭州:浙江大学出版社,2012.)

### 1. 直接注射盐酸与碳酸氢钠构建酸碱中毒的基础研究

➢ JAVAHERI S, DE HEMPTINNE A, VANHEEL B, et al. Changes in brain ECF pH during metabolic acidosis and alkalosis: a microelectrode study[J]. J Appl Physiol Respir Environ Exerc Physiol, 1983,55(6):1849 – 1853.

➢ FRANS A, CLERBAUX T, WILLEMS E, et al. Effect of metabolic acidosis on pulmonary gas exchange of artificially ventilated dogs[J]. J Appl Physiol, 1993,74(5):2301 – 2308.

➢ STENGL M, LEDVINOVA L, CHVOJKA J, et al. Effects of clinically relevant acute hypercapnic and metabolic acidosis on the cardiovascular system: an experimental porcine study[J]. Crit Care, 2013,17(6):R303.

➢ LÓPEZ I, AGUILERA-TEJERO E, ESTEPA J C, et al. Role of acidosis-induced increases in calcium on PTH secretion in acute metabolic and respiratory acidosis in the dog[J]. Am J Physiol Endocrinol Metab, 2004,286(5):E780 – 785.

➢ ANG R C, HOOP B, KAZEMI H. Brain glutamate metabolism during metabolic alkalosis and acidosis[J]. J Appl Physiol , 1992,73(6):2552 – 2558.

➢ PAVLIN E G, HORNBEIN T F. Distribution of $H^+$ and $HCO_3^-$ between CSF and blood during metabolic alkalosis in dogs[J]. Am J Physiol, 1975,228(4):1141 – 1144.

➢ LEMIEUX G, KISS A L, LEMIEUX C, et al. Renal tubular biochemistry during acute and chronic metabolic alkalosis in the dog[J]. Kidney Int, 1985,27(6):908 – 918.

➢ NISHIO I. Changes in respiratory system resistance and reactance following acute respiratory and metabolic alkalosis in dogs[J]. J Anesth, 1996,10(4):282 – 288.

2. 临床案例与临床研究

➢ JURISIC D, SAMARDZIC J, HRECKOVSKI B, et al. Massive necrosis of the upper gastrointestinal tract with acute gastric perforation and metabolic acidosis after hydrochloric acid (HCl) ingestion[J]. Zentralbl Chir, 2011,136(3):289 – 290.

➢ LINFORD S M, JAMES H D. Sodium bicarbonate abuse:a case report[J]. Br J Psychiatry, 1986,149:502 – 503.

➢ MENNEN M, SLOVIS C M. Severe metabolic alkalosis in the emergency department [J]. Ann Emerg Med, 1988,17(4):354 – 357.

➢ GREEN S, SIEGLER J C. Empirical modeling of metabolic alkalosis induced by sodium bicarbonate ingestion[J]. Appl Physiol Nutr Metab, 2016,41(10):1092 – 1095.

➢ ZOLADZ J A, SZKUTNIK Z, DUDA K, et al. Preexercise metabolic alkalosis induced via bicarbonate ingestion accelerates $VO_2$ kinetics at the onset of a high-power-output exercise in humans[J]. J Appl Physiol, 2005,98(3):895 – 904.

思考题:

(1) 家兔发生代谢性酸碱平衡紊乱时血气变化是什么?

(2) 实验中可通过哪些实验指标来确定动物发生了代酸或代碱?

(3) 动物和人在发生代酸或代碱时,呼吸与循环系统有哪些改变? 改变的机制是什么?

［拓展实验］

1. 运动、饮食、药物/化合物以及疾病相关的代谢性酸中毒动物模型与临床研究

➢ ROBERGS R A, GHIASVAND F, PARKER D. Biochemistry of exercise-induced metabolic acidosis[J]. Am J Physiol Regul Integr Comp Physiol, 2004,287(3):R502 – 516.

➢ DILGER R N, BAKER D H. Excess dietary L-cysteine causes lethal metabolic acidosis in chicks[J]. J Nutr, 2008,138(9):1628 – 1633.

➢ SAFIRSTEIN R, GLASSMAN V P, DISCALA V A. Effects of an $NH_4Cl$-induced metabolic acidosis on salt and water reabsorption in dog kidney[J]. Am J Physiol, 1973, 225(4):805 – 809.

➢ SABBOH H, BESSON C, TRESSOL J C, et al. Excess casein in the diet is not the unique cause of low-grade metabolic acidosis:role of a deficit in potassium citrate in a rat model[J]. Ann Nutr Metab, 2006,50(3):229 – 236.

➤ PHAM A Q, XU L H, MOE O W. Drug-induced metabolic acidosis[J]. F1000Res, 2015,4 (F1000 Faculty Rev):1460.

➤ MIRSKY I A, NELSON N, ELGART S. Diabetic acidosis and coma in the monkey [J]. Science, 1941,93(2424):576.

➤ LÓPEZ-CAYUQUEO K I, CHAVEZ-CANALES M, PILLOT A, et al. A mouse model of pseudohypoaldosteronism type Ⅱ reveals a novel mechanism of renal tubular acidosis [J]. Kidney Int, 2018,94(3):514 – 523.

➤ HARRIS A N, GRIMM P R, LEE H W, et al. Mechanism of hyperkalemia-induced metabolic acidosis[J]. J Am Soc Nephrol, 2018,29(5):1411 – 1425.

➤ WAGNER C A. Metabolic acidosis: new insights from mouse models[J]. Curr Opin Nephrol Hypertens, 2007,16(5):471 – 476.

## 2. 手术与饮食诱发的代谢性碱中毒动物模型

➤ GINGERICH D A, MURDICK P W. Experimentally induced intestinal obstruction in sheep: paradoxical aciduria in metabolic alkalosis[J]. Am J Vet Res, 1975,36(5):663 – 668.

➤ HULTER H N, TOTO R D, ILNICKI L P, et al. Metabolic alkalosis in models of primary and secondary hyperparathyroid states[J]. Am J Physiol, 1983,245(4):F450 – 461.

➤ BORKAN S, NORTHRUP T E, COHEN J J, et al. Renal response to metabolic alkalosis induced by isovolemic hemofiltration in the dog[J]. Kidney Int, 1987,32(3):322 – 328.

➤ WESSON D E. Augmented bicarbonate reabsorption by both the proximal and distal nephron maintains chloride-deplete metabolic alkalosis in rats[J]. J Clin Invest, 1989, 84(5):1460 – 1469.

➤ SMITH D F, LUNN D P, ROBINSON G M, et al. Experimental model of hypochloremic metabolic alkalosis caused by diversion of abomasal outflow in sheep[J]. Am J Vet Res, 1990,51(11):1715 – 1722.

➤ LEVINE D Z, IACOVITTI M, HARRISON V. Bicarbonate secretion in vivo by rat distal tubules during alkalosis induced by dietary chloride restriction and alkali loading[J]. J Clin Invest, 1991,87(5):1513 – 1518.

➤ PRADERVAND S, WANG Q, BURNIER M, et al. A mouse model for Liddle's syndrome[J]. J Am Soc Nephrol, 1999,10(12):2527 – 2533.

思考题：

(1) 各种代酸与代碱实验模型的发病机理是什么？

(2) 各种代酸与代碱实验模型与临床的相似度如何？

（郑　栋　赵　颖）

# 第四章　发　热

## ［拓展实验］

### 1. 关于发热的"新""老"观点

➢ WALTER E J, HANNA-JUMMA S, CARRARETTO M, et al. The pathophysiological basis and consequences of fever[J]. Crit Care, 2016, 20(1):200.

➢ HARDEN L M, KENT S, PITTMAN Q J, et al. Fever and sickness behavior: friend or foe? [J]. Brain Behav Immun, 2015, 50:322 – 333.

➢ BECKER J H, WU S C. Fever—an update[J]. J Am Podiatr Med Assoc, 2010, 100(4):281 – 290.

➢ BERNHEIM H A, BLOCK L H, ATKINS E. Fever: pathogenesis, pathophysiology, and purpose[J]. Ann Intern Med, 1979, 91(2):261 – 270.

### 2. 发热对中枢神经系统影响的文献

➢ BURKE S, HANANI M. The actions of hyperthermia on the autonomic nervous system: central and peripheral mechanisms and clinical implications[J]. Auton Neurosci, 2012, 168(1 – 2):4 – 13.

➢ DIETRICH W D, BRAMLETT H M. Hyperthermia and central nervous system injury[J]. Prog Brain Res, 2007, 162:201 – 217.

➢ SMINIA P, HULSHOF M C. Hyperthermia and the central nervous system[J]. Prog Brain Res, 1998, 115:337 – 350.

### 3. 关于临床上热疗法的一些研究

➢ WALTER E J, CARRARETTO M. The neurological and cognitive consequences of hyperthermia[J]. Crit Care, 2016, 20(1):199.

➢ DIETRICH W D, BRAMLETT H M. Hyperthermia and central nervous system injury[J]. Prog Brain Res, 2007, 162:201 – 217.

➢ TISHIN A M, SHTIL A A, PYATAKOV A P, et al. Developing antitumor magnetic hyperthermia: principles, materials and devices[J]. Recent Pat Anticancer Drug Discov, 2016, 11(4):360 – 375.

思考题：

（1）如果让你去设计发热实验的话，可以如何进行呢？

（2）关于发热引起中枢神经系统症状的机制可以通过何种模型及技术展开研究？

（3）热疗法适用于何种患者？用热疗法进行肿瘤治疗的可能机制是什么？

（孙丽娜）

# 第五章　应　激

[课程实验]：应激对小鼠行为及学习记忆能力的影响

（选自：王建枝,钱睿哲.病理生理学实验指导[M].北京:人民卫生出版社,2017.）

## 1. 早期临床前研究及综述分析

➢ MITCHELL D, OSBORNE E W, O'BOYLE M W. Habituation under stress：shocked mice show nonassociative learning in a T-maze[J]. Behav Neural Biol, 1985, 43(2): 212 – 217.

➢ DE WIED D, CROISET G. Stress modulation of learning and memory processes[J]. Methods Achiev Exp Pathol, 1991, 15:167 – 199.

➢ BANGASSER D A, SHORS T J. Critical brain circuits at the intersection between stress and learning[J]. Neurosci Biobehav Rev, 2010, 34(8):1223 – 1233.

➢ LUKSYS G, SANDI C. Neural mechanisms and computations underlying stress effects on learning and memory[J]. Curr Opin Neurobiol, 2011, 21(3):502 – 508.

## 2. 人群研究

➢ KALISH H I, GARMEZY N, RODNICK E H, et al. The effects of anxiety and experimentally-induced stress on verbal learning[J]. J Gen Psychol, 1958, 59(1):87 – 95.

➢ DOWD S B. Stress in clinical learning：a transactional approach[J]. Radiol Technol, 1985, 56(3):154 – 158.

➢ PAUL M, BELLEBAUM C, GHIO M, et al. Stress effects on learning and feedback-related neural activity depend on feedback delay[J]. Psychophysiology, 2020, 57(2):e13471.

➢ CARVALHEIRO J, CONCEIÇÃO V A, MESQUITA A, et al. Acute stress impairs reward learning in men[J]. Brain Cogn, 2021, 147:105657.

思考题：

（1）实验中可通过哪些指标来明确动物的应激反应？

（2）急性应激对动物学习能力的影响机制有哪些？是否与人类相似？

（3）如何明确应激时神经体液反应对动物学习能力的影响？

[拓展实验]

### 1. 抑郁症研究

近年来由于发病率逐渐增高,抑郁症已成为影响人类身心健康的常见疾病之一。抑郁

症的发病过程与应激密不可分,以下是一些关于抑郁症研究中常用的实验方法以及研究现状的文献:

> HAO Y, GE H, SUN M, et al. Selecting an appropriate animal model of depression [J]. Int J Mol Sci, 2019, 20(19):4827.

> MÉNARD C, HODES G E, RUSSO S J. Pathogenesis of depression:insights from human and rodent studies[J]. Neuroscience, 2016, 321:138 – 162.

> CZÉH B, FUCHS E, WIBORG O, et al. Animal models of major depression and their clinical implications [J]. Prog Neuropsychopharmacol Biol Psychiatry, 2016, 64:293 – 310.

> PLANCHEZ B, SURGET A, BELZUNG C. Animal models of major depression:drawbacks and challenges[J]. J Neural Transm (Vienna), 2019, 126(11):1383 – 1408.

### 2. 热休克蛋白研究

热休克蛋白是最早发现的细胞应激反应蛋白,它们的表达高低与应激状态直接相关。热休克蛋白能够有效地增强细胞应对有害刺激的抗损伤能力,对细胞产生非特异性的保护作用。以下是关于热休克蛋白的研究文献:

> JACOB P, HIRT H, BENDAHMANE A. The heat-shock protein/chaperone network and multiple stress resistance[J]. Plant Biotechnol J, 2017, 15(4):405 – 414.

> CHEN B, FEDER M E, KANG L. Evolution of heat-shock protein expression underlying adaptive responses to environmental stress[J]. Mol Ecol, 2018, 27(15):3040 – 3054.

> GARBUZ D G. Regulation of heat shock gene expression in response to stress[J]. Mol Biol (Mosk), 2017, 51(3):400 – 417.

> BEERE H M, GREEN D R. Stress management-heat shock protein-70 and the regulation of apoptosis[J]. Trends Cell Biol, 2001, 11(1):6 – 10.

### 3. 心身疾病研究

在社会心理因素的刺激下,以躯体症状表现为主的一类心身疾病逐渐增多。心身疾病与躯体遭受长期或过强的应激有密切关系,以下是关于一些心身疾病的文献:

> PETRIE J R, GUZIK T J, TOUYZ R M. Diabetes, hypertension, and cardiovascular disease:clinical insights and vascular mechanisms[J]. Can J Cardiol, 2018, 34(5):575 – 584.

> BOONE J L. Stress and hypertension[J]. Prim Care, 1991, 18(3):623 – 649.

> HAMMEN C. Stress and depression[J]. Annu Rev Clin Psychol, 2005, 1:293 – 319.

> BURGESS C. Stress and cancer[J]. Cancer Surv, 1987, 6(3):403 – 416.

> ZILAEE M, SHIRALI S. Heat shock proteins and diabetes[J]. Can J Diabetes, 2016, 40(6):594 – 602.

**思考题:**

(1) 应激时机体内酸碱平衡是否会被打破?可能发生哪种酸碱平衡紊乱?如何设计实验进行检测?

（2）关于应激可以设计何种动物实验？如何对动物的状态进行评价？

（3）应激时细胞反应的调节机制有哪些？如何在实验室条件下进行检测？

（4）请尝试设计一个应激与心身疾病的实验。

（孙丽娜）

# 第六章　缺　氧

## ［课程实验］：不同类型缺氧对小鼠的影响

（选自：谢可鸣，王国卿，蒋星红，等.机能学实验［M］.北京：高等教育出版社，2014.）

### 1. 低张性缺氧基础与临床研究

➢ LENFANT C, WAYS P, AUCUTT C, et al. Effect of chronic hypoxic hypoxia on the $O_2$-Hb dissociation curve and respiratory gas transport in man［J］. Respir Physiol, 1969, 7(1): 7 – 29.

➢ HONIG A. Electrolytes, body fluid volumes and renal function in acute hypoxic hypoxia ［J］. Acta Physiol Pol, 1979, 30(18 Suppl): 93 – 125.

➢ KOZNIEWSKA E, WELLER L, HÖPER J, et al. Cerebrocortical microcirculation in different stages of hypoxic hypoxia［J］. J Cereb Blood Flow Metab, 1987, 7(4): 464 – 470.

➢ DANNENBERG R, KLIMA S. Effects of short-term hypoxic hypoxia on the sodium and potassium homoeostasis in humans［J］. Biomed Biochim Acta, 1989, 48(2 – 3): S274 – 278.

➢ MANKOVSKAYA I N, LYABAKH K G. Oxygen transport to muscular tissue under adaptation to hypoxic hypoxia［J］. Adv Exp Med Biol, 1999, 471: 295 – 306.

➢ LU G, DING D, SHI M. Acute adaptation of mice to hypoxic hypoxia［J］. Biol Signals Recept, 1999, 8(4 – 5): 247 – 255.

➢ JONES J G, BAKEWELL S E, HENEGHAN C P, et al. Profound hypoxemia in pulmonary patients in airline-equivalent hypoxia: roles of $V_A$/Q and shunt［J］. Aviat Space Environ Med, 2008, 79(2): 81 – 86.

➢ PETRASSI F A, HODKINSON P D, WALTERS P L, et al. Hypoxic hypoxia at moderate altitudes: review of the state of the science［J］. Aviat Space Environ Med, 2012, 83(10): 975 – 984.

### 2. 血液性缺氧基础与临床研究

➢ WESTPHAL R G, AZEN E A. Experimental enterogenous cyanosis and anaemia［J］.

Br J Haematol, 1972, 22(5):609 – 616.

➤ BAUMEL I P, PITTERMAN A, PATEL G, et al. Mechanisms underlying potentiation of barbiturate action by sodium nitrite in the mouse: the role of methemoglobin-induced hypoxia[J]. J Pharmacol Exp Ther, 1974, 188(2):481 – 489.

➤ BRADBERRY S M, GAZZARD B, VALE J A. Methemoglobinemia caused by the accidental contamination of drinking water with sodium nitrite[J]. J Toxicol Clin Toxicol, 1994, 32(2):173 – 178.

➤ LEE S S, CHOI I S, SONG K S. Hematologic changes in acute carbon monoxide intoxication[J]. Yonsei Med J, 1994, 35(3):245 – 251.

➤ GABRIELLI A, LAYON A J. Carbon monoxide intoxication during pregnancy: a case presentation and pathophysiologic discussion, with emphasis on molecular mechanisms [J]. J Clin Anesth, 1995, 7(1):82 – 87.

➤ LEE A C, OU Y, LAM S Y, et al. Non-accidental carbon monoxide poisoning from burning charcoal in attempted combined homicide-suicide[J]. J Paediatr Child Health, 2002, 38(5):465 – 468.

➤ SKOLD A, COSCO D L, KLEIN R. Methemoglobinemia: pathogenesis, diagnosis, and management[J]. South Med J, 2011, 104(11):757 – 761.

### 3. 组织性缺氧临床案例及机制研究

➤ BAIN J T, KNOWLES E L. Successful treatment of cyanide poisoning[J]. Br Med J, 1967, 2(5554):763.

➤ PIANTADOSI C A, SYLVIA A L, JÖBSIS F F. Cyanide-induced cytochrome a, a3 oxidation-reduction responses in rat brain in vivo[J]. J Clin Invest, 1983, 72(4):1224 – 1233.

➤ JEEVARATNAM K, VIDYA S, VAIDYANATHAN C S. In vitro and in vivo effect of methyl isocyanate on rat liver mitochondrial respiration[J]. Toxicol Appl Pharmacol, 1992, 117(2):172 – 179

➤ ABOUL-ENEIN F, LASSMANN H. Mitochondrial damage and histotoxic hypoxia: a pathway of tissue injury in inflammatory brain disease? [J]. Acta Neuropathol, 2005, 109(1):49 – 55.

➤ BERLING I, BUCKLEY N A, MOSTAFA A, et al. 2-Methyl-4-chlorophenoxyacetic acid and bromoxynil herbicide death[J]. Clin Toxicol (Phila), 2015, 53(5):486 – 488.

**思考题：**

（1）不同类型缺氧的发生机制有何不同？

（2）通过浓硫酸和甲酸产 CO 实现血液性缺氧的实验设计有何缺陷？有何改进的方法？

（3）还可以用什么方法构建组织性缺氧模型？其机制又是什么？请简单描述其解救方法。

（4）缺氧与哪种水、电解质紊乱和酸碱平衡紊乱有关？

## ［拓展实验］

### 1. 缺氧对于中枢神经系统影响的文献

➢ CERVÓS-NAVARRO J, SAMPAOLO S, HAMDORF G. Brain changes in experimental chronic hypoxia[J]. Exp Pathol, 1991, 42(4):205 – 212.

➢ HIRANO S, HASEGAWA M, KAMEI A, et al. Responses of cerebral blood volume and oxygenation to carotid ligation and hypoxia in young rabbits: near-infrared spectroscopy study[J]. J Child Neurol, 1993, 8(3):237 – 241.

➢ GOLAN H, HULEIHEL M. The effect of prenatal hypoxia on brain development: short- and long-term consequences demonstrated in rodent models[J]. Dev Sci, 2006, 9(4):338 – 349.

➢ ADHAMI F, LIAO G, MOROZOV Y M, et al. Cerebral ischemia-hypoxia induces intravascular coagulation and autophagy[J]. Am J Pathol, 2006, 169(2):566 – 583.

➢ RODRIGO J, FERNÁNDEZ A P, SERRANO J, et al. The role of free radicals in cerebral hypoxia and ischemia[J]. Free Radic Biol Med, 2005, 39(1):26 – 50.

➢ DEKOSKY S T, KOCHANEK P M, VALADKA A B, et al. Blood biomarkers for detection of brain injury in COVID-19 patients[J]. J Neurotrauma, 2021, 38(1):1 – 43.

### 2. 关于临床上氧疗的一些研究综述

➢ CHOUDHURY R. Hypoxia and hyperbaric oxygen therapy: a review[J]. Int J Gen Med, 2018, 11:431 – 442.

➢ ALLARDET-SERVENT J, SICARD G, METZ V, et al. Benefits and risks of oxygen therapy during acute medical illness: just a matter of dose! [J]. Rev Med Interne, 2019, 40(10):670 – 676.

➢ TRETTER V, ZACH M L, BÖHME S, et al. Investigating disturbances of oxygen homeostasis: from cellular mechanisms to the clinical practice[J]. Front Physiol, 2020, 11:947.

➢ FISCHER I, BARAK B. Molecular and therapeutic aspects of hyperbaric oxygen therapy in neurological conditions[J]. Biomolecules, 2020, 10(9):1247.

➢ JIANG B, WEI H. Oxygen therapy strategies and techniques to treat hypoxia in COVID-19 patients[J]. Eur Rev Med Pharmacol Sci, 2020, 24(19):10239 – 10246.

➢ SEN S, SEN S. Therapeutic effects of hyperbaric oxygen: integrated review[J]. Med Gas Res, 2021, 11(1):30 – 33.

**思考题:**

（1）机体细胞如何调节氧平衡?

（2）大脑对于缺氧的适应性调节有哪些? 其机制是什么?

（3）氧疗的危害有哪些? 其机制什么?

（孙丽娜）

# 第七章　休　克

[课程实验]：家兔失血性休克

（选自：谢可鸣，王国卿，蒋星红，等．机能学实验[M]．北京：高等教育出版社，2014．）

**失血性休克动物模型综述分析**

➢ FÜLÖP A, TURÓCZI Z, GARBAISZ D, et al. Experimental models of hemorrhagic shock：a review[J]. Eur Surg Res, 2013, 50(2)：57 – 70.

➢ MOOCHHALA S, WU J, LU J. Hemorrhagic shock：an overview of animal models [J]. Front Biosci (Landmark Ed), 2009, 14(12)：4631 – 4639.

➢ LOMAS-NIERA J L, PERL M, CHUNG C S, et al. Shock and hemorrhage：an overview of animal models[J]. Shock, 2005, 24 (suppl 1)：33 – 39.

思考题：

（1）在复制家兔休克模型实验中如何判断休克的发生？

（2）除了家兔，还有哪些实验动物可用于复制失血性休克动物模型？

（3）请分析各种实验动物制作失血性休克模型的优缺点。

[拓展实验]

1．过敏性休克动物模型

➢ BARSAN W G, HEDGES J R, SYVERUD S A, et al. A hemodynamic model for anaphylactic shock[J]. Ann Emerg Med, 1985, 14(9)：834 – 839.

➢ HIEDA Y, KAGEURA M, HARA K, et al. An experimental model of death from anaphylactic shock with compound 48/80 and postmortem changes in levels of histamine in blood[J]. Forensic Sci Int, 1990, 45(1 – 2)：159 – 169.

➢ GREENBERG M I, ROBERTS J R, KRUSZ J C, et al. Endotracheal epinephrine in a canine anaphylactic shock model[J]. JACEP, 1979, 8(12)：500 – 503.

2．脓毒性休克动物模型

➢ LILLEY E, ARMSTRONG R, CLARK N, et al. Refinement of animal models of sepsis and septic shock[J]. Shock, 2015, 43(4)：304 – 316.

➢ VILLA P, GHEZZI P. Animal models of endotoxic shock[J]. Methods Mol Med, 2004, 98：199 – 206.

思考题：

（1）上述拓展实验模型中引发休克的机制各是什么？

（2）上述拓展实验动物模型存在哪些优缺点？

（赵丽梅）

# 第八章 凝血与抗凝血平衡紊乱

**［课程实验］：家兔实验性弥散性血管内凝血**

（选自：王建枝，钱睿哲. 病理生理学实验指导［M］. 北京：人民卫生出版社，2017.）

**1. 早期临床前研究及最新有关发病机制的综述**

➤ MENACHE D，BEHRE H E，ORTHNER C L，et al. Coagulation Factor Ⅸ concentrate：method of preparation and assessment of potential *in vivo* thrombogenicity in animal models［J］. Blood，1984，64（6）：1220 – 1227.

➤ HARRISON J，ABILDGAARD C，LAZERSON J，et al. Assessment of thrombogenicity of prothrombin complex concentrates in a porcine model［J］. Thromb Res，1985，38（2）：173 – 188.

➤ LEVI M，SIVAPALARATNAM S. Disseminated intravascular coagulation：an update on pathogenesis and diagnosis［J］. Expert Rev Hematol，2018，11（8）：663 – 672.

**2. 临床案例**

➤ OHGA S，SAITO M，MATSUKAZI A，et al. Disseminated intravascular coagulation in a patient with haemophilia B during factor Ⅸ replacement therapy［J］. Br J Haematol，1993，84（2）：343 – 345.

➤ EDWARDS R L，RICKLES F R，CRONLUND M. Abnormalities of blood coagulation in patients with cancer. Mononuclear cell tissue factor generation［J］. J Lab Clin Med，1981，98（6）：917 – 928.

**思考题：**

（1）本实验模型中引发 DIC 的病因与机制分别是什么？

（2）除了教材中的检测指标，哪些指标能更好地判断 DIC 的进展？

（3）DIC 动物模型还有哪些？

**［拓展实验］**

**1. 脓毒血症及组织因子引发的 DIC**

➤ SUGA Y，KUBO A，KATSURA H，et al. Detailed exploration of pathophysiology involving inflammatory status and bleeding symptoms between lipopolysaccharide- and tissue factor-induced disseminated intravascular coagulation in rats［J］. Int J Hematol，

2021，114（2）：172－178.

> SOERENSEN K E, OLSEN H G, SKOVGAARD K, et al. Disseminated intravascular coagulation in a novel porcine model of severe Staphylococcus aureus sepsis fulfills human clinical criteria［J］. J Comp Pathol，2013，149（4）：463－474.

## 2. 有关动物模型与临床 DIC 相关性的综述

> ASAKURA H. Classifying types of disseminated intravascular coagulation：clinical and animal models［J］. J Intensive Care，2014，2（1）：20.

> BERTHELSEN L O, KRISTENSEN A T, TRANHOLM M. Animal models of DIC and their relevance to human DIC：a systematic review［J］. Thromb Res，2011，128（2）：103－116.

思考题：

（1）不同疾病引发的 DIC 有何不同？

（2）目前动物模型与临床 DIC 的相关性如何？

（3）目前的临床前研究为临床 DIC 的治疗提供了哪些治疗思路？

（刘立民　赵丽梅）

# 第九章　缺血-再灌注损伤

**［课程实验］：大鼠心脏缺血-再灌注损伤**

（选自：王建枝，钱睿哲. 病理生理学实验指导［M］. 北京：人民卫生出版社，2017.）

## 1. 早期临床前研究及综述

> MURRY C E, JENNINGS R B, REIMER K A. Preconditioning with ischemia：a delay of lethal cell injury in ischemic myocardium［J］. Circulation，1986，74（5）：1124－1136.

> FRANK A, BONNEY M, BONNEY S, et al. Myocardial ischemia reperfusion injury：from basic science to clinical bedside［J］. Semin Cardiothorac Vasc Anesth，2012，16（3）：123－132.

## 2. 临床案例

> TANAKA K, SATO N, YASUTAKE M, et al. Clinical course，timing of rupture and relationship with coronary recanalization therapy in 77 patients with ventricular free wall rupture following acute myocardial infarction［J］. J Nippon Med Sch，2002，69（5）：481－488.

> TANAKA R, NAKAMURA T, KUMAMOTO H, et al. Detection of stunned myocardi-

um in post-reperfusion cases of acute myocardial infarction［J］. Ann Nucl Med，2003，17（1）:53－60.

**思考题:**

（1）心肌缺血-再灌注后会出现哪些功能和结构变化？

（2）可以采取哪些措施减轻缺血-再灌注损伤？

（3）缺血-再灌注造成的损伤是可逆的还是不可逆的？为什么？

## ［拓展实验］

### 1. 肠缺血-再灌注损伤

➤ GONZALEZ L M，MOESER A J，BLIKSLAGER A T. Animal models of ischemia-reperfusion-induced intestinal injury: progress and promise for translational research［J］. Am J Physiol Gastrointest Liver Physiol，2015，308（2）:G63－75.

### 2. 肾缺血-再灌注损伤

➤ SHIVA N，SHARMA N，KULKARNI Y A，et al. Renal ischemia/reperfusion injury: an insight on *in vitro* and *in vivo* models［J］. Life Sci，2020，256:117860.

### 3. 脑缺血-再灌注损伤

➤ MA R，XIE Q，LI Y，et al. Animal models of cerebral ischemia: a review［J］. Biomed Pharmacother，2020，131:110686.

### 4. 肺缺血-再灌注损伤

➤ FARD N，SAFFARI A，EMAMI G，et al. Acute respiratory distress syndrome induction by pulmonary ischemia-reperfusion injury in large animal models［J］. J Surg Res，2014，189（2）:274－284.

➤ FERRARI R S，ANDRADE C F. Oxidative stress and lung ischemia-reperfusion injury［J］. Oxid Med Cell Longev，2015，2015:590987.

### 5. 肝缺血-再灌注损伤

➤ YANG W，CHEN J，MENG Y，et al. Novel targets for treating ischemia-reperfusion injury in the liver［J］. Int J Mol Sci，2018，19（5）:1302.

➤ ZHOU J，CHEN J，WEI Q，et al. The role of ischemia/reperfusion injury in early hepatic allograft dysfunction［J］. Liver Transpl，2020，26（8）:1034－1048.

**思考题:**

（1）不同器官缺血-再灌注损伤的普遍机制与器官特异性机制有哪些？

（2）评判不同器官缺血-再灌注损伤的主要指标有哪些？

（3）临床上预防缺血-再灌注损伤的方案有哪些？

（刘立民　赵丽梅）

# 第十章  心功能不全

## ［课程实验］：  肺栓塞所致急性右心衰竭

（选自：谢可鸣，王国卿，蒋星红，等.机能学实验［M］.北京：高等教育出版社，2014.）

### 1. 临床案例

➤ SHARMA M, SUERO-ABREU G A, NEUPANE R, et al. Role of phosphodiesterase-5 inhibitors in acute right ventricular failure due to pulmonary embolism［J］. Am J Case Rep, 2019, 20：1144 – 1147.

### 2. 右心衰竭动物模型的相关文献

➤ GUPTA S C, VARIAN K D, BAL N C, et al. Pulmonary artery banding alters the expression of $Ca^{2+}$ transport proteins in the right atrium in rabbits［J］. Am J Physiol Heart Circ Physiol, 2009, 296(6)：H1933 – 1939.

➤ ANDERSEN A, FEEN D, ANDERSEN S, et al. Animal models of right heart failure ［J］. Cardiovasc Diagn Ther, 2020, 10(5)：1561 – 1579.

思考题：

（1）实验中可通过哪些实验指标和现象来确定动物发生急性右心衰竭？

（2）肺栓塞诱导急性右心衰竭的机制是什么？

（3）除了课程实验中所用的家兔，还有哪些实验动物可以用于诱导急性右心衰竭？

（4）诱导右心衰竭的方法还有哪些？

## ［拓展实验］：左心衰竭

### 左心衰竭动物模型的相关文献

➤ LIU Y H, YANG X P, NASS O, et al. Chronic heart failure induced by coronary artery ligation in Lewis inbred rats［J］. Am J Physiol, 1997, 272(2)：H722 – 727.

➤ MAGID N M, OPIO G, WALLERSON D C, et al. Heart failure due to chronic experimental aortic regurgitation［J］. Am J Physiol, 1994, 267(2)：H556 – 562.

➤ SABBAH H N, STEIN P D, KONO T, et al. A canine model of chronic heart failure produced by multiple sequential coronary microembolizations［J］. Am J Physiol, 1991, 260(4)：H1379 – 1384.

➤ WEINHEIMER C J, LAI L, KELLY D P, et al. Novel mouse model of left ventricular pressure overload and infarction causing predictable ventricular remodelling and progression to heart failure［J］. Clin Exp Pharmacol Physiol, 2015, 42(1)：33 – 40.

➢ COPS J, HAESEN S, DE MOOR B, et al. Current animal models for the study of congestion in heart failure：an overview[J]. Heart Fail Rev, 2019, 24(3):387-397.

➢ RIEHLE C, BAUERSACHS J. Small animal models of heart failure[J]. Cardiovasc Res, 2019, 115(13):1838-1849.

➢ SILVA K, EMTER C A. Large animal models of heart failure：a translational bridge to clinical success[J]. JACC Basic Transl Sci, 2020, 5(8):840-856.

**思考题：**

（1）用于复制左心衰竭模型的大动物和小动物分别有哪些？各自的优缺点是什么？

（2）复制慢性左心衰竭的方法有哪些？

（3）哪些方法复制的心力衰竭模型更接近人体的病理状况？

（赵丽梅）

# 第十一章 肺功能不全

## ［课程实验］：家兔的肺通气功能障碍

（选自：谢可鸣，王国卿，蒋星红，等.机能学实验[M].北京：高等教育出版社,2014.）

**临床案例与病理综述**

➢ GEORGE R B, HERBERT S J, SHAMES J M, et al. Pneumothorax complicating pulmonary emphysema[J]. JAMA, 1975, 234(4):389-393.

➢ REES P J, HAY J G, WEBB J R. Acute exacerbation of upper airway obstruction in acromegaly[J]. Postgrad Med J, 1982, 58(681):429-430.

➢ RAJU P, MANTHOUS C A. The pathogenesis of respiratory failure：an overview[J]. Respir Care Clin N Am, 2000, 6(2):195-212.

**思考题：**

（1）阻塞性通气障碍根据阻塞部位如何分类？本实验属于哪一种？会出现何种呼吸困难？

（2）部分夹闭气道流出道造成阻塞性通气不足的具体机制是什么？

（3）在诱导阻塞性通气障碍时,家兔的血压、呼吸、窦反射有何变化？发生变化的机制是什么？

（4）限制性通气障碍的原因有哪些？本实验造成限制性通气不足的具体机制是什么？

（5）严重限制性通气不足时,家兔的血压、呼吸、窦反射有何变化？发生变化的机制是什么？

**[拓展实验]**

1. 慢性阻塞性肺疾病与呼吸功能衰竭的基础研究与临床案例

➢ SERBAN K A, PETRACHE I. Mouse models of COPD[J]. Methods Mol Biol, 2018, 1809:379 – 394.

➢ JONES B, DONOVAN C, LIU G, et al. Animal models of COPD: what do they tell us? [J]. Respirology, 2017, 22(1):21 – 32.

➢ O'DONNELL D E, MILNE K M, JAMES M D, et al. Dyspnea in COPD: new mechanistic insights and management implications[J]. Adv Ther, 2020, 37(1):41 – 60.

2. 急性呼吸窘迫综合征与呼吸功能衰竭的基础研究与临床案例

➢ AEFFNER F, BOLON B, DAVIS I C. Mouse models of acute respiratory distress syndrome: a review of analytical approaches, pathologic features, and common measurements[J]. Toxicol Pathol, 2015, 43(8):1074 – 1092.

➢ D'ALESSIO F R. Mouse models of acute lung injury and ARDS[J]. Methods Mol Biol, 2018, 1809:341 – 350.

➢ GOH K J, CHOONG M C, CHEONG E H, et al. Rapid progression to acute respiratory distress syndrome: review of current understanding of critical illness from COVID-19 infection[J]. Ann Acad Med Singap, 2020, 49(3):108 – 118.

思考题:

(1) COPD 和 ARDS 实验模型中引发呼吸衰竭的机制分别是什么?

(2) COPD 和 ARDS 实验模型中可选用哪些指标明确呼吸衰竭的发生?

(3) COPD 和 ARDS 实验模型的发病机制还有哪些不清楚?

(孙晓东　赵　颖)

# 第十二章　肝功能不全

**[课程实验]:家兔肝功能不全**

（选自:谢可鸣,王国卿,蒋星红,等.机能学实验[M].北京:高等教育出版社,2014.）

肝性脑病临床案例与动物模型制备

➢ FENTON J C, KNIGHT E J, HUMPHERSON P L. Milk-and-cheese diet in portal-systemic encephalopathy[J]. Lancet, 1966, 1(7430):164 – 166.

➢ RUSSELL D M, KELLER F S, WHITAKER J N. Episodic confusion and tremor associated with extrahepatic portacaval shunting in cirrhotic liver disease[J]. Neurology,

1989，39（3）：403 – 405.

➤ LEE Y L，PANG S，ONG C. Non-cirrhotic hyperammonaemia：are we missing the diagnosis？［J］. BMJ Case Rep，2020，13（3）：e233218.

➤ MARDINI H，RECORD C. Pathogenesis of hepatic encephalopathy：lessons from nitrogen challenges in man［J］. Metab Brain Dis，2013，28（2）：201 – 207.

➤ DEMORROW S，CUDALBU C，DAVIES N，et al. 2021 ISHEN guidelines on animal models of hepatic encephalopathy［J］. Liver Int，2021，26.

思考题：

（1）肾上腺素改变血压与呼吸的机制是什么？请比较耳缘静脉与肠系膜静脉给药后家兔血压、呼吸变化的差异并分析出现差异的原因。

（2）本实验中，家兔发生肝性脑病的具体机制是什么？配制本实验所用的氯化铵混合液时为何要加 $NaHCO_3$？

（3）家兔发生肝性脑病时，血压、呼吸发生了哪些变化？为什么会出现这些变化？

（4）请问正常组与肝功能不全组家兔引发肝性脑病时所需的氯化铵用量有什么不同？为什么？

［拓展实验］

**肝性脑病的动物模型、病理机制及临床现状**

➤ MULLEN K D，BIRGISSON S，GACAD R C，et al. Animal models of hepatic encephalopathy and hyperammonemia［J］. Adv Exp Med Biol，1994，368：1 – 10.

➤ DEMORROW S，CUDALBU C，DAVIES N，et al. 2021 ISHEN guidelines on animal models of hepatic encephalopathy［J］. Liver Int，2021，41（7）：1474 – 1488.

➤ WEISSENBORN K. Hepatic encephalopathy：definition，clinical grading and diagnostic principles［J］. Drugs，2019，79（Suppl 1）：5 – 9.

➤ GONZÁLEZ-REGUEIRO J A，HIGUERA-DE LA TIJERA M F，MORENO-ALCÁNTAR R，et al. Pathophysiology of hepatic encephalopathy and future treatment options［J］. Rev Gastroenterol Mex（Engl Ed），2019，84（2）：195 – 203.

思考题：

（1）肝性脑病动物模型可以用来研究哪些科学问题？

（2）动物模型在研究肝性脑病上有哪些优缺点？

（孙晓东 赵 颖）

# 第十三章　肾功能不全

[课程实验]：家兔急性中毒性肾衰竭

（选自：王建枝，钱睿哲.病理生理学实验指导[M].北京：人民卫生出版社，2017.）

1. 早期临床前研究

➤ HSU C H, KURTZ T W, ROSENZWEIG J, et al. Renal hemodynamics in HgCl$_2$-induced acute renal failure[J]. Nephron, 1977, 18(6):326 – 332.

➤ HSU C H, KURTZ T W, WELLER J M. The role of tubular necrosis in the pathophysiology of acute renal failure[J]. Nephron, 1976, 17(3):204 – 214.

➤ STACCHIOTTI A, BORSANI E, RODELLA L, et al. Dose-dependent mercuric chloride tubular injury in rat kidney[J]. Ultrastruct Pathol, 2003, 27(4):253 – 259.

2. 临床案例

➤ MURPHY M J, CULLIFORD E J, PARSONS V. A case of poisoning with mercuric chloride[J]. Resuscitation, 1979, 7(1):35 – 44.

➤ LAI K N, PUGSLEY D J, BLACK R B. Acute renal failure after peritoneal lavage with mercuric chloride[J]. Med J Aust, 1983, 1(1):37 – 38.

➤ DHANAPRIYA J, GOPALAKRISHNAN N, ARUN V, et al. Acute kidney injury and disseminated intravascular coagulation due to mercuric chloride poisoning[J]. Indian J Nephrol, 2016, 26(3):206 – 208.

思考题：

（1）本实验模型中引发急性肾衰竭的机制是什么？

（2）除了教材中的检测指标，哪些指标的检测能更好地判断急性肾衰竭的进展？

（3）中毒性急性肾衰竭还可以在哪些实验动物中构建？不同类型动物间病程的差异有哪些？

[拓展实验]

1. 脓毒症急性肾损伤模型

➤ DEJAGER L, PINHEIRO I, DEJONCKHEERE E, et al. Cecal ligation and puncture：the gold standard model for polymicrobial sepsis？[J]. Trends in Microbiology, 2011, 19(4):198 – 208.

2. 缺血-再灌注引起的急性肾损伤模型

➤ HESKETH E E, CZOPEK A, CLAY M, et al. Renal ischaemia reperfusion injury：a mouse model of injury and regeneration[J]. J Vis Exp, 2014, (88):51816.

➢ WEI Q, DONG Z. Mouse model of ischemic acute kidney injury: technical notes and tricks[J]. Am J Physiol Renal Physiol, 2012, 303(11): F1487 – 1494.

### 3. 单侧输尿管结扎诱导的急性肾损伤模型

➢ BANDER S J, BUERKERT J E, MARTIN D, et al. Long-term effects of 24-hr unilateral ureteral obstruction on renal function in the rat[J]. Kidney Int, 1985, 28(4): 614 – 620.

➢ CHEVALIER R L, FORBES M S, THORNHILL B A. Ureteral obstruction as a model of renal interstitial fibrosis and obstructive nephropathy [J]. Kidney Int, 2009, 75 (11):1145 – 1152.

➢ UCERO A C, BENITO-MARTIN A, IZQUIERDO M C, et al. Unilateral ureteral obstruction: beyond obstruction[J]. Int Urol Nephrol, 2014, 46(4):765 – 776.

### 4. 药物引起的急性肾损伤模型

➢ HOLDITCH S J, BROWN C N, LOMBARDI A M, et al. Recent advances in models, mechanisms, biomarkers, and interventions in cisplatin-induced acute kidney injury[J]. Int J Mol Sci, 2019, 20(12):3011.

➢ PABLA N, DONG Z. Cisplatin nephrotoxicity: mechanisms and renoprotective strategies[J]. Kidney Int, 2008, 73(9):994 – 1007.

➢ MATSUI K, KAMIJO-IKEMORIF A, SUGAYA T, et al. Renal liver-type fatty acid binding protein (L-FABP) attenuates acute kidney injury in aristolochic acid nephrotoxicity[J]. Am J Pathol, 2011, 178(3):1021 – 1032.

➢ WU J, LIU X H, FAN J J, et al. Bardoxolone methyl (BARD) ameliorates aristolochic acid (AA)-induced acute kidney injury through Nrf2 pathway[J]. Toxicology, 2014, 318:22 – 31.

➢ WEN X Y, PENG Z Y, LI Y J, et al. One dose of cyclosporine A is protective at initiation of folic acid-induced acute kidney injury in mice[J]. Nephrol Dial Transplant, 2012, 27(8):3100 – 3109.

➢ GENG Y Q, ZHANG L, FU B, et al. Mesenchymal stem cells ameliorate rhabdomyolysis-induced acute kidney injury via the activation of M2 macrophages[J]. Stem Cell Res Ther, 2014, 5(3):80.

**思考题:**

(1) 不同急性肾衰竭模型的发病机制差异是什么?

(2) 各种模型构建急性肾损伤的评估指标有哪些?

(3) 为何要构建不同的急性肾损伤模型,对临床工作有什么指导意义?

(郑 栋 赵 颖)

# 第十四章　脑功能不全

**[拓展实验]：乙醇对小鼠学习记忆能力的影响**

**临床前及临床研究与综述**

➢ BRADY M L, ALLAN A M, CALDWELL K K. A limited access mouse model of pre-natal alcohol exposure that produces long-lasting deficits in hippocampal-dependent learn-ing and memory[J]. Alcohol Clin Exp Res, 2012, 36(3):457 – 466.

➢ SPEAR L P. Effects of adolescent alcohol consumption on the brain and behaviour[J]. Nat Rev Neurosci, 2018, 19(4):197 – 214.

➢ BRUMBACK T, CAO D, MCNAMARA P, et al. Alcohol-induced performance im-pairment：a 5-year re-examination study in heavy and light drinkers[J]. Psychopharma-cology (Berl), 2017, 234(11):1749 – 1759.

➢ LOHESWARAN G, BARR M S, ZOMORRODI R, et al. Impairment of neuroplasticity in the dorsolateral prefrontal cortex by alcohol[J]. Sci Rep, 2017, 7(1):5276.

**思考题：**

（1）除了上述文献报道的实验方法以外,测定学习记忆能力的方法还有哪些？

（2）本实验中,可用哪些指标来测定动物的学习记忆能力？

（3）学习记忆有哪些分类？乙醇所引起的学习记忆能力改变属于哪一类？

（4）有哪些疾病会影响学习记忆能力？

（5）在临床上,医生如何检测患者的学习记忆能力？

（单立冬）

English Version

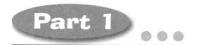

# Learning Objectives and Mind Map

## Chapter 1　Introduction to Disease

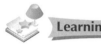 **Learning Objectives**

（1）To master concepts of disease, health and sub-health.

（2）To master causes, predisposing factors, precipitating factors and risk factors in etiology.

（3）To be familiar with the classification of causes.

（4）To master the general principle and fundamental mechanisms for pathogenesis of disease.

（5）To be familiar with outcomes of disease.

（6）To master the concept and criteria of brain death.

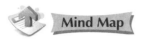 **Mind Map**

■ Health(H)：a state of complete well-being (physiological/psychological/social)

■ Subhealth(S)：the intermediate state between health and disease

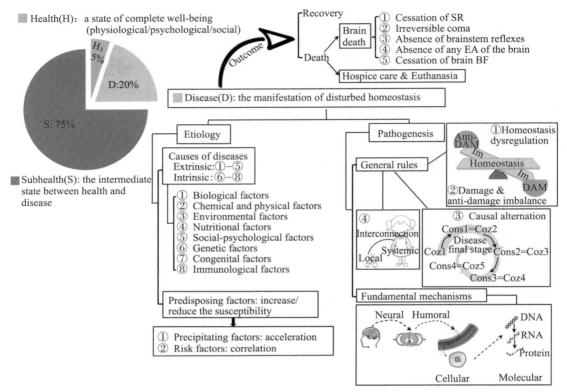

Recovery

Death

Brain death
① Cessation of SR
② Irreversible coma
③ Absence of brainstem reflexes
④ Absence of any EA of the brain
⑤ Cessation of brain BF

Hospice care & Euthanasia

Outcome

■ Disease(D): the manifestation of disturbed homeostasis

Etiology

Causes of diseases
Extrinsic：①—⑤
Intrinsic：⑥—⑧
① Biological factors
② Chemical and physical factors
③ Environmental factors
④ Nutritional factors
⑤ Social-psychological factors
⑥ Genetic factors
⑦ Congenital factors
⑧ Immunological factors

Predisposing factors: increase/ reduce the susceptibility

① Precipitating factors: acceleration
② Risk factors: correlation

Pathogenesis

General rules

① Homeostasis dysregulation

② Damage & anti-damage imbalance

③ Causal alternation
Cons1=Coz2
Coz1 Disease final stage Cons2=Coz3
Cons4=Coz5
Cons3=Coz4

④ Interconnection
Systemic
Local

Fundamental mechanisms
Neural Humoral
DNA
RNA
Protein
Cellular Molecular

（BF：blood flow；Cons：consequence；Coz：cause；DAM：damage；EA：electrical activity；Im：imbalance；SR：spontaneous respiration）

（赵　颖）

# Chapter 2　　Fluid and Electrolyte Imbalance

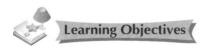 **Learning Objectives**

（1）To understand metabolisms of water, sodium, potassium, magnesium, calcium, and phosphorus and their metabolic regulation.

（2）To master the concept, etiology, pathogenesis and metabolic changes of hypo/ hypertonic dehydration.

（3）To be familiar with the concept, etiology, pathogenesis and metabolic changes of water/sodium intoxication.

（4）To master the concept and pathogenesis of edema, and be familiar with the classifications and features of edema fluids and associated metabolic changes.

（5）To master the concept, etiology, pathogenesis and metabolic changes of hypo/hyperkalemia.

（6）To be familiar with the concept, etiology, pathogenesis and metabolic changes of hypo/hypermagnesemia.

（7）To be familiar with the concept, etiology, pathogenesis and metabolic changes of hypo/hypercalcemia and hypo/hyperphosphatemia.

（8）To be familiar with the principle of prevention and treatment for all kinds of metabolic disorders.

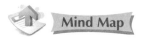

**Mind Map**

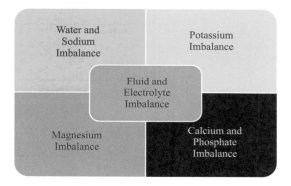

## ◇ **Water and Sodium Imbalance**

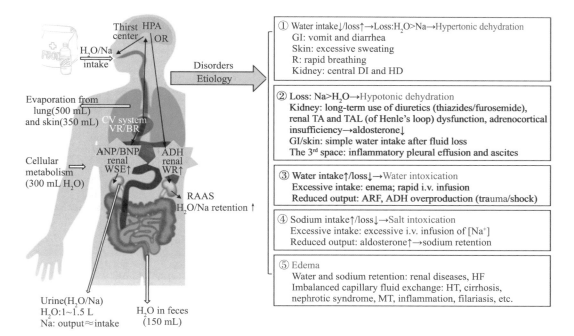

① Water intake↓/loss↑→Loss:$H_2O$>Na→Hypertonic dehydration
GI: vomit and diarrhea
Skin: excessive sweating
R: rapid breathing
Kidney: central DI and HD

② Loss: Na>$H_2O$→Hypotonic dehydration
Kidney: long-term use of diuretics (thiazides/furosemide), renal TA and TAL (of Henle's loop) dysfunction, adrenocortical insufficiency→aldosterone↓
GI/skin: simple water intake after fluid loss
The 3$^{rd}$ space: inflammatory pleural effusion and ascites

③ Water intake↑/loss↓→Water intoxication
Excessive intake: enema; rapid i.v. infusion
Reduced output: ARF, ADH overproduction (trauma/shock)

④ Sodium intake↑/loss↓→Salt intoxication
Excessive intake: excessive i.v. infusion of [$Na^+$]
Reduced output: aldosterone↑→sodium retention

⑤ Edema
Water and sodium retention: renal diseases, HF
Imbalanced capillary fluid exchange: HT, cirrhosis, nephrotic syndrome, MT, inflammation, filariasis, etc.

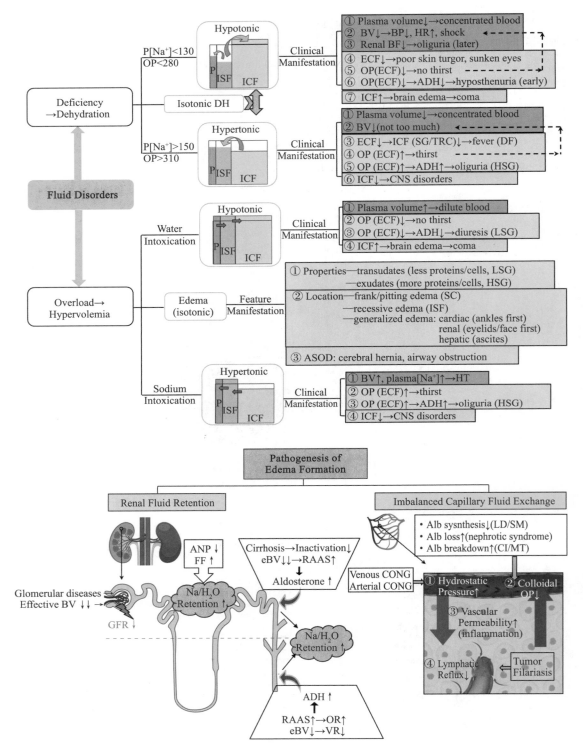

(ADH：antidiuretic hormone；Alb：albumin；ANP/BNP：atrial/brain natriuretic peptide；ARF：acute renal failure；ASOD：acute severe organ dysfunction；BF: blood flow；BP: blood pressure；BR: baroreceptor；BV: blood volume；CI: chronic inflammation；CNS: central nervous system；CONG: congestion；CV: cardiovascular；DF: dehydration fever；

DH: dehydration; DI: diabetes insipidus; eBV: effective blood volume; FF: filtration fraction; GFR: glomerular filtration rate; GI: gastrointestine; HD: hypertonic diuresis; HF: heart failure; HPA: hypothalamus; HR: heart rate; HSG: high specific gravity; HT: hypertension; ICF: intracellular fluid; LD: liver disease; ISF: interstitial fluid; LSG: low specific gravity; MT: malignant tumor; OP: osmotic pressure; OR: osmoreceptor; P: plasma; R: respiration; RAAS: renin-angiotensin-aldosterone system; SC: subcutaneous; SG: sweat gland; SM: severe malnutrition; TA: tubular acidosis; TAL: thick ascending limb; TRC: thermoregulatory center; VR: volume receptor; WR: water retention; WSE: water and sodium excretion)

# ◇ **Potassium Imbalance**

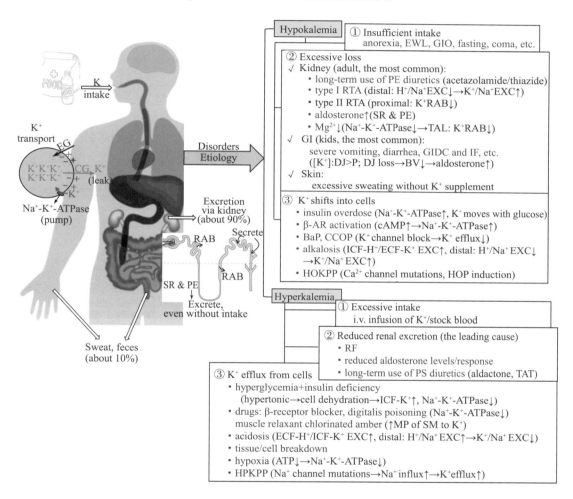

**Hypokalemia**

① Insufficient intake
  anorexia, EWL, GIO, fasting, coma, etc.

② Excessive loss
  √ Kidney (adult, the most common):
    • long-term use of PE diuretics (acetazolamide/thiazide)
    • type I RTA (distal: H⁺/Na⁺EXC↓→K⁺/Na⁺EXC↑)
    • type II RTA (proximal: K⁺RAB↓)
    • aldosterone↑(SR & PE)
    • Mg²⁺↓(Na⁺-K⁺-ATPase↓→TAL: K⁺RAB↓)
  √ GI (kids, the most common):
    severe vomiting, diarrhea, GIDC and IF, etc.
    ([K⁺]:DJ>P; DJ loss→BV↓→aldosterone↑)
  √ Skin:
    excessive sweating without K⁺ supplement

③ K⁺ shifts into cells
  • insulin overdose (Na⁺-K⁺-ATPase↑, K⁺ moves with glucose)
  • β-AR activation (cAMP↑→Na⁺-K⁺-ATPase↑)
  • BaP, CCOP (K⁺ channel block→K⁺ efflux↓)
  • alkalosis (ICF-H⁺/ECF-K⁺ EXC↑, distal: H⁺/Na⁺ EXC↓→K⁺/Na⁺EXC↑)
  • HOKPP (Ca²⁺ channel mutations, HOP induction)

**Hyperkalemia**

① Excessive intake
  i.v. infusion of K⁺/stock blood

② Reduced renal excretion (the leading cause)
  • RF
  • reduced aldosterone levels/response
  • long-term use of PS diuretics (aldactone, TAT)

③ K⁺ efflux from cells
  • hyperglycemia+insulin deficiency
    (hypertonic→cell dehydration→ICF-K⁺↑, Na⁺-K⁺-ATPase↓)
  • drugs: β-receptor blocker, digitalis poisoning (Na⁺-K⁺-ATPase↓)
    muscle relaxant chlorinated amber (↑MP of SM to K⁺)
  • acidosis (ECF-H⁺/ICF-K⁺ EXC↑, distal: H⁺/Na⁺ EXC↑→K⁺/Na⁺ EXC↓)
  • tissue/cell breakdown
  • hypoxia (ATP↓→Na⁺-K⁺-ATPase↓)
  • HPKPP (Na⁺ channel mutations→Na⁺ influx↑→K⁺efflux↑)

K intake

K⁺ transport

EG

K⁺K⁺K⁺
K⁺K⁺K⁺
CG K⁺ (leak)
K⁺
Na⁺-K⁺-ATPase (pump)

Disorders Etiology

Excretion via kidney (about 90%)

RAB   Secrete

RAB

SR & PE   Excrete, even without intake

Sweat, feces (about 10%)

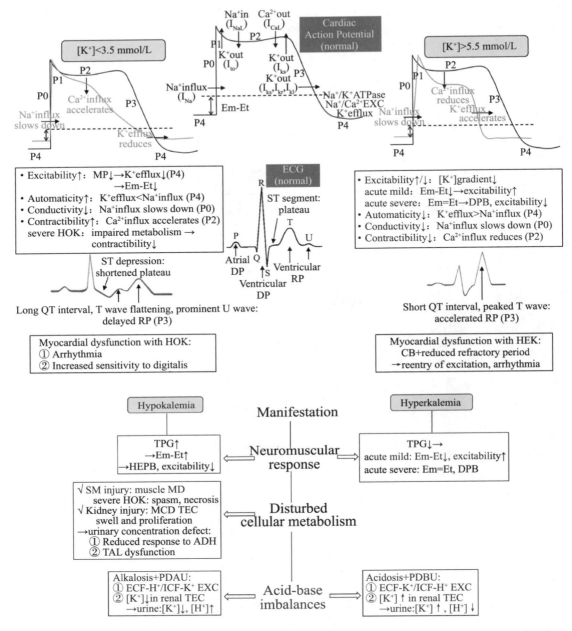

（ADH：antidiuretic hormone；AR：adrenergic receptor；BaP：barium poisoning；CB：conduction block；CG：concentration gradient；CCOP：crude cottonseed oil poisoning；DJ：digestive juice；DP：depolarization；DPB：depolarization block；ECF：extracellular fluid；EG：electrical gradient；EXC：exchange；EWL：excessive weight loss；GI：gastrointestine；GIDC：gastrointestinal decompression；GIO：gastrointestinal obstruction；HEK：hyperkalemia；HEPB：hyperpolarization block；HOK：hypokalemia；HOKPP：hypokalemic periodic paralysis；HPKPP：hyperkalemic periodic paralysis；ICF：intracellular fluid；IF：intestinal fistula；MCD：medullary collecting ducts；MD：metabolic disorder；MP：membrane permeability；P：plasma；P0-P4：Phase 0-4；PDAU：paradoxical aciduria；PDBU：paradoxical baseuria；PE：potassium excretion；PS：potassium sparing；RAB：reabsorption；RTA：renal tubular acidosis；RP：repolarization；TAL：thick ascending limb；TAT：triamterene；TEC：tubular epithelial cell；TPG：transmembrane potassium gradient；SM：skeletal muscle；SR：sodium retention；VSMC：vascular smooth muscle cell）

# ◇ **Magnesium Imbalance**

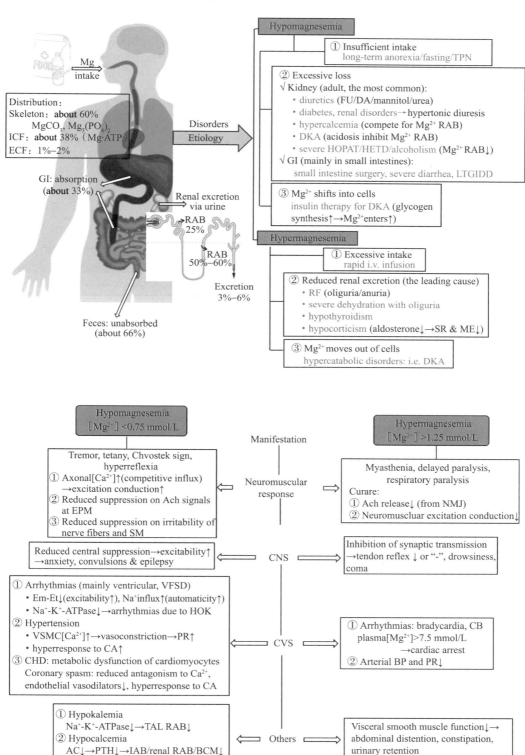

**Hypomagnesemia**

① Insufficient intake
long-term anorexia/fasting/TPN

② Excessive loss
√ Kidney (adult, the most common):
 · diuretics (FU/DA/mannitol/urea)
 · diabetes, renal disorders→ hypertonic diuresis
 · hypercalcemia (compete for $Mg^{2+}$ RAB)
 · DKA (acidosis inhibit $Mg^{2+}$ RAB)
 · severe HOPAT/HETD/alcoholism ($Mg^{2+}$ RAB↓)
√ GI (mainly in small intestines):
 small intestine surgery, severe diarrhea, LTGIDD

③ $Mg^{2+}$ shifts into cells
insulin therapy for DKA (glycogen
synthesis↑→$Mg^{2+}$enters↑)

**Hypermagnesemia**

① Excessive intake
rapid i.v. infusion

② Reduced renal excretion (the leading cause)
 · RF (oliguria/anuria)
 · severe dehydration with oliguria
 · hypothyroidism
 · hypocorticism (aldosterone↓→SR & ME↓)

③ $Mg^{2+}$ moves out of cells
hypercatabolic disorders: i.e. DKA

Mg intake

Distribution：
Skeleton：**about** 60%
 $MgCO_3$, $Mg_3(PO_4)_2$
ICF：**about** 38%（$Mg\cdot ATP$）
ECF：1%–2%

Disorders
Etiology

GI: absorption
(**about** 33%)

Renal excretion
via urine
RAB
25%
RAB
50%–60%

Excretion
3%–6%

Feces: unabsorbed
(about 66%)

---

**Hypomagnesemia**
$[Mg^{2+}] < 0.75$ mmol/L

Tremor, tetany, Chvostek sign,
hyperreflexia
① Axonal$[Ca^{2+}]$↑(competitive influx)
→excitation conduction↑
② Reduced suppression on Ach signals
at EPM
③ Reduced suppression on irritability of
nerve fibers and SM

Manifestation

Neuromuscular
response

**Hypermagnesemia**
$[Mg^{2+}] > 1.25$ mmol/L

Myasthenia, delayed paralysis,
respiratory paralysis
Curare:
① Ach release↓ (from NMJ)
② Neuromuscluar excitation conduction↓

Reduced central suppression→excitability↑
→anxiety, convulsions & epilepsy

CNS

Inhibition of synaptic transmission
→tendon reflex ↓ or "-", drowsiness,
coma

① Arrhythmias (mainly ventricular, VFSD)
 · Em-Et↓(excitability↑), $Na^+$influx↑(automaticity↑)
 · $Na^+$-$K^+$-ATPase↓→arrhythmias due to HOK
② Hypertension
 · VSMC$[Ca^{2+}]$↑→vasoconstriction→PR↑
 · hyperresponse to CA↑
③ CHD: metabolic dysfunction of cardiomyocytes
Coronary spasm: reduced antagonism to $Ca^{2+}$,
endothelial vasodilators↓, hyperresponse to CA

CVS

① Arrhythmias: bradycardia, CB
plasma$[Mg^{2+}]$>7.5 mmol/L
→cardiac arrest
② Arterial BP and PR↓

① Hypokalemia
 $Na^+$-$K^+$-ATPase↓→TAL RAB↓
② Hypocalcemia
 AC↓→PTH↓→IAB/renal RAB/BCM↓

Others

Visceral smooth muscle function↓→
abdominal distention, constipation,
urinary retention

（AC：adenylate cyclase；Ach：acetylcholine；BCM：bone calcium mobilization；BP：blood pressure；CA：catecholamine；CB：conduction block；CHD：coronary heart disease；CNS：central nervous system；CVS：cardiovascular system；DA：diuretic acid；DKA：diabetic ketoacidosis；ECF：extracellular fluid；EPM：end-plate membrane；FU：furosemide；GI：gastrointestine；HETD：hyperthyroidism；HOK：hypokalemia；HOPAT：hypoparathyroidism；IAB：intestinal absorption；ICF：intracellular fluid；LTGIDD：long-term gastrointestinal decompression and drainage；ME：magnesium excretion；NMJ：neuromuscular junction；PR：peripheral resistance；RAB：reabsorption；RF：renal failure；SR：sodium retention；TAL：thick ascending limb；TPN：total parenteral nutrition；VFSD：ventricular fibrillation and sudden death；VSMC：vascular smooth muscle cell）

# ◇ Calcium and Phosphate Imbalance

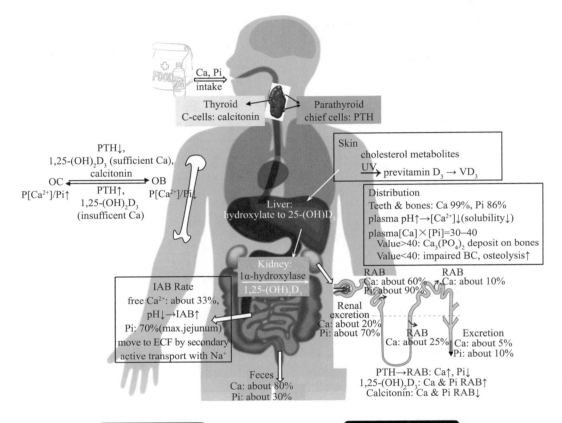

| Hypocalcemia<br>$[Ca^{2+}]$ <1.0 mmol/L | Hypercalcemia<br>$[Ca^{2+}]$ >1.4 mmol/L |
|---|---|
| Etiology:<br>① Insufficient UV/IAB: active $VD_3$↓, hepatic/renal disorders<br>② PTH deficiency/resistance: HOP, pseudo-HOP<br>③ IAB↓, PTH sensitivity↓: CRF, AP<br>④ PTH↓, $Ca^{2+}$-$Mg^{2+}$ EXC↓ (bones): HOM | Etiology:<br>① Osteolysis↑:<br> • hyperparathyroidism:<br> primary: PA, hyperplasia, adenocarcinoma<br> secondary: vitamin D deficiency, CRF<br> • MT with bone metastasis, HT<br>② IAB↑: vitamin D poisoning<br>③ Renal RAB↑: Addison disease, EVAI, thiazides |
| Manifestation:<br>① NM: tremor, tetany, laryngeal stridor, convulsions<br>② Myocardium:<br> • $Na^+$ influx ↑ →excitability/conductivity↑<br> • $Ca^{2+}$ influx↓(plateau)→QT/ST prolongation, flattened/inverted T wave<br>③ Skeleton: rickets (kids)/osteoporosis (adults)<br>④ Infant: immunity↓, dry skin, brittle nails | Manifestation:<br>① NM: excitability↓→fatigue, tendon reflex↓, MD<br>② Myocardium:<br> • $Na^+$influx ↓ →excitability/conductivity↓<br> • $Ca^{2+}$influx↑ (plateau) →QT shortening<br>③ Kidney: RTI→urine concentration↓ (early)<br>④ Vessels & Organs: ectopic calcification |

| Hypophosphatemia [Pi] <0.8 mmol/L |
| --- |
| Etiology: |
| ① Impaired IAB: starve, vomit, MABS, 1,25-(OH)$_2$D$_3$ deficiency, phosphate binders |
| ② Urine output↑: diuretics, acute alcoholism, VD$_3$ resistance, hyperparathyroidism, RTA, metabolic acidosis |
| ③ Pi shifts into cells: insulin, glucose, androgen, RFS, respiratory alkalosis (carbohydrate phosphorylation↑) |
| Manifestation (no typical symptom): |
| ① ATP synthesis↓→myasthenia, MD |
| ② 2,3-DPG↓→Hb oxygen affinity↑ |

| Hyperphosphatemia [Pi] >1.6/1.9 mmol/L (Adult/Kid) |
| --- |
| Etiology: |
| ① Renal excretion↓: ARI & CRI, HOP, acromegaly (GH↑→urine Pi output↓) |
| ② Osteolysis↑: hyperthyroidism |
| ③ IAB & RAB↑: VD$_3$ poisoning |
| ④ Pi moves out of cells: acute acidosis, rhabdomyolysis, high fever, LL, MT (chemical therapy) |
| ⑤ Intake↑: PCL, phosphate infusion |
| Manifestation: |
| ① Hypocalcemia: 1α-hydroxylase↓, bone RAB↓ |
| ② Vessels/Organs: ectopic calcification |

(2,3-DPG: 2,3 diphosphoglyceric acid; AP: acute pancreatitis; ARI: acute renal insufficiency; BC: bone calcification; CRF: chronic renal failure; CRI: chronic renal insufficiency; ECF: extracellular fluid; EVAI: excessive vitamin A intake; EXC: exchange; GH: growth hormone; Hb: hemoglobin; HOM: hypomagnesemia; HOP: hypoparathyroidism; HT: hyperthyroidism; IAB: intestinal absorption; LL: lymphocytic leukemia; MABS: malabsorption syndrome; MD: mental disorder; MT: malignant tumor; NM: neuromuscle; PA: parathyroid adenoma; PCL: phosphorus-containing laxatives; Pi: inorganic phosphorus; PTH: parathyroid hormone; RAB: renal absorption; RFS: refeeding syndrome; RTA: renal tubalar acidosis; RTI: renal tubular injury; UV: ultraviolet; VD$_3$: vitamin D$_3$)

(赵丽梅　赵　颖)

# Chapter 3　Acid-base Disturbance

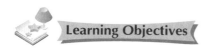

**Learning Objectives**

(1) To master the concept of acid-base disturbance as well as the interpretation and significance of acid-base parameters.

(2) To be familiar with the generation of acids and bases as well as the regulation of acid-base balance *in vivo*.

(3) To master the concept, pathogenesis, compensation, and manifestations of metabolic acidosis, respiratory acidosis, metabolic alkalosis and respiratory alkalosis.

(4) To be familiar with the etiology and classification of metabolic acidosis, respiratory acidosis, metabolic alkalosis and respiratory alkalosis.

(5) To master the types, etiology and characteristics of mixed acid-base disturbances and a systemic approach to analyze acid-base disturbances.

(6) To understand the pathophysiological basis of the prevention and treatment for metabolic acidosis, respiratory acidosis, metabolic alkalosis and respiratory alkalosis.

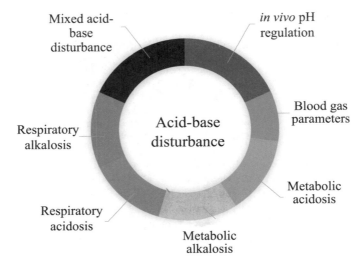

Mind Map

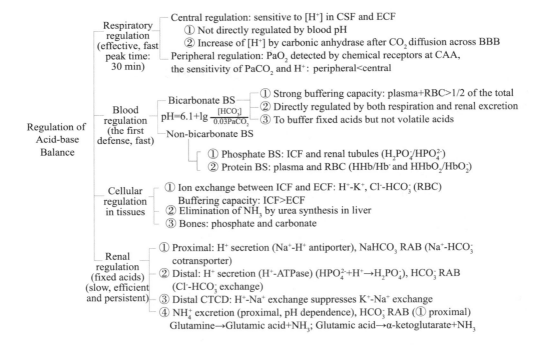

Regulation of Acid-base Balance

**Respiratory regulation (effective, fast peak time: 30 min)**
Central regulation: sensitive to [H⁺] in CSF and ECF
① Not directly regulated by blood pH
② Increase of [H⁺] by carbonic anhydrase after $CO_2$ diffusion across BBB
Peripheral regulation: $PaO_2$ detected by chemical receptors at CAA, the sensitivity of $PaCO_2$ and H⁺: peripheral<central

**Blood regulation (the first defense, fast)**
Bicarbonate BS
$pH=6.1+lg\dfrac{[HCO_3^-]}{0.03PaCO_2}$
① Strong buffering capacity: plasma+RBC>1/2 of the total
② Directly regulated by both respiration and renal excretion
③ To buffer fixed acids but not volatile acids
Non-bicarbonate BS
① Phosphate BS: ICF and renal tubules ($H_2PO_4^-/HPO_4^{2-}$)
② Protein BS: plasma and RBC ($HHb/Hb^-$ and $HHbO_2/HbO_2^-$)

**Cellular regulation in tissues**
① Ion exchange between ICF and ECF: H⁺-K⁺, Cl⁻-$HCO_3^-$ (RBC)
Buffering capacity: ICF>ECF
② Elimination of $NH_3$ by urea synthesis in liver
③ Bones: phosphate and carbonate

**Renal regulation (fixed acids) (slow, efficient and persistent)**
① Proximal: H⁺ secretion (Na⁺-H⁺ antiporter), $NaHCO_3$ RAB (Na⁺-$HCO_3^-$ cotransporter)
② Distal: H⁺ secretion (H⁺-ATPase) ($HPO_4^{2-}+H^+→H_2PO_4^-$), $HCO_3^-$ RAB (Cl⁻-$HCO_3^-$ exchange)
③ Distal CTCD: H⁺-Na⁺ exchange suppresses K⁺-Na⁺ exchange
④ $NH_4^+$ excretion (proximal, pH dependence), $HCO_3^-$ RAB (① proximal)
Glutamine→Glutamic acid+$NH_3$; Glutamic acid→α-ketoglutarate+$NH_3$

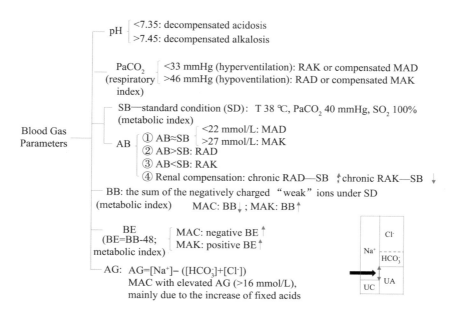

Blood Gas Parameters
- pH
  - <7.35: decompensated acidosis
  - >7.45: decompensated alkalosis
- $PaCO_2$ (respiratory index)
  - <33 mmHg (hyperventilation): RAK or compensated MAD
  - >46 mmHg (hypoventilation): RAD or compensated MAK
- SB—standard condition (SD): T 38 ℃, $PaCO_2$ 40 mmHg, $SO_2$ 100% (metabolic index)
- AB
  - ① AB≈SB
    - <22 mmol/L: MAD
    - >27 mmol/L: MAK
  - ② AB>SB: RAD
  - ③ AB<SB: RAK
  - ④ Renal compensation: chronic RAD—SB ↑; chronic RAK—SB ↓
- BB: the sum of the negatively charged "weak" ions under SD (metabolic index)　MAC: BB↓; MAK: BB↑
- BE (BE=BB-48; metabolic index)
  - MAC: negative BE ↑
  - MAK: positive BE ↑
- AG: AG=[$Na^+$]− ([$HCO_3^-$]+[$Cl^-$])
  MAC with elevated AG (>16 mmol/L), mainly due to the increase of fixed acids

Metabolic Acidosis (MAD)

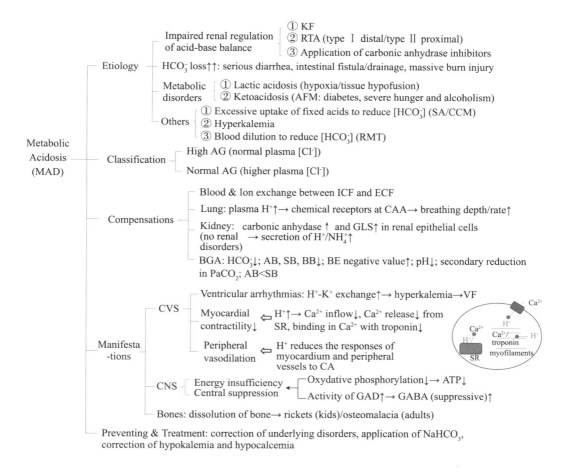

- Etiology
  - Impaired renal regulation of acid-base balance
    - ① KF
    - ② RTA (type Ⅰ distal/type Ⅱ proximal)
    - ③ Application of carbonic anhydrase inhibitors
  - $HCO_3^-$ loss↑↑: serious diarrhea, intestinal fistula/drainage, massive burn injury
  - Metabolic disorders
    - ① Lactic acidosis (hypoxia/tissue hypofusion)
    - ② Ketoacidosis (AFM: diabetes, severe hunger and alcoholism)
  - Others
    - ① Excessive uptake of fixed acids to reduce [$HCO_3^-$] (SA/CCM)
    - ② Hyperkalemia
    - ③ Blood dilution to reduce [$HCO_3^-$] (RMT)
- Classification
  - High AG (normal plasma [$Cl^-$])
  - Normal AG (higher plasma [$Cl^-$])
- Compensations
  - Blood & Ion exchange between ICF and ECF
  - Lung: plasma $H^+$↑→ chemical receptors at CAA→ breathing depth/rate↑
  - Kidney: carbonic anhydase ↑ and GLS↑ in renal epithelial cells (no renal disorders) → secretion of $H^+$/$NH_4^+$↑
  - BGA: $HCO_3^-$↓; AB, SB, BB↓; BE negative value↑; pH↓; secondary reduction in $PaCO_2$; AB<SB
- Manifesta-tions
  - CVS
    - Ventricular arrhythmias: $H^+$-$K^+$ exchange↑→ hyperkalemia→VF
    - Myocardial contractility↓ ⇐ $H^+$↑→ $Ca^{2+}$ inflow↓, $Ca^{2+}$ release↓ from SR, binding in $Ca^{2+}$ with troponin↓
    - Peripheral vasodilation ⇐ $H^+$ reduces the responses of myocardium and peripheral vessels to CA
  - CNS
    - Energy insufficiency
    - Central suppression
      - Oxydative phosphorylation↓→ ATP↓
      - Activity of GAD↑→ GABA (suppressive)↑
  - Bones: dissolution of bone→ rickets (kids)/osteomalacia (adults)
- Preventing & Treatment: correction of underlying disorders, application of $NaHCO_3$, correction of hypokalemia and hypocalcemia

**Respiratory Acidosis (RAD)**

- Etiology
  - Expired $CO_2$ ↓ — Respiratory depression (RD); airway obstruction (AO); respiratory paralysis (RP); thoracic disorders; lung diseases; improper use of ventilators
  - Inspired $CO_2$ ↑ (seldom): environmental $[CO_2]$ ↑
- Classification
  - Acute: mainly due to acute AO or apnea (RD/RP)
  - Chronic: $PaCO_2$ elevation > 24 h, developed in COPD/massive PF/atelectasis
- Compensations
  - Acute
    - ① Transmembrane exchange of $H^+$-$K^+$, buffered by phosphates and proteins in ICF
    - ② Diffusion of $CO_2$ into RBC, buffered by Hb/$HbO_2$ systems
  - Chronic: renal CAH&GLS ↑ → $H^+$/$NH_4^+$ secretion ↑
  - BGA
    - ① Acute: $PaCO_2$ ↑, pH ↓
    - ② Chronic with renal compensation: AB/SB/BB ↑, AB>SB, BE positive value ↑

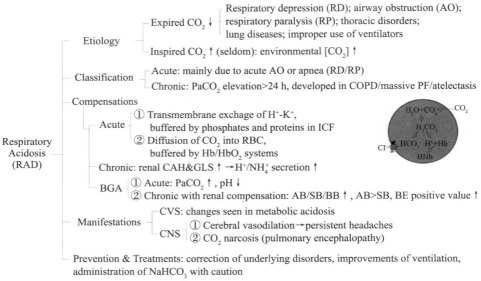

- Manifestations
  - CVS: changes seen in metabolic acidosis
  - CNS
    - ① Cerebral vasodilation → persistent headaches
    - ② $CO_2$ narcosis (pulmonary encephalopathy)
- Prevention & Treatments: correction of underlying disorders, improvements of ventilation, administration of $NaHCO_3$ with caution

**Metabolic Alkalosis (MAK)**

- Etiology
  - Hypokalemia
    - ① $H^+$-$K^+$ exchange(EXC), $H^+$ transfers into cells
    - ② $K^+$-$Na^+$ EXC(distal RT)↓→$H^+$-$Na^+$ EXC↑→$HCO_3^-$RAB↑
  - Excessive acid loss
    - Via stomach (severe vomit, gastric drainage)
      - ① Gastric $H^+$ loss, intestinal $HCO_3^-$ accumulation
      - ② Gastric $Cl^-$ loss→hypochloremia
      - ③ Effective CV↓→aldosterone↑→hypokalemia
    - Via kidney
      - ① Loop diuretics→active RAB of $Cl^-$ in TAL↓→$Cl^-$ excretion↑ →passive RAB of $Na^+$↓→distal secretion of $H^+$↑
      - ② Adrenal cortex hormones↑→aldosterone↑ →hypokalemia/$H^+$-ATPase↑ in CD→$H^+$ secretion↑
  - Hepatic failure
    - ① Aldosterone inactivation↓→hypokalemia
    - ② Urea synthesis↓→plasma ammonia↑
  - Excessive intake of $HCO_3^-$(iatrogenic): overdose of $NaHCO_3$ for peptic ulcer and metabolic acidosis
- Classification
  - Saline-responsive: alleviation by infusion of NS/half NS (vomiting/gastric drainage/diuretics)
  - Saline-resistant: no alleviation by NS (generalized edema/primary aldosteronism/hypokalemia/Cushing's syndrome)
- Compensation
  - pH buffers in the blood and ion exchange between ECF and ICF
  - Lung: respiratory depression→$PaCO_2$ or plasma $H_2CO_3$↑
  - Kidney: epithelial CAH and GLS↓→$H^+$/$NH_4^+$ secretion↓→$HCO_3^-$ reabsorption↓ (Note: hypochloremia/hypokalemia/excessive secretion of aldosterone →renal $H^+$ secretion↑, renal compensation↓→paradoxical aciduria)
  - BGA: pH↑; AB, SB, BB↑; AB>SB; BE positive value↑; $PaCO_2$↑ (secondary)
- Manifestations
  - CNS
    - GABA transaminase ↑→GABA↓→CNS excitation
    - The leftward shift of oxygen Hb dissociation curve→hypoxia →neurological signs including coma
  - NMS: plasma $[Ca^{2+}]$ ↓→irritability↑→tendon reflex↑, myoclonus, tetany
  - Hypokalemia
    - ① $H^+$-$K^+$ exchange↑
    - ② RTECs: $H^+$-$Na^+$↓→$K^+$-$Na^+$↑
- Prevention & Treatment
  - Saline-responsive
    - NS
      - ① ECF↑→correction of contraction alkalosis
      - ② $Cl^-$ supplement→urinal $HCO_3^-$ excretion↑
    - KCl→correct severe hypokalemia
    - HCl (HCl+$NaHCO_3$→NaCl+$H_2CO_3$)→correct severe alkalosis
  - Saline-resistant
    - CAH inhibitors→renal $H^+$ secretion↓, $HCO_3^-$ reabsorption↓
    - Treatment with aldosterone antagonists and potassium supplements

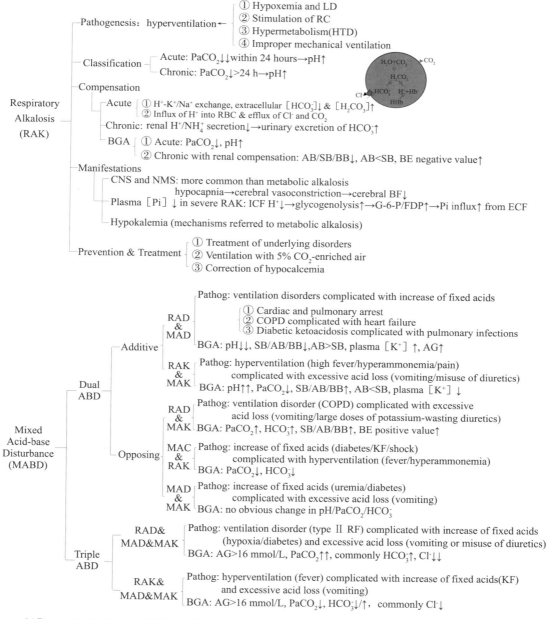

Respiratory Alkalosis (RAK)

- Pathogenesis: hyperventilation ←
  - ① Hypoxemia and LD
  - ② Stimulation of RC
  - ③ Hypermetabolism(HTD)
  - ④ Improper mechanical ventilation
- Classification
  - Acute: $PaCO_2\downarrow\downarrow$ within 24 hours→pH↑
  - Chronic: $PaCO_2\downarrow$>24 h→pH↑
- Compensation
  - Acute
    - ① $H^+$-$K^+$/$Na^+$ exchange, extracellular $[HCO_3^-]\downarrow$ & $[H_2CO_3]\uparrow$
    - ② Influx of $H^+$ into RBC & efflux of $Cl^-$ and $CO_2$
  - Chronic: renal $H^+$/$NH_4^+$ secretion↓→urinary excretion of $HCO_3^-\uparrow$
- BGA
  - ① Acute: $PaCO_2\downarrow$, pH↑
  - ② Chronic with renal compensation: AB/SB/BB↓, AB<SB, BE negative value↑
- Manifestations
  - CNS and NMS: more common than metabolic alkalosis
    hypocapnia→cerebral vasoconstriction→cerebral BF↓
  - Plasma $[Pi]$ ↓ in severe RAK: ICF $H^+\downarrow$→glycogenolysis↑→G-6-P/FDP↑→Pi influx↑ from ECF
  - Hypokalemia (mechanisms referred to metabolic alkalosis)
- Prevention & Treatment
  - ① Treatment of underlying disorders
  - ② Ventilation with 5% $CO_2$-enriched air
  - ③ Correction of hypocalcemia

Mixed Acid-base Disturbance (MABD)

- Dual ABD
  - Additive
    - RAD & MAD
      - Pathog: ventilation disorders complicated with increase of fixed acids
        - ① Cardiac and pulmonary arrest
        - ② COPD complicated with heart failure
        - ③ Diabetic ketoacidosis complicated with pulmonary infections
      - BGA: pH↓↓, SB/AB/BB↓,AB>SB, plasma $[K^+]$ ↑, AG↑
    - RAK & MAK
      - Pathog: hyperventilation (high fever/hyperammonemia/pain) complicated with excessive acid loss (vomiting/misuse of diuretics)
      - BGA: pH↑↑, $PaCO_2\downarrow$, SB/AB/BB↑, AB<SB, plasma $[K^+]$ ↓
  - Opposing
    - RAD & MAK
      - Pathog: ventilation disorder (COPD) complicated with excessive acid loss (vomiting/large doses of potassium-wasting diuretics)
      - BGA: $PaCO_2\uparrow$, $HCO_3^-\uparrow$, SB/AB/BB↑, BE positive value↑
    - MAC & RAK
      - Pathog: increase of fixed acids (diabetes/KF/shock) complicated with hyperventilation (fever/hyperammonemia)
      - BGA: $PaCO_2\downarrow$, $HCO_3^-\downarrow$
    - MAD & MAK
      - Pathog: increase of fixed acids (uremia/diabetes) complicated with excessive acid loss (vomiting)
      - BGA: no obvious change in pH/$PaCO_2$/$HCO_3^-$
- Triple ABD
  - RAD & MAD&MAK
    - Pathog: ventilation disorder (type Ⅱ RF) complicated with increase of fixed acids (hypoxia/diabetes) and excessive acid loss (vomiting or misuse of diuretics)
    - BGA: AG>16 mmol/L, $PaCO_2\uparrow\uparrow$, commonly $HCO_3^-\uparrow$, $Cl^-\downarrow\downarrow$
  - RAK & MAD&MAK
    - Pathog: hyperventilation (fever) complicated with increase of fixed acids(KF) and excessive acid loss (vomiting)
    - BGA: AG>16 mmol/L, $PaCO_2\downarrow$, $HCO_3^-\downarrow/\uparrow$, commonly $Cl^-\downarrow$

（AB：actual bicarbonate；ABD：acid-base disturbance；AFM：abnormal fat metabolism；AG：anion gap；BB：buffer base；BBB：blood brain barrier；BF：blood flow；BGA：blood gas analysis；BS：buffer system；CA：catecholamine；CAA：the carotid artery and aorta；CAH：carbonic anhydrase；CCM：chlorine-containing medicine；CD：collecting duct；CNS：central nerve system；COPD：chronic obstructive pulmonary disease；CSF：cerebrospinal fluid；CTCD：convoluted tubules and collecting ducts；CV：circulatory volume；CVS：cadiovascular system；ECF：extracellular fluid；GABA：γ-aminobutyric acid；GAD：glutamic acid decarboxylase；GE：generalized edema；GLS：glutaminase；Hb：hemoglobin；HTD：hyperthyroidism；ICF：intracellular fluid；KF：kidney failure；LD：lung diseases；MAD：metabolic acidosis；MAK：metabolic alkalosis；NMS：neuromuscular system；NS：normal saline；Pathog：pathogenesis；PF：pulmonary fibrosis；Pi：inorganic phosphate；RAB：reabsorption；RAD：respiratory acidosis；RAK：respiratory alkalosis；RBC：red blood cell；RC：respiratory center；RF：respiratory failure；RMT：rapid and massive transfusion；RT：renal tubule；RTA：renal tubular acidosis；RTECs：renal tubular epithelial cells；SA：salicylic acid；SB：standard bicarbonate；SR：sarcoplasmic reticulum；TAL：thick ascending limb；VF：ventricular fibrillation）

（郑　栋　赵丽梅）

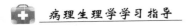
# Chapter 4    Fever

 **Learning Objectives**

(1) To master the concepts of fever, hyperthermia, pyrogenic activators, endogenous pyrogens and hyperthermic ceiling.

(2) To master the etiology and pathogenesis of fever.

(3) To be familiar with the classification of high body temperature as well as the classification and functions of pyrogenic activators, endogenous pyrogens, and central positive (negative) regulatory mediators.

(4) To be familiar with the effects of fever on metabolism and function.

(5) To be familiar with three stages of fever and associated thermometabolism.

(6) To understand the set-point theory.

(7) To understand the pathophysiological basis of prevention and treatment for fever.

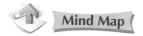

**Mind Map**

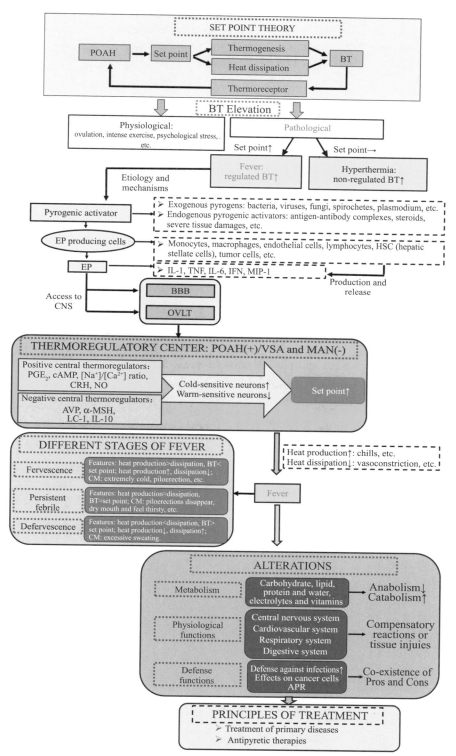

SET POINT THEORY

POAH → Set point → Thermogenesis / Heat dissipation → BT

Thermoreceptor

BT Elevation

Physiological:
ovulation, intense exercise, psychological stress, etc.

Pathological

Set point↑

Set point→

Fever:
regulated BT↑

Hyperthermia:
non-regulated BT↑

Etiology and mechanisms

Pyrogenic activator

➤ Exogenous pyrogens: bacteria, viruses, fungi, spirochetes, plasmodium, etc.
➤ Endogenous pyrogenic activators: antigen-antibody complexes, steroids, severe tissue damages, etc.

EP producing cells

➤ Monocytes, macrophages, endothelial cells, lymphocytes, HSC (hepatic stellate cells), tumor cells, etc.

EP

➤ IL-1, TNF, IL-6, IFN, MIP-1

Production and release

Access to CNS

BBB

OVLT

THERMOREGULATORY CENTER: POAH(+)/VSA and MAN(-)

Positive central thermoregulators:
$PGE_2$, cAMP, $[Na^+]/[Ca^{2+}]$ ratio, CRH, NO

Negative central thermoregulators:
AVP, α-MSH, LC-1, IL-10

Cold-sensitive neurons↑
Warm-sensitive neurons↓

Set point↑

DIFFERENT STAGES OF FEVER

Fervescence — Features: heat production>dissipation, BT< set point; heat production↑, dissipation↓; CM: extremely cold, piloerection, etc.

Persistent febrile — Features: heat production=dissipation, BT≈set point; CM: piloerections disappear, dry mouth and feel thirsty, etc.

Defervescence — Features: heat production<dissipation, BT> set point; heat production↓, dissipation↑; CM: excessive sweating.

Heat production↑: chills, etc.
Heat dissipation↓: vasoconstriction, etc.

Fever

ALTERATIONS

Metabolism — Carbohydrate, lipid, protein and water, electrolytes and vitamins → Anabolism↓ Catabolism↑

Physiological functions — Central nervous system, Cardiovascular system, Respiratory system, Digestive system → Compensatory reactions or tissue injuries

Defense functions — Defense against infections↑ Effects on cancer cells APR → Co-existence of Pros and Cons

PRINCIPLES OF TREATMENT
➤ Treatment of primary diseases
➤ Antipyretic therapies

165

（APR：acute phase response；AVP：arginine vasopressin；BBB：blood brain barrier；BT：body temperature；cAMP：cyclic adenosine monophosphate；CM：clinical manifestation；CRH：corticotropin releasing hormone；EP：endogenous pyrogen；IFN：interferon；IL-1：interleukin-1；IL-6：interleukin-6；IL-10：interleukin-10；LC-1：lipocortin-1；LPS：lipopolysaccharide；MAN：medial amygdaloid nucleus；MIP-1：macrophage inflammatory protein-1；α-MSH：α-melanocyte stimulating hormone；NO：nitric oxide；OVLT：organum vasculosum of lamina terminalis；$PGE_2$：prostaglandin $E_2$；POAH：preoptic anterior hypothalamus；TNF：tumor necrosis factor；VSA：ventral septal area）

（孙丽娜）

# Chapter 5　Stress

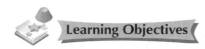 **Learning Objectives**

（1）To master the concept of stress and stressor, as well as the concept and stages of general adaptation syndrome.

（2）To master the neuroendocrine responses of stress and underlying mechanisms, acute phase response and acute phase proteins, as well as cellular heat shock response and heat shock proteins.

（3）To master the concept and pathogenesis of stress ulcer.

（4）To be familiar with the classification of the stress response, as well as stress-induced metabolic and functional changes.

（5）To be familiar with the psychological responses to stress.

（6）To be familiar with the relationships of cardiovascular diseases, mental and neurological diseases, immunological diseases, endocrine and metabolic diseases to stress.

（7）To understand other endocrine and immunological responses to stress, as well as the concept and mechanisms of oxidative stress.

（8）To understand the principles of prevention and treatment for stress.

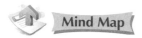

**Mind Map**

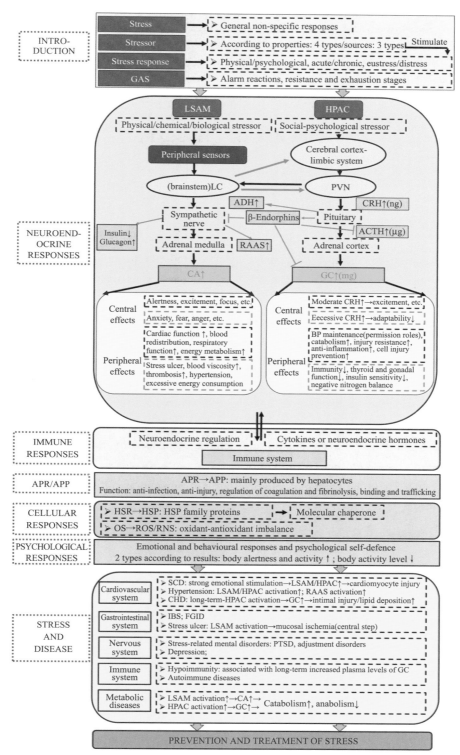

| INTRODUCTION | Stress → General non-specific responses |
| Stressor → According to properties: 4 types/sources: 3 types — Stimulate |
| Stress response → Physical/psychological, acute/chronic, eustress/distress |
| GAS → Alarm reactions, resistance and exhaustion stages |

LSAM / HPAC

Physical/chemical/biological stressor / Social-psychological stressor

Peripheral sensors / Cerebral cortex-limbic system

(brainstem)LC ⇄ PVN

ADH↑ / CRH↑(ng)

Sympathetic nerve — β-Endorphins — Pituitary

Insulin↓/Glucagon↑

ACTH↑(μg)

**NEUROENDOCRINE RESPONSES**

Adrenal medulla — RAAS↑ / Adrenal cortex

CA↑ / GC↑(mg)

Central effects:
- Alertness, excitement, focus, etc.
- Anxiety, fear, anger, etc.

Peripheral effects:
- Cardiac function↑, blood redistribution, respiratory function↑, energy metabolism↑
- Stress ulcer, blood viscosity↑, thrombosis↑, hypertension, excessive energy consumption

Central effects:
- Moderate CRH↑→excitement, etc.
- Eecessive CRH↑→adaptability↓

Peripheral effects:
- BP maintenance(permission roles), catabolism↑, injury resistance↑, anti-inflammation↑, cell injury prevention↑
- Immunity↓, thyroid and gonadal function↓, insulin sensitivity↓, negative nitrogen balance

**IMMUNE RESPONSES**

Neuroendocrine regulation / Cytokines or neuroendocrine hormones

Immune system

**APR/APP**

APR→APP: mainly produced by hepatocytes
Function: anti-infection, anti-injury, regulation of coagulation and fibrinolysis, binding and trafficking

**CELLULAR RESPONSES**

- HSR→HSP: HSP family proteins → Molecular chaperone
- OS→ROS/RNS: oxidant-antioxidant imbalance

**PSYCHOLOGICAL RESPONSES**

Emotional and behavioural responses and psychological self-defence
2 types according to results: body alertness and activity↑; body activity level↓

**STRESS AND DISEASE**

| Cardiovascular system |
- SCD: strong emotional stimulation→LSAM/HPAC↑→cardiomyocyte injury
- Hypertension: LSAM/HPAC activation↑; RAAS activation↑
- CHD: long-term-HPAC activation→GC↑→intimal injury/lipid deposition↑

| Gastrointestinal system |
- IBS; FGID
- Stress ulcer: LSAM activation→mucosal ischemia(central step)

| Nervous system |
- Stress-related mental disorders: PTSD, adjustment disorders
- Depression;

| Immune system |
- Hypoimmunity: associated with long-term increased plasma levels of GC
- Autoimmune diseases

| Metabolic diseases |
- LSAM activation↑→CA↑→
- HPAC activation↑→GC↑→ Catabolism↑, anabolism↓

**PREVENTION AND TREATMENT OF STRESS**

（ACTH：adrenocorticotropic hormone；ADH：antidiuretic hormone；APP：acute phase protein；APR：acute phase response；CA：catecholamine；CHD：coronary heart disease；CRH：corticotropin releasing hormone；FGID：functional gastrointestinal disease；GAS：general adaptation syndrome；GC：glucocorticoid；HPAC：hypothalamus-pituitary-adrenal cortex system；HSR：heat shock response；HSP：heat shock protein；IBS：irritable bowel syndrome；LC：locus ceruleus；LSAM：locus ceruleus-sympathetic-adrenal medulla system；RAAS：renin-angiotensin-aldosterone system；PTSD：posttraumatic stress disorder；PVN：paraventricular nucleus；SCD：sudden cardiac death）

（孙丽娜）

# Chapter 6　Hypoxia

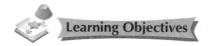 **Learning Objectives**

（1）To master the concepts of hypoxia, cyanosis and enterogenous cyanosis.

（2）To master the concepts of all blood oxygen parameters including partial pressure of oxygen（$PO_2$）, oxygen binding capacity of hemoglobin（$CO_2 max$）, oxygen content（$CO_2$）and oxygen saturation（$SO_2$）, as well as the interpretation of abnormal parameters.

（3）To master the classification of hypoxia as well as the etiology and pathogenesis of different types of hypoxia.

（4）To master the changes of blood oxygen parameters in different types of hypoxia.

（5）To master the compensatory reactions and tissue damage of respiratory, circulatory, and hematological system in hypoxia.

（6）To be familiar with the central and cellular compensatory reactions, central nervous system alterations, and cell damage in hypoxia.

（7）To understand the pathophysiological basis of prevention and treatment for hypoxia.

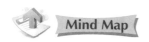
**Mind Map**

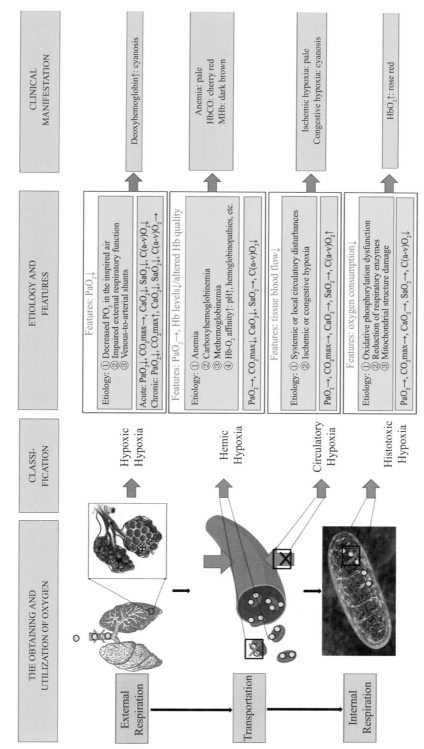

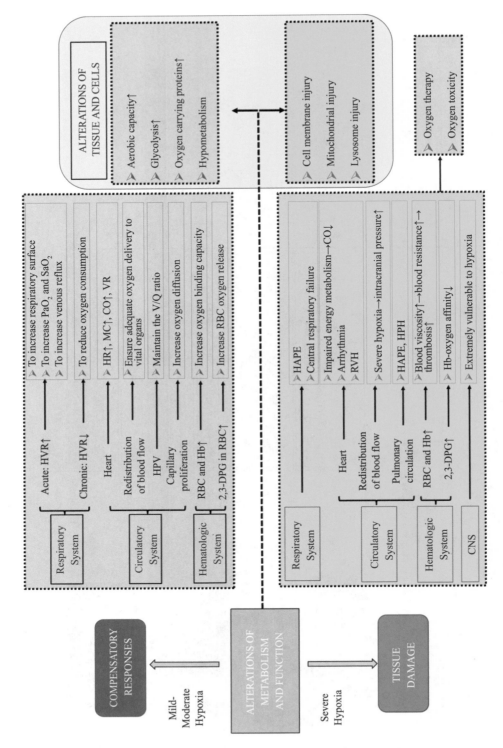

［CO：cardiac output；CO$_2$max：oxygen binding capacity of hemoglobin；CO$_2$：oxygen content；CaO$_2$：arterial oxygen content；C（a-v）O$_2$：arterial-to-venous oxygen content difference；CNS：central nervous system；EPO：erythropoietin；HAPE：high altitude pulmonary edema；Hb：hemoglobin；HbCO：carboxyhemoglobin；HPH：hypoxic pulmonary hypertension；HPV：hypoxic pulmonary vasoconstriction；HVR：hypoxia ventilation reaction；HR：heart rate；

MC: myocardial contractility; MHb: methemoglobin; RVH: right ventricular hypertrophy; PaO$_2$: the arterial partial pressure of oxygen; PO$_2$: partial pressure of oxygen; RBC: red blood cells; SO$_2$: oxygen saturation of hemoglobin; VR: ventricular remodeling]

（孙丽娜）

# Chapter 7   Shock

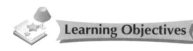
**Learning Objectives**

（1）To master the concept of shock, and the primum movens of different types of shock.

（2）To master the microcirculatory mechanisms of shock and the alterations at different stages.

（3）To be familiar with the etiology and classification of shock.

（4）To be familiar with the cellular and molecular mechanisms of shock.

（5）To be familiar with the functional and metabolic changes in shock.

（6）To understand the characteristics and pathogenesis of hemorrhagic, septic, anaphylactic, and cardiogenic shock.

（7）To understand the pathophysiological basis of the prevention and treatment for shock.

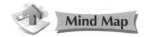

## 1. The causes and primum movens of shock

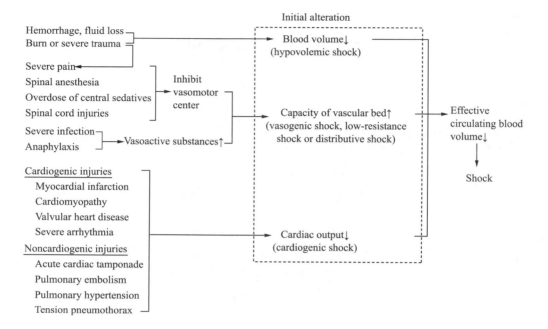

## 2. Mechanisms of microcirculatory disturbances at different stages of shock

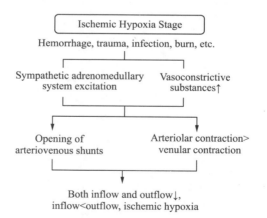

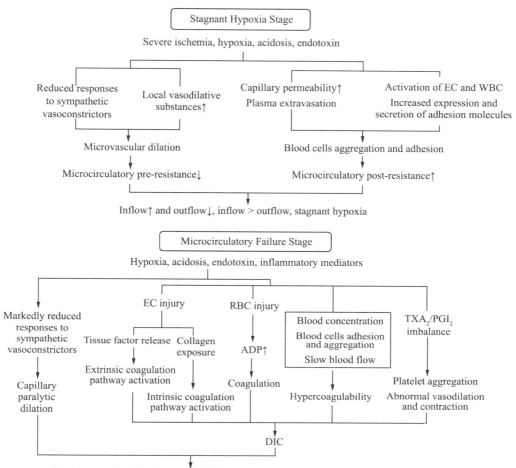

( ADP: adenosine diphosphate; DIC: disseminated intravascular coagulation; EC: endothelial cell; PGI$_2$: prostaglandin I$_2$; RBC: red blood cells; TXA$_2$: thromboxane A$_2$; WBC: white blood cells )

## 3. The influence of microcirculatory disturbance at different stages of shock

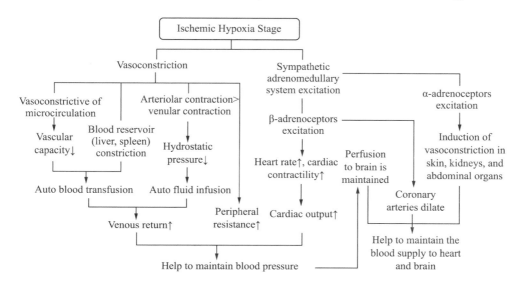

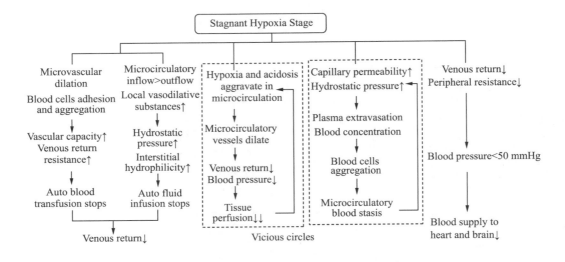

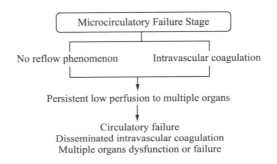

（赵丽梅）

# Chapter 8　Disturbances of Hemostasis

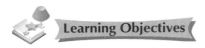 **Learning Objectives**

（1）To master the basic concept, pathogenesis, function and metabolic changes of disseminated intravascular coagulation（DIC）.

（2）To be familiar with the common causes of DIC and the factors affecting the occurrence and development of DIC.

（3）To be familiar with the functions of coagulation, anticoagulation and fibrinolysis systems and the causes of their imbalance.

（4）To understand the classification and staging of DIC and the pathophysiological basis of DIC prevention and treatment.

**Mind Map**

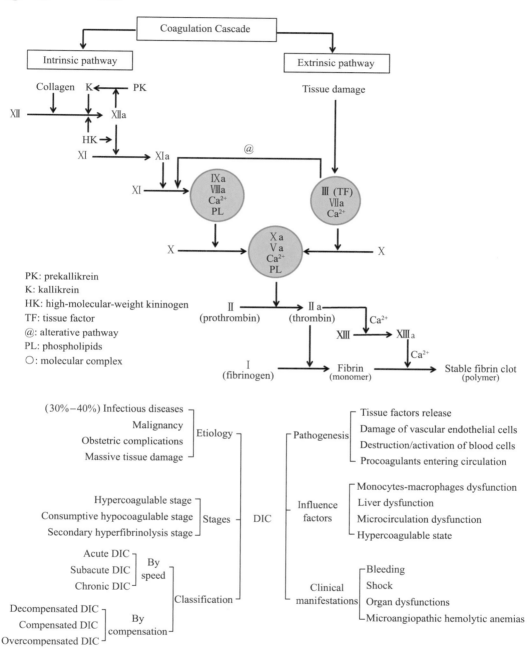

PK: prekallikrein
K: kallikrein
HK: high-molecular-weight kininogen
TF: tissue factor
@: alterative pathway
PL: phospholipids
○: molecular complex

（刘立民　赵丽梅）

# Chapter 9    Ischemia-reperfusion Injury

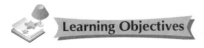 **Learning Objectives**

（1）To master the concept and pathogenesis of ischemia-reperfusion injury.

（2）To be familiar with the causes and involved factors of ischemia-reperfusion injury.

（3）To be familiar with the functional and metabolic changes of various organs with ischemia-reperfusion injury.

（4）To understand the pathophysiological basis of prevention and treatment for ischemia-reperfusion injury.

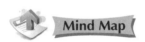 **Mind Map**

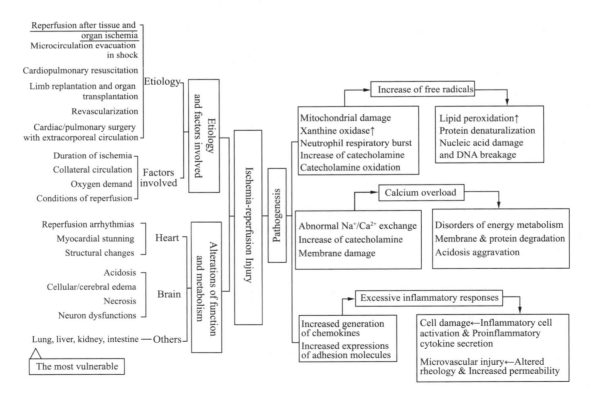

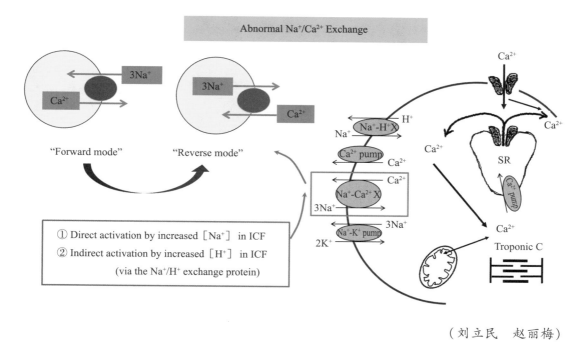

Abnormal Na⁺/Ca²⁺ Exchange

"Forward mode"　"Reverse mode"

① Direct activation by increased $[Na^+]$ in ICF
② Indirect activation by increased $[H^+]$ in ICF
　　(via the $Na^+/H^+$ exchange protein)

（刘立民　赵丽梅）

# Chapter 10　Cardiac Insufficiency

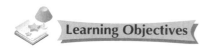 **Learning Objectives**

（1）To master the concepts of cardiac insufficiency and heart failure.

（2）To master compensatory responses to cardiac insufficiency and the pathogenesis of cardiac insufficiency.

（3）To master the mechanisms underlying the manifestations of cardiac insufficiency.

（4）To be familiar with the etiology, precipitating factors and classification of cardiac insufficiency.

（5）To be familiar with the neurohumoral mechanisms underlying compensatory responses to cardiac insufficiency.

（6）To understand the pathophysiological basis of prevention and treatment for cardiac insufficiency.

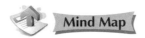

# 1. Causes of cardiac insufficiency

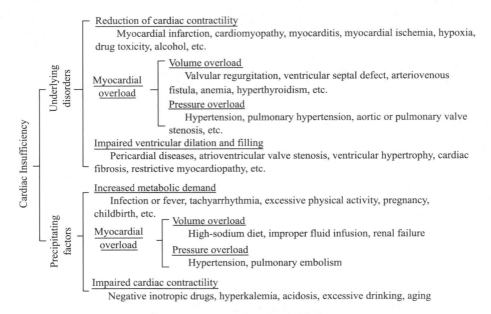

# 2. Compensatory responses to cardiac insufficiency

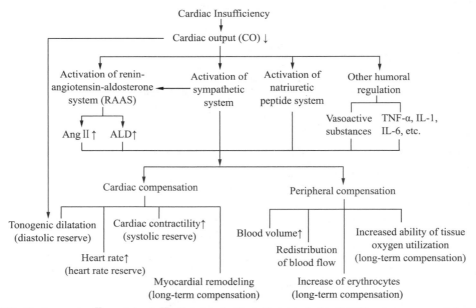

(ALD: aldosterone; Ang II: angiotensin II; IL-1: interleukin-1; IL-6: interleukin-6; TNF-α: tumour necrosis factor-α)

Beneficial effects: CO↑, BP and blood perfusion to vital organs maintained, oxygen supply and ultilizing to tissues↑.
Adverse effects: cardiac workloads↑, myocardial oxygen consumption↑, coronary perfusion↓, ventricular filling↓, arrhythmia, peripheral tissues and organs ischemia, cardiac function decompensates eventually.

## 3. Mechanisms of cardiac insufficiency

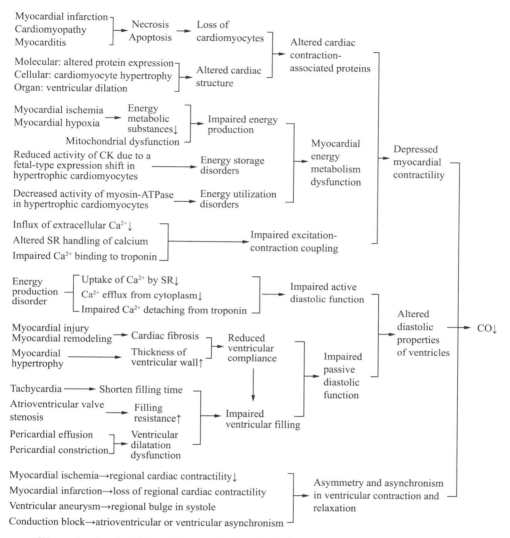

(CK: creatine phosphate kinase; SR: sarcoplasmic reticulum)

## 4. Mechanisms underlying manifestations in cardiac insufficiency

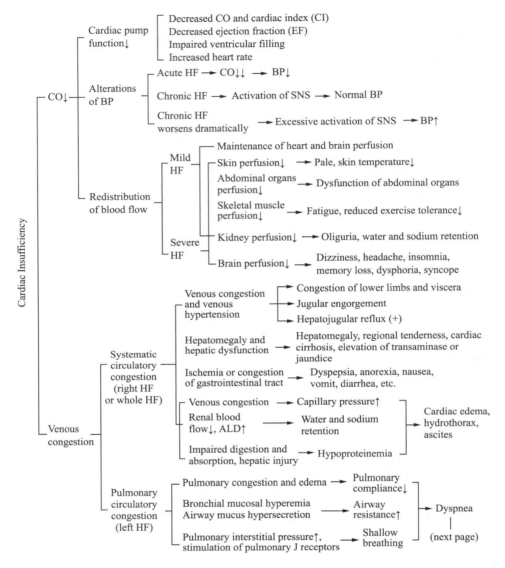

(HF: heart failure)

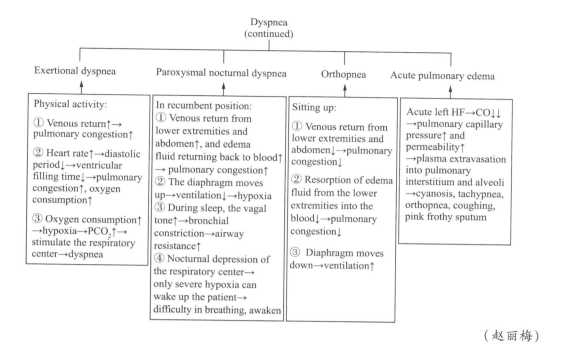

Dyspnea
(continued)

**Exertional dyspnea**

Physical activity:

① Venous return↑→pulmonary congestion↑

② Heart rate↑→diastolic period↓→ventricular filling time↓→pulmonary congestion↑, oxygen consumption↑

③ Oxygen consumption↑→hypoxia→$PCO_2$↑→stimulate the respiratory center→dyspnea

**Paroxysmal nocturnal dyspnea**

In recumbent position:

① Venous return from lower extremities and abdomen↑, and edema fluid returning back to blood↑→ pulmonary congestion↑

② The diaphragm moves up→ventilation↓→hypoxia

③ During sleep, the vagal tone↑→bronchial constriction→airway resistance↑

④ Nocturnal depression of the respiratory center→only severe hypoxia can wake up the patient→difficulty in breathing, awaken

**Orthopnea**

Sitting up:

① Venous return from lower extremities and abdomen↓→pulmonary congestion↓

② Resorption of edema fluid from the lower extremities into the blood↓→pulmonary congestion↓

③ Diaphragm moves down→ventilation↑

**Acute pulmonary edema**

Acute left HF→CO↓↓→pulmonary capillary pressure↑ and permeability↑→plasma extravasation into pulmonary interstitium and alveoli→cyanosis, tachypnea, orthopnea, coughing, pink frothy sputum

（赵丽梅）

# Chapter 11   Pulmonary Insufficiency

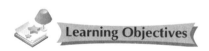

**Learning Objectives**

（1）To master the concept, etiology, pathogenesis as well as functional and metabolic changes of respiratory failure.

（2）To be familiar with the changes of blood oxygen parameters in respiratory failure.

（3）To be familiar with the concept, etiology and pathogenesis of acute respiratory distress syndrome（ARDS）.

（4）To be familiar with the concept, etiology and pathogenesis of chronic obstructive pulmonary disease（COPD）.

（5）To understand the pathophysiological basis for prevention and treatment of respiratory failure.

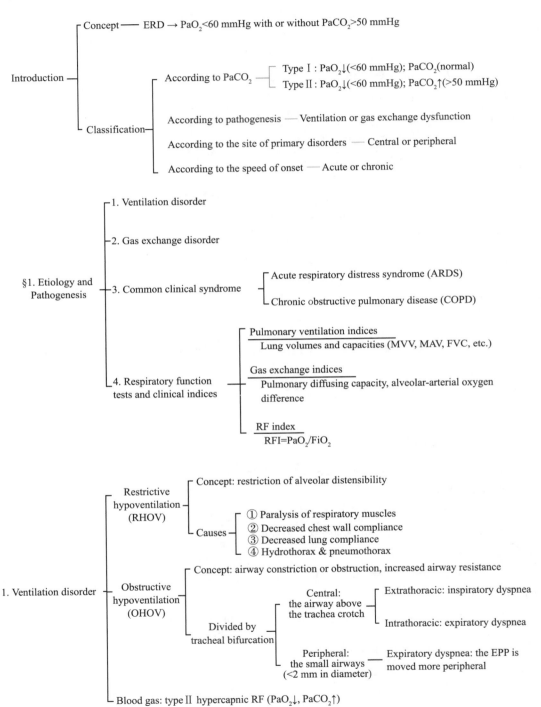

**Mind Map**

Introduction
- Concept —— ERD → $PaO_2$<60 mmHg with or without $PaCO_2$>50 mmHg
- Classification
  - According to $PaCO_2$
    - Type I: $PaO_2$↓(<60 mmHg); $PaCO_2$(normal)
    - Type II: $PaO_2$↓(<60 mmHg); $PaCO_2$↑(>50 mmHg)
  - According to pathogenesis —— Ventilation or gas exchange dysfunction
  - According to the site of primary disorders —— Central or peripheral
  - According to the speed of onset —— Acute or chronic

§1. Etiology and Pathogenesis
- 1. Ventilation disorder
- 2. Gas exchange disorder
- 3. Common clinical syndrome
  - Acute respiratory distress syndrome (ARDS)
  - Chronic obstructive pulmonary disease (COPD)
- 4. Respiratory function tests and clinical indices
  - Pulmonary ventilation indices
    Lung volumes and capacities (MVV, MAV, FVC, etc.)
  - Gas exchange indices
    Pulmonary diffusing capacity, alveolar-arterial oxygen difference
  - RF index
    $RFI=PaO_2/FiO_2$

1. Ventilation disorder
- Restrictive hypoventilation (RHOV)
  - Concept: restriction of alveolar distensibility
  - Causes
    - ① Paralysis of respiratory muscles
    - ② Decreased chest wall compliance
    - ③ Decreased lung compliance
    - ④ Hydrothorax & pneumothorax
- Obstructive hypoventilation (OHOV)
  - Concept: airway constriction or obstruction, increased airway resistance
  - Divided by tracheal bifurcation
    - Central: the airway above the trachea crotch
      - Extrathoracic: inspiratory dyspnea
      - Intrathoracic: expiratory dyspnea
    - Peripheral: the small airways (<2 mm in diameter)
      - Expiratory dyspnea: the EPP is moved more peripheral
- Blood gas: type II hypercapnic RF ($PaO_2$↓, $PaCO_2$↑)

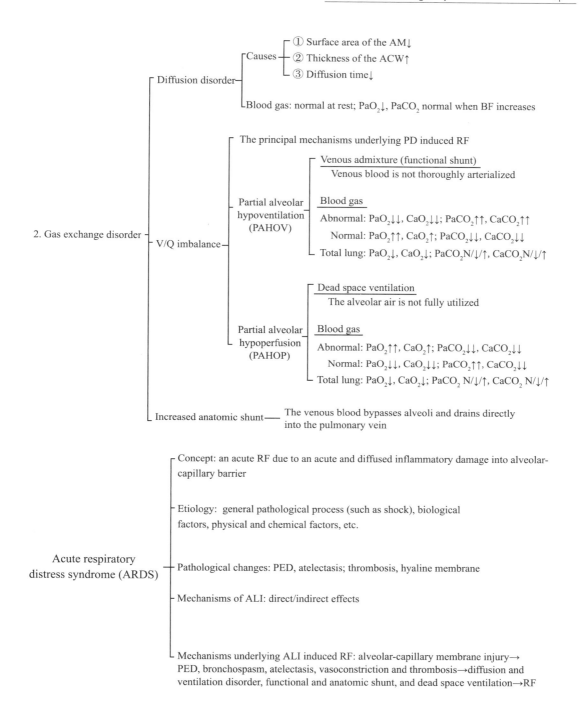

Diffusion disorder
  Causes
    ① Surface area of the AM↓
    ② Thickness of the ACW↑
    ③ Diffusion time↓
  Blood gas: normal at rest; $PaO_2$↓, $PaCO_2$ normal when BF increases

2. Gas exchange disorder

V/Q imbalance
  The principal mechanisms underlying PD induced RF

  Partial alveolar hypoventilation (PAHOV)
    Venous admixture (functional shunt)
      Venous blood is not thoroughly arterialized
    Blood gas
      Abnormal: $PaO_2$↓↓, $CaO_2$↓↓; $PaCO_2$↑↑, $CaCO_2$↑↑
      Normal: $PaO_2$↑↑, $CaO_2$↑; $PaCO_2$↓↓, $CaCO_2$↓↓
      Total lung: $PaO_2$↓, $CaO_2$↓; $PaCO_2$N/↓/↑, $CaCO_2$N/↓/↑

  Partial alveolar hypoperfusion (PAHOP)
    Dead space ventilation
      The alveolar air is not fully utilized
    Blood gas
      Abnormal: $PaO_2$↑↑, $CaO_2$↑; $PaCO_2$↓↓, $CaCO_2$↓↓
      Normal: $PaO_2$↓↓, $CaO_2$↓↓; $PaCO_2$↑↑, $CaCO_2$↓↓
      Total lung: $PaO_2$↓, $CaO_2$↓; $PaCO_2$ N/↓/↑, $CaCO_2$ N/↓/↑

Increased anatomic shunt
  The venous blood bypasses alveoli and drains directly into the pulmonary vein

Acute respiratory distress syndrome (ARDS)

  Concept: an acute RF due to an acute and diffused inflammatory damage into alveolar-capillary barrier

  Etiology: general pathological process (such as shock), biological factors, physical and chemical factors, etc.

  Pathological changes: PED, atelectasis; thrombosis, hyaline membrane

  Mechanisms of ALI: direct/indirect effects

  Mechanisms underlying ALI induced RF: alveolar-capillary membrane injury→PED, bronchospasm, atelectasis, vasoconstriction and thrombosis→diffusion and ventilation disorder, functional and anatomic shunt, and dead space ventilation→RF

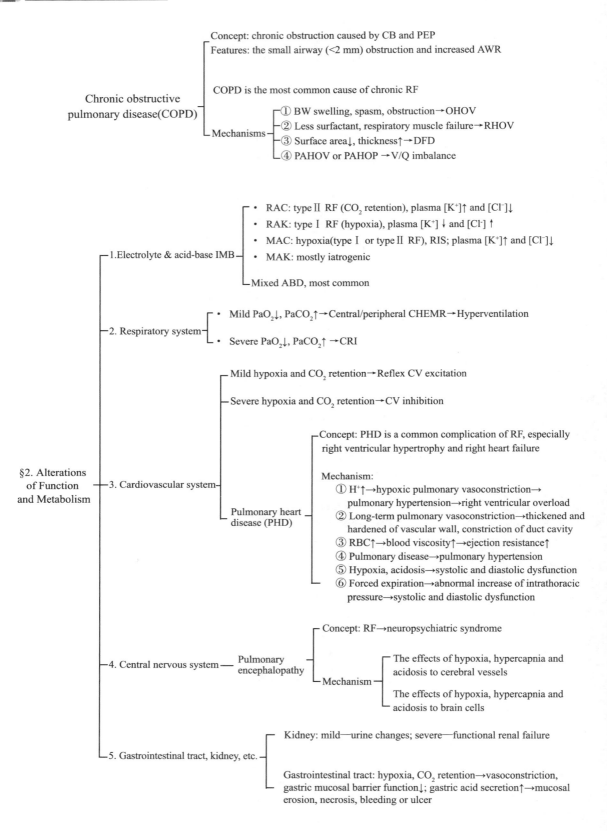

Chronic obstructive pulmonary disease(COPD)
- Concept: chronic obstruction caused by CB and PEP
- Features: the small airway (<2 mm) obstruction and increased AWR
- COPD is the most common cause of chronic RF
- Mechanisms
  - ① BW swelling, spasm, obstruction→OHOV
  - ② Less surfactant, respiratory muscle failure→RHOV
  - ③ Surface area↓, thickness↑→DFD
  - ④ PAHOV or PAHOP →V/Q imbalance

§2. Alterations of Function and Metabolism

1. Electrolyte & acid-base IMB
   - RAC: type II RF (CO$_2$ retention), plasma [K$^+$]↑ and [Cl$^-$]↓
   - RAK: type I RF (hypoxia), plasma [K$^+$]↓ and [Cl$^-$]↑
   - MAC: hypoxia(type I or type II RF), RIS; plasma [K$^+$]↑ and [Cl$^-$]↓
   - MAK: mostly iatrogenic
   - Mixed ABD, most common

2. Respiratory system
   - Mild PaO$_2$↓, PaCO$_2$↑→Central/peripheral CHEMR→Hyperventilation
   - Severe PaO$_2$↓, PaCO$_2$↑→CRI

3. Cardiovascular system
   - Mild hypoxia and CO$_2$ retention→Reflex CV excitation
   - Severe hypoxia and CO$_2$ retention→CV inhibition
   - Pulmonary heart disease (PHD)
     - Concept: PHD is a common complication of RF, especially right ventricular hypertrophy and right heart failure
     - Mechanism:
       - ① H$^+$↑→hypoxic pulmonary vasoconstriction→pulmonary hypertension→right ventricular overload
       - ② Long-term pulmonary vasoconstriction→thickened and hardened of vascular wall, constriction of duct cavity
       - ③ RBC↑→blood viscosity↑→ejection resistance↑
       - ④ Pulmonary disease→pulmonary hypertension
       - ⑤ Hypoxia, acidosis→systolic and diastolic dysfunction
       - ⑥ Forced expiration→abnormal increase of intrathoracic pressure→systolic and diastolic dysfunction

4. Central nervous system — Pulmonary encephalopathy
   - Concept: RF→neuropsychiatric syndrome
   - Mechanism
     - The effects of hypoxia, hypercapnia and acidosis to cerebral vessels
     - The effects of hypoxia, hypercapnia and acidosis to brain cells

5. Gastrointestinal tract, kidney, etc.
   - Kidney: mild—urine changes; severe—functional renal failure
   - Gastrointestinal tract: hypoxia, CO$_2$ retention→vasoconstriction, gastric mucosal barrier function↓; gastric acid secretion↑→mucosal erosion, necrosis, bleeding or ulcer

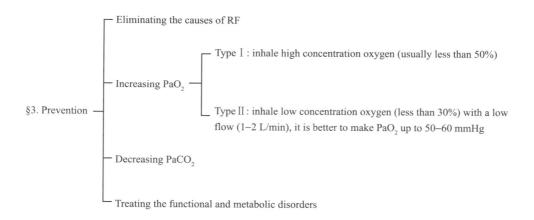

§3. Prevention
- Eliminating the causes of RF
- Increasing $PaO_2$
  - Type I : inhale high concentration oxygen (usually less than 50%)
  - Type II : inhale low concentration oxygen (less than 30%) with a low flow (1–2 L/min), it is better to make $PaO_2$ up to 50–60 mmHg
- Decreasing $PaCO_2$
- Treating the functional and metabolic disorders

(ABD: acid-base disturbances; ACW: alveolar capillary wall; AM: alveolar membrane; AWR: airway resistance; BW: bronchial wall; CB: chronic bronchitis; CHEMR: chemoreceptor; CRI: central respiratory inhibition; CV: cardiovascular; DFD: diffusion disorder; EPP: equal pressure point; ERD: external respiratory dysfunction; FVC: forced vital capacity; IMB: imbalance; MAC: metabolic acidosis; MAK: metabolic alkalosis; MAV: minute alveolar ventilation; MVV: minute ventilation volume; PD: pulmonary diseases; PED: pulmonary edema; PEP: pulmonary emphysema; RAC: respiratory acidosis; RAK: respiratory alkalosis; RF: respiratory failure; RIS: renal insufficiency)

(孙晓东　孙丽娜)

# Chapter 12　Hepatic Insufficiency

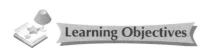

（1）To master the concept as well as functional and metabolic alterations of hepatic insufficiency.

（2）To master the concept, pathogenesis and precipitating factors of hepatic encephalopathy.

（3）To be familiar with the etiology and classification of hepatic insufficiency.

（4）To be familiar with the stages and clinical manifestations of hepatic encephalopathy.

（5）To be familar with the concept, etiology and pathogenesis of hepatorenal syndrome.

（6）To understand the principles of prevention and treatment for hepatic insufficiency.

Mind Map

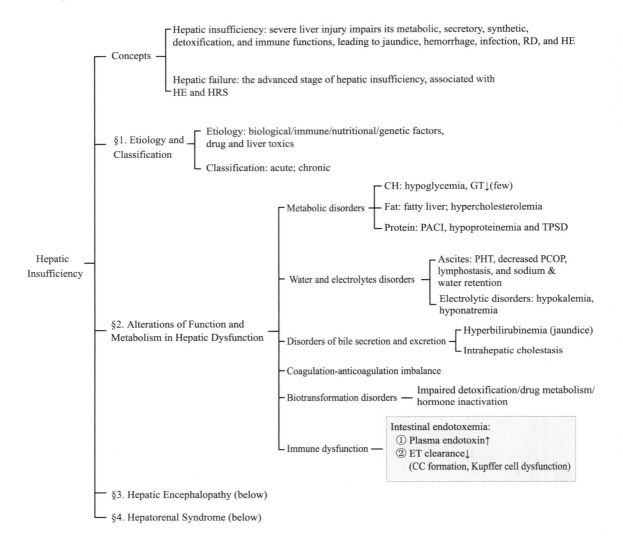

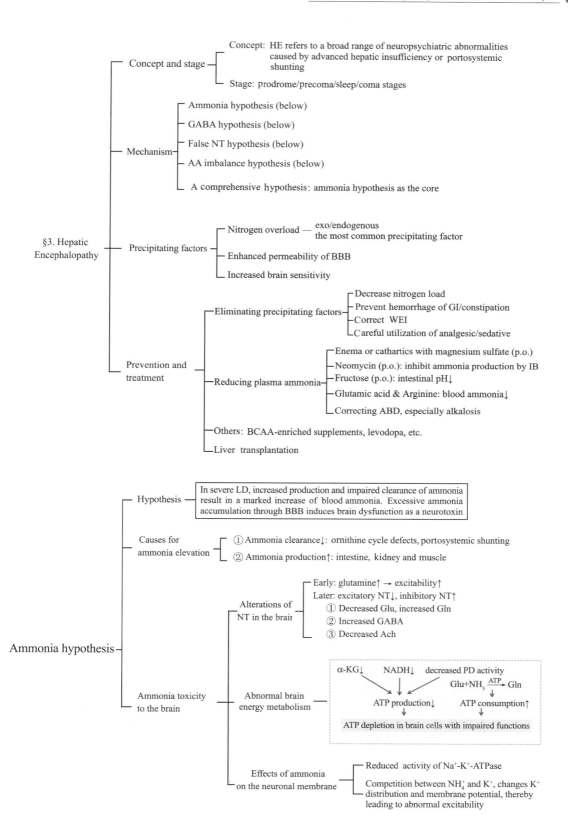

§3. Hepatic Encephalopathy

Concept and stage
- Concept: HE refers to a broad range of neuropsychiatric abnormalities caused by advanced hepatic insufficiency or portosystemic shunting
- Stage: prodrome/precoma/sleep/coma stages

Mechanism
- Ammonia hypothesis (below)
- GABA hypothesis (below)
- False NT hypothesis (below)
- AA imbalance hypothesis (below)
- A comprehensive hypothesis: ammonia hypothesis as the core

Precipitating factors
- Nitrogen overload — exo/endogenous the most common precipitating factor
- Enhanced permeability of BBB
- Increased brain sensitivity

Prevention and treatment
- Eliminating precipitating factors
  - Decrease nitrogen load
  - Prevent hemorrhage of GI/constipation
  - Correct WEI
  - Careful utilization of analgesic/sedative
- Reducing plasma ammonia
  - Enema or cathartics with magnesium sulfate (p.o.)
  - Neomycin (p.o.): inhibit ammonia production by IB
  - Fructose (p.o.): intestinal pH↓
  - Glutamic acid & Arginine: blood ammonia↓
  - Correcting ABD, especially alkalosis
- Others: BCAA-enriched supplements, levodopa, etc.
- Liver transplantation

Ammonia hypothesis

Hypothesis
- In severe LD, increased production and impaired clearance of ammonia result in a marked increase of blood ammonia. Excessive ammonia accumulation through BBB induces brain dysfunction as a neurotoxin

Causes for ammonia elevation
- ① Ammonia clearance↓: ornithine cycle defects, portosystemic shunting
- ② Ammonia production↑: intestine, kidney and muscle

Ammonia toxicity to the brain
- Alterations of NT in the brain
  - Early: glutamine↑ → excitability↑
  - Later: excitatory NT↓, inhibitory NT↑
    - ① Decreased Glu, increased Gln
    - ② Increased GABA
    - ③ Decreased Ach
- Abnormal brain energy metabolism

  $\alpha$-KG↓    NADH↓    decreased PD activity

  $Glu + NH_3 \xrightarrow{ATP} Gln$

  ATP production↓    ATP consumption↑

  ATP depletion in brain cells with impaired functions

- Effects of ammonia on the neuronal membrane
  - Reduced activity of $Na^+$-$K^+$-ATPase
  - Competition between $NH_4^+$ and $K^+$, changes $K^+$ distribution and membrane potential, thereby leading to abnormal excitability

GABA hypothesis

— GABA is the major inhibitory NT in the brain

Postsynaptic inhibition (POSSI)
    After presynaptic excitation, GABA, released from the vesicles, binds to the GABA receptor on postsynaptic neurons, resulting in a hyperpolarization by increasing its membrane permeability to Cl⁻ and Cl⁻ influx

Presynaptic inhibition (PRESI)
    When GABA acts on presynaptic terminals, it increases membrane permeability to Cl⁻ and results in the outflow of Cl⁻ and a depolarization, thereby reducing the release of NT when the nerve impulse reaches the end of axon

During HE, GABA inhibition is enhanced
    The plasma levels of GABA are increased
    Postsynaptic GABA-A receptor activity↑, enhanced binding capacity

False NT hypothesis

The neural basis of consciousness
    Structural: ascending reticular activating system
    Material: NT like DA and NE

False NT（FNT）
    Phenylethanolamine and octopamine, which are similar in chemical structure to true NT, manifest weak actions on the ascending reticular activating system

Reasons for the increase of false NT in HF
    Normally, amines transported to the liver via the portal vein can be oxidatively decomposed by monoamine oxidase
    During HF: food spoilage↑→PEA & TYR↑, hepatic detoxification↓; portosystemic shunting→ PEA and TA bypass the liver and directly enter the brain to generate PETA and OA, respectively by β-hydroxylase

Effects of false NT

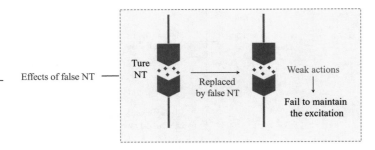

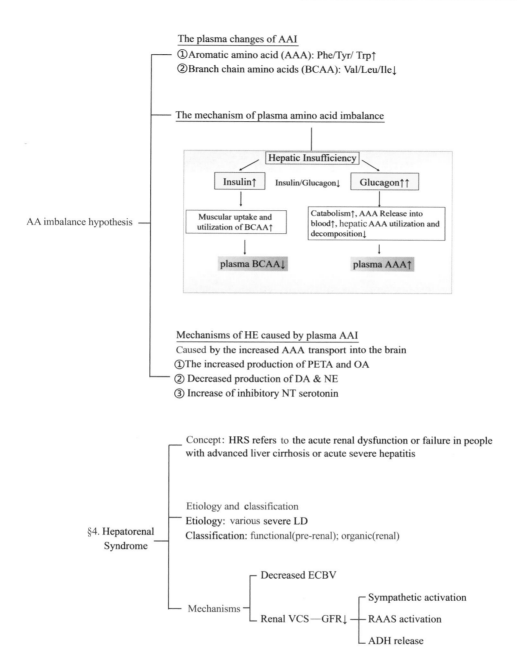

The plasma changes of AAI
①Aromatic amino acid (AAA): Phe/Tyr/ Trp↑
②Branch chain amino acids (BCAA): Val/Leu/Ile↓

The mechanism of plasma amino acid imbalance

Hepatic Insufficiency

Insulin↑　　Insulin/Glucagon↓　　Glucagon↑↑

Muscular uptake and utilization of BCAA↑

Catabolism↑, AAA Release into blood↑, hepatic AAA utilization and decomposition↓

plasma BCAA↓　　　plasma AAA↑

AA imbalance hypothesis

Mechanisms of HE caused by plasma AAI
Caused by the increased AAA transport into the brain
①The increased production of PETA and OA
② Decreased production of DA & NE
③ Increase of inhibitory NT serotonin

§4. Hepatorenal Syndrome

Concept: HRS refers to the acute renal dysfunction or failure in people with advanced liver cirrhosis or acute severe hepatitis

Etiology and classification
Etiology: various severe LD
Classification: functional(pre-renal); organic(renal)

Mechanisms —
Decreased ECBV
Renal VCS—GFR↓ —
Sympathetic activation
RAAS activation
ADH release

（AA：amino acid；AAI：amino acid imbalance；ABD：acid-base disturbance；Ach：acetylcholine；BBB：blood brain barrier；BCAA：branched chain amino acid；CC：collateral circulation；CH：carbohydrate；DA：dopamine；DM：drug metabolism；ECBV：effective circulating blood volume；ET：endotoxin；GABA：gamma aminobutyric acid；GI：gastrointestinal；Gln：glutamine；Glu：glutamate；GT：glucose tolerance；HE：hepatic encephalopathy；HF：hepatic failure；HIA：hormone inactivation；HRS：hepatorenal syndrome；IB：intestinal bacteria；Ile：isoleucine；LD：liver disorders；Leu：leucine；α-KG：α-ketoglutarate；NE：norepinephrine；NT：neurotransmitter；OA：octopamine；PACI：plasma amino acid imbalance；PCOP：plasma colloidal osmotic pressure；PD：pyruvate decarboxylase；PEA：phenylethylamine；PETA：phenylethanolamine；Phe：

phenylalanine；PHT：portal hypertension；RD：renal dysfunction；TA：tyramine；TPSD：transport protein synthesis dysfunction；Trp：tryptophan；Tyr：tyrosine；WEI：water and electrolyte imbalance；Val：valine；VCS：vasoconstriction）

（孙晓东　孙丽娜）

# Chapter 13　Renal Insufficiency

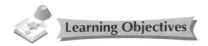

**Learning Objectives**

（1）To master the concept，classification，etiology，pathogenesis，disease course as well as functional and metabolic alterations of acute renal failure.

（2）To master the concept，etiology，pathogenesis as well as functional and metabolic alterations of chronic renal failure.

（3）To be familiar with the basic pathological process of renal insufficiency，the disease course and stages of chronic renal insufficiency，as well as the concept and toxins of uremia.

（4）To understand the principles for the prevention and treatment of acute and chronic renal insufficiency.

（5）To understand the functional and metabolic alternations as well as the principles for the prevention and treatment of uremia.

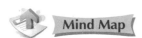

**Mind Map**

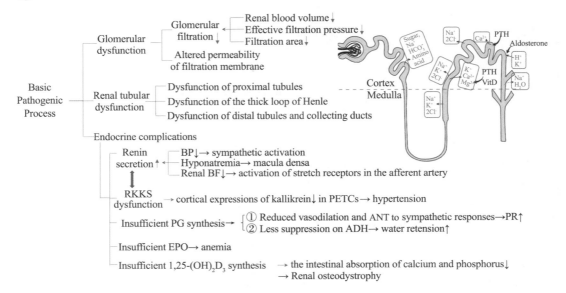

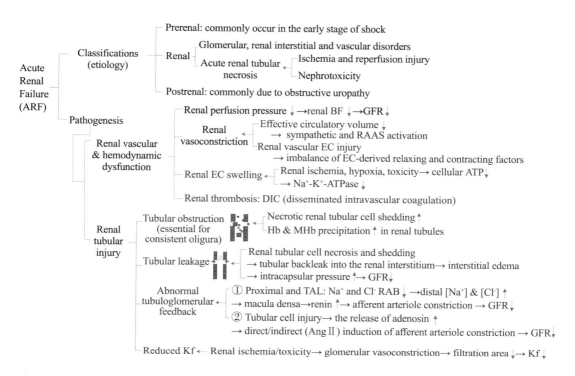

Acute Renal Failure (ARF)

- Classifications (etiology)
  - Prerenal: commonly occur in the early stage of shock
  - Renal
    - Glomerular, renal interstitial and vascular disorders
    - Acute renal tubular necrosis
      - Ischemia and reperfusion injury
      - Nephrotoxicity
  - Postrenal: commonly due to obstructive uropathy
- Pathogenesis
  - Renal vascular & hemodynamic dysfunction
    - Renal perfusion pressure ↓ →renal BF ↓→GFR↓
    - Renal vasoconstriction
      - Effective circulatory volume ↓ → sympathetic and RAAS activation
      - Renal vascular EC injury → imbalance of EC-derived relaxing and contracting factors
    - Renal EC swelling ← Renal ischemia, hypoxia, toxicity→ cellular ATP↓ → Na⁺-K⁺-ATPase ↓
    - Renal thrombosis: DIC (disseminated intravascular coagulation)
  - Renal tubular injury
    - Tubular obstruction (essential for consistent oligura)
      - Necrotic renal tubular cell shedding ↑
      - Hb & MHb precipitation ↑ in renal tubules
    - Tubular leakage ←
      - Renal tubular cell necrosis and shedding → tubular backleak into the renal interstitium→ interstitial edema → intracapsular pressure ↑→ GFR↓
    - Abnormal tubuloglomerular feedback ←
      - ① Proximal and TAL: Na⁺ and Cl⁻ RAB ↓ →distal [Na⁺] & [Cl⁻] ↑ → macula densa→renin ↑→ afferent arteriole constriction → GFR↓
      - ② Tubular cell injury→ the release of adenosin ↑ → direct/indirect (Ang Ⅱ) induction of afferent arteriole constriction → GFR↓
    - Reduced Kf ← Renal ischemia/toxicity→ glomerular vasoconstriction→ filtration area ↓→ Kf ↓

$Na^+$-$K^+$-ATPase

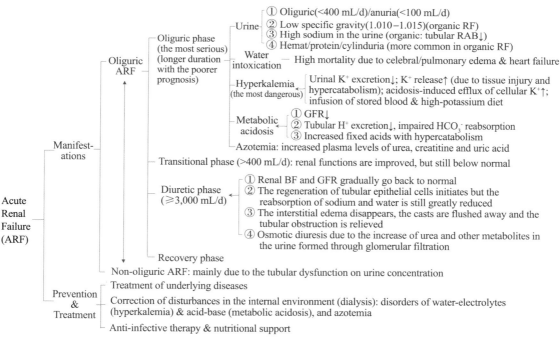

Acute Renal Failure (ARF)

- Manifestations
  - Oliguric ARF
    - Oliguric phase (the most serious) (longer duration with the poorer prognosis)
      - Urine
        - ① Oliguric(<400 mL/d)/anuria(<100 mL/d)
        - ② Low specific gravity(1.010–1.015)(organic RF)
        - ③ High sodium in the urine (organic: tubular RAB↓)
        - ④ Hemat/protein/cylinduria (more common in organic RF)
      - Water intoxication — High mortality due to celebral/pulmonary edema & heart failure
      - Hyperkalemia (the most dangerous) ← Urinal K⁺ excretion↓; K⁺ release↑ (due to tissue injury and hypercatabolism); acidosis-induced efflux of cellular K⁺↑; infusion of stored blood & high-potassium diet
      - Metabolic acidosis
        - ① GFR↓
        - ② Tubular H⁺ excretion↓, impaired HCO₃⁻ reabsorption
        - ③ Increased fixed acids with hypercatabolism
      - Azotemia: increased plasma levels of urea, creatitine and uric acid
    - Transitional phase (>400 mL/d): renal functions are improved, but still below normal
    - Diuretic phase (≥3,000 mL/d) ←
      - ① Renal BF and GFR gradually go back to normal
      - ② The regeneration of tubular epithelial cells initiates but the reabsorption of sodium and water is still greatly reduced
      - ③ The interstitial edema disappears, the casts are flushed away and the tubular obstruction is relieved
      - ④ Osmotic diuresis due to the increase of urea and other metabolites in the urine formed through glomerular filtration
    - Recovery phase
  - Non-oliguric ARF: mainly due to the tubular dysfunction on urine concentration
- Prevention & Treatment
  - Treatment of underlying diseases
  - Correction of disturbances in the internal environment (dialysis): disorders of water-electrolytes (hyperkalemia) & acid-base (metabolic acidosis), and azotemia
  - Anti-infective therapy & nutritional support

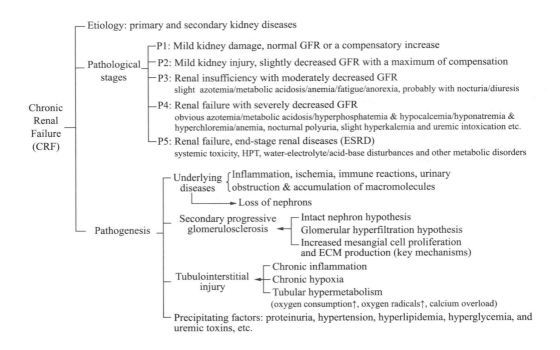

Chronic Renal Failure (CRF)
— Etiology: primary and secondary kidney diseases
— Pathological stages
  — P1: Mild kidney damage, normal GFR or a compensatory increase
  — P2: Mild kidney injury, slightly decreased GFR with a maximum of compensation
  — P3: Renal insufficiency with moderately decreased GFR
    slight azotemia/metabolic acidosis/anemia/fatigue/anorexia, probably with nocturia/diuresis
  — P4: Renal failure with severely decreased GFR
    obvious azotemia/metabolic acidosis/hyperphosphatemia & hypocalcemia/hyponatremia & hyperchloremia/anemia, nocturnal polyuria, slight hyperkalemia and uremic intoxication etc.
  — P5: Renal failure, end-stage renal diseases (ESRD)
    systemic toxicity, HPT, water-electrolyte/acid-base disturbances and other metabolic disorders
— Pathogenesis
  — Underlying diseases { Inflammation, ischemia, immune reactions, urinary obstruction & accumulation of macromolecules
    → Loss of nephrons
  — Secondary progressive glomerulosclerosis ← { Intact nephron hypothesis / Glomerular hyperfiltration hypothesis / Increased mesangial cell proliferation and ECM production (key mechanisms)
  — Tubulointerstitial injury ← { Chronic inflammation / Chronic hypoxia / Tubular hypermetabolism
    (oxygen consumption↑, oxygen radicals↑, calcium overload)
  — Precipitating factors: proteinuria, hypertension, hyperlipidemia, hyperglycemia, and uremic toxins, etc.

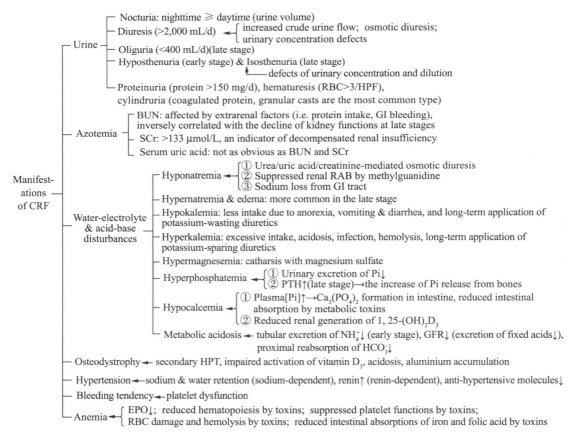

Manifestations of CRF
— Urine
  — Nocturia: nighttime ≥ daytime (urine volume)
  — Diuresis (>2,000 mL/d) ← { increased crude urine flow; osmotic diuresis; urinary concentration defects
  — Oliguria (<400 mL/d)(late stage)
  — Hyposthenuria (early stage) & Isosthenuria (late stage)
    ↑ — defects of urinary concentration and dilution
  — Proteinuria (protein >150 mg/d), hematuresis (RBC>3/HPF), cylindruria (coagulated protein, granular casts are the most common type)
— Azotemia
  — BUN: affected by extrarenal factors (i.e. protein intake, GI bleeding), inversely correlated with the decline of kidney functions at late stages
  — SCr: >133 μmol/L, an indicator of decompensated renal insufficiency
  — Serum uric acid: not as obvious as BUN and SCr
— Water-electrolyte & acid-base disturbances
  — Hyponatremia ← { ① Urea/uric acid/creatinine-mediated osmotic diuresis / ② Suppressed renal RAB by methylguanidine / ③ Sodium loss from GI tract
  — Hypernatremia & edema: more common in the late stage
  — Hypokalemia: less intake due to anorexia, vomiting & diarrhea, and long-term application of potassium-wasting diuretics
  — Hyperkalemia: excessive intake, acidosis, infection, hemolysis, long-term application of potassium-sparing diuretics
  — Hypermagnesemia: catharsis with magnesium sulfate
  — Hyperphosphatemia ← { ① Urinary excretion of Pi↓ / ② PTH↑(late stage)→the increase of Pi release from bones
  — Hypocalcemia ← { ① Plasma[Pi]↑→$Ca_3(PO_4)_2$ formation in intestine, reduced intestinal absorption by metabolic toxins / ② Reduced renal generation of 1, 25-$(OH)_2D_3$
  — Metabolic acidosis ← tubular excretion of $NH_4^+$↓ (early stage), GFR↓ (excretion of fixed acids↓), proximal reabsorption of $HCO_3^-$↓
— Osteodystrophy ← secondary HPT, impaired activation of vitamin $D_3$, acidosis, aluminium accumulation
— Hypertension ← sodium & water retention (sodium-dependent), renin↑ (renin-dependent), anti-hypertensive molecules↓
— Bleeding tendency ← platelet dysfunction
— Anemia ← { EPO↓; reduced hematopoiesis by toxins; suppressed platelet functions by toxins; RBC damage and hemolysis by toxins; reduced intestinal absorptions of iron and folic acid by toxins

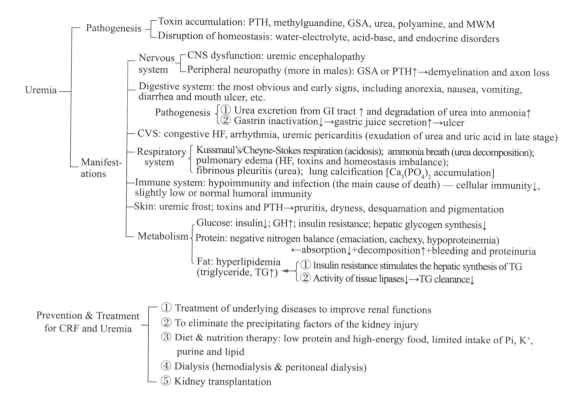

Uremia

Pathogenesis
- Toxin accumulation: PTH, methylguandine, GSA, urea, polyamine, and MWM
- Disruption of homeostasis: water-electrolyte, acid-base, and endocrine disorders

Manifestations
- Nervous system
  - CNS dysfunction: uremic encephalopathy
  - Peripheral neuropathy (more in males): GSA or PTH↑→demyelination and axon loss
- Digestive system: the most obvious and early signs, including anorexia, nausea, vomiting, diarrhea and mouth ulcer, etc.
  - Pathogenesis ① Urea excretion from GI tract ↑ and degradation of urea into anmonia↑
  - ② Gastrin inactivation↓→gastric juice secretion↑→ulcer
- CVS: congestive HF, arrhythmia, uremic pericarditis (exudation of urea and uric acid in late stage)
- Respiratory system: Kussmaul's/Cheyne-Stokes respiration (acidosis); ammonia breath (urea decomposition); pulmonary edema (HF, toxins and homeostasis imbalance); fibrinous pleuritis (urea); lung calcification [$Ca_3(PO_4)_2$ accumulation]
- Immune system: hypoimmunity and infection (the main cause of death) — cellular immunity↓, slightly low or normal humoral immunity
- Skin: uremic frost; toxins and PTH→pruritis, dryness, desquamation and pigmentation
- Metabolism
  - Glucose: insulin↓; GH↑; insulin resistance; hepatic glycogen synthesis↓
  - Protein: negative nitrogen balance (emaciation, cachexy, hypoproteinemia) ←absorption↓+decomposition↑+bleeding and proteinuria
  - Fat: hyperlipidemia (triglyceride, TG↑) ① Insulin resistance stimulates the hepatic synthesis of TG ② Activity of tissue lipases↓→TG clearance↓

Prevention & Treatment for CRF and Uremia
- ① Treatment of underlying diseases to improve renal functions
- ② To eliminate the precipitating factors of the kidney injury
- ③ Diet & nutrition therapy: low protein and high-energy food, limited intake of Pi, $K^+$, purine and lipid
- ④ Dialysis (hemodialysis & peritoneal dialysis)
- ⑤ Kidney transplantation

（ADH：antidiuretic；Ang Ⅱ：angiotensin Ⅱ；ANT：antagonism；BF：blood flow；BP：blood pressure；BUN：blood urea nitrogen；BV：blood volume；CNS：central nervous system；CVS：cardiovascular system；EC：endothelial cells；EPO：erythropoietin；GFR：glomerular filtration rate；GH：growth hormone；GI：gastrointestine；GSA：guanidinosuccinic acid；Hb：hemoglobin；HF：heart failure；HPF：high-power field；HPT：hyperparathyroidism；Kf：filtration coefficient；MHb：myohemoglobin；MVM：middle-weight molecules；$P_{1-5}$：Phase 1 – 5；PETCs：proximal tubular epithelial cells；PG：prostaglandin；Pi：inorganic phosphate；PR：peripheral resistance；PTH：parathyroid hormone；RAAS：renin-angiotensin-aldosterone system；RAB：reabsorption；RBC：red blood cell；RF：renal failure；RKKS：renal kallikrein-kinin system；SCr：serum creatinine；TAL：thick ascending limb）

（郑　栋　赵丽梅）

# Chapter 14　Brain Dysfunction

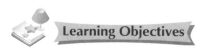

## Learning Objectives

（1）To master the concepts of brain dysfunction, cognitive and consciousness disorders.

（2）To master the pathogenesis of learning and memory impairment.

（3）To master the pathogenesis of consciousness disorders.

（4）To be familiar with the etiology, manifestations, and functional and metabolic alterations of cognitive disorders.

（5）To be familiar with the etiology, manifestations, functional and metabolic alterations of consciousness disorders.

（6）To understand the pathophysiological basis of prevention and treatment for cognitive and consciousness disorders.

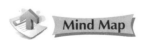

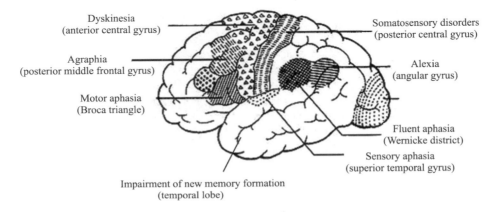

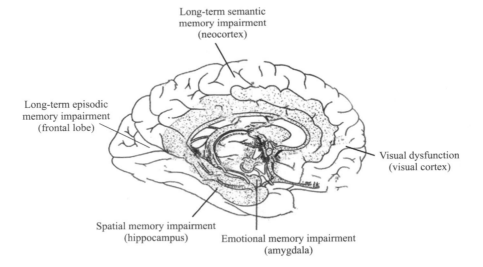

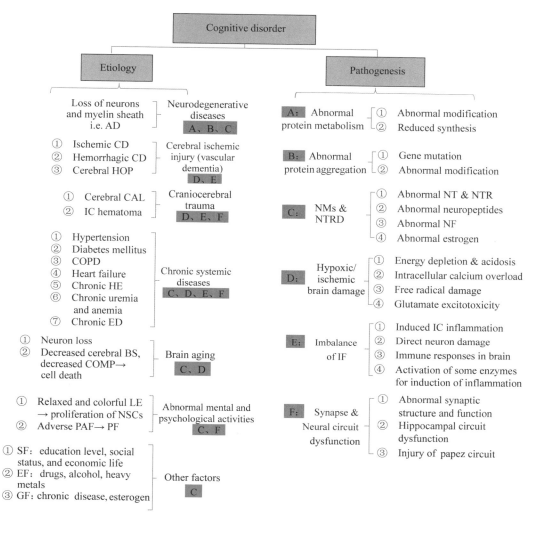

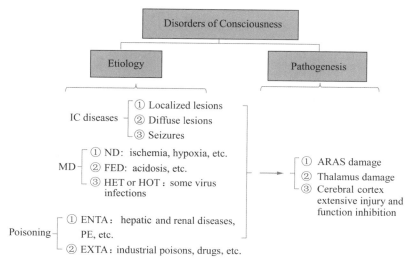

（AD：Alzheimer's disease；ARAS：ascending reticular activating system；BS：blood supply；CAL：contusion and laceration；CD：cerebrovascular disease；COMP：clearance of metabolites and poisons；COPD：chronic obstructive pulmonary disease；ED：electrolyte disorders；EF：environmental factors；ENTA：endogenous toxin accumulation；EXTA：exogenous toxin accumulation；FED：fluid and electrolyte disorders；GF：gender factors；HE：hepatic encephalopathy；HOP：hypoperfusion；HOT：hypothermia；HET：hyperthermia；IC：intracranial；IF：inflammatory factors；LE：living environment；MD：metabolic disorders；ND：nutrient deficiency；NF：neurotrophic factor；NMs：neuromodulators；NSCs：neural stem cells；NTRD：neurotransmitter receptor disorders；PAF：psychological and social factors；PE：pulmonary encephalopathy；PF：precipitating factor；SF：social factors）

（单立冬）

# Chapter 15　Multiple Organ Dysfunction Syndrome

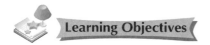
## Learning Objectives

（1）To master the concept and fundamental pathogenesis of multiple organ dysfunction syndrome（MODS）.

（2）To be familiar with the etiology, classification, as well as the functional and metabolic changes of MODS.

（3）To understand the pathophysiological basis of prevention and treatment for MODS.

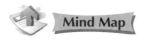
## Mind Map

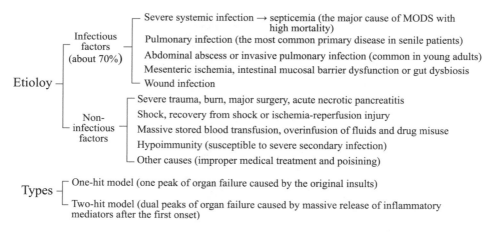

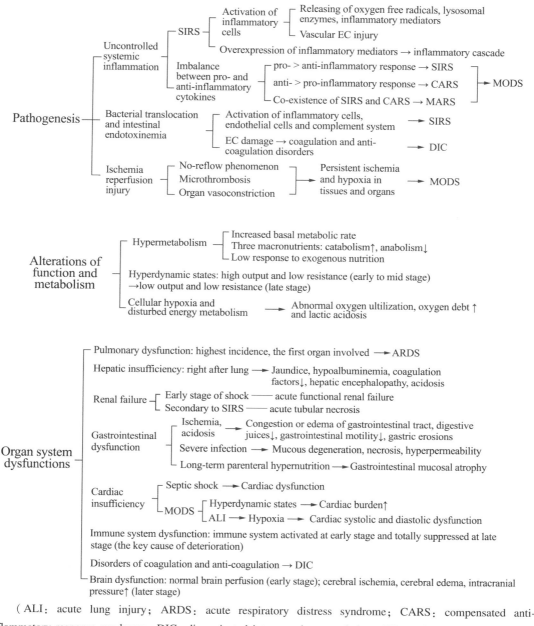

( ALI：acute lung injury；ARDS：acute respiratory distress syndrome；CARS：compensated anti-inflammatory response syndrome；DIC：disseminated intravascular coagulation；EC：endothelial cells；MARS：mixed antagonist response syndrome；MODS：multiple organ dysfunction syndrome；SIRS：systemic inflammatory response syndrome）

（赵丽梅）

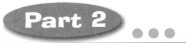

## Part 2

# Case Analysis

## Chapter 1   Introduction to Disease

### Case-based multiple choice questions (single answer)

**1. A 60-yr-old man was hospitalized due to pneumonia. He had a 40-year history of smoking.**

(1) Which of the following caused the development of pneumonia in this patient?

    A. Chemical agent/physical factors      B. Biological agents

    C. Nutrition imbalance      D. Congenital factors

    E. Genetic factors

(2) Which of the following is the predisposing factor for the development of pneumonia in this patient?

    A. Bacteria infection      B. Virus infection

    C. Smoking      D. Elevation of blood pressure

    E. Arrhythmias

(3) Which one of the following rules is involved in the development of pneumonia?

    A. Damage and anti-damage imbalance      B. Systemic and local interconnection

    C. Vicious circle      D. Interrelation

    E. Transformation

(4) Which one of the following aging changes does NOT affect the development of pneumonia?

    A. Declined functional reserve

    B. Declined homeostatic regulation

    C. Increased reaction time

    D. Declined adaptation to external environment

    E. Stable and lasting immunity

（5）Which of the following is the possible disease outcome in this patient?

    A.  Recovery

    B.  Health

    C.  Disease

    D.  Recovery/death

    E.  Death

**2. A 60-yr-old lady presented with obesity, hypertension, and hyperlipidemia. She had acute myocardial infarction several years ago and developed the chronic heart failure.**

（1）Which of the following caused the development of chronic heart failure in this patient?

    A.  Chemical agent/physical factors

    B.  Biological agents

    C.  Nutrition imbalance

    D.  Congenital factors

    E.  Genetic factors

（2）Which one of the following disorders is the cause of chronic heart failure in this patient?

    A.  Obesity

    B.  Hypertension

    C.  Myocardial infarction

    D.  Hyperlipidemia

    E.  Aging

（3）Which one of the following is NOT the role of obesity, hypertension, hyperlipidemia in the development of acute myocardial infarction?

    A.  Cause

    B.  Predisposing factor

    C.  Precipitating factor

    D.  Risk factor

    E.  Result

（4）What's the role of myocardial infarction in the development of chronic heart failure?

    A.  Cause

    B.  Predisposing factor

    C.  Precipitating factor

    D.  Common factor

    E.  Result

（5）Which one of the following mechanisms is NOT involved in the development of chronic heart failure?

    A.  Soft tissue dysfunction

    B.  Neural dysfunction

    C.  Humoral dysfunction

    D.  Cellular dysfunction

    E.  Molecular dysfunction

**3. A 35-yr-old lady who drinks and smokes regularly got pregnant accidently and delivered a baby girl with cleft lip.**

（1）Which of the following caused the development of cleft lip in the baby girl?

    A.  Social-psychological factors

    B.  Immunological factors

    C.  Nutrition imbalance

    D.  Congenital factors

    E.  Genetic factors

（2）Studies have shown that smoking (including secondhand one) doubled the risk of cleft lip. Thus, what is the role of smoking in cleft lip?

    A.  Cause

    B.  Predisposing factor

    C.  Precipitating factor

    D.  Risk factor

    E.  Result

（3）Animal studies have demonstrated that fibroblast growth factor and bone morphogenetic protein pathway might be involved in the development of cleft lip. Which one of the following mechanisms is revealed by these findings?

    A. Immunological dysfunction
    B. Neural dysfunction
    C. Humoral dysfunction
    D. Cellular dysfunction
    E. Molecular dysfunction

**4. A 15-yr-old girl had a bone marrow transplantation with haploidentical umbilical cord blood stem cells due to beta thalassemia and unfortunately died of graft rejection and infection one month later.**

（1）Which of the following caused the development of beta thalassemia in this girl?

    A. Social-psychological factors
    B. Immunological factors
    C. Nutrition imbalance
    D. Congenital factors
    E. Genetic factors

（2）Which one of the following rules is involved in the development of beta thalassemia?

    A. Damage and anti-damage imbalance
    B. Systemic and local interconnection
    C. Vicious cycle
    D. Homeostasis dysfunction
    E. Transformation

（3）Which of the following caused the development of graft rejection in this girl?

    A. Chemical agents/physical factors
    B. Biological agents
    C. Immunological factors
    D. Environmental-ecological factors
    E. Social-psychological factors

（4）Which one of the following rules is involved in the development of graft rejection and infection after bone marrow transplantation?

    A. Damage and anti-damage imbalance
    B. Systemic and local interconnection
    C. Causal alteration
    D. Transformation
    E. None of the above

**5. A mid-aged married lady was delivered to hospital due to severe burning. She had elevated WBC and high fever with local infection. Despite recovered, she changed a lot in temper with facial disfigurement and got depression after a divorce.**

（1）Which one of the following rules is involved in the development of high fever with local infection?

    A. Transformation
    B. Homeostasis dysfunction
    C. Systemic and local interconnection
    D. Causal alternation
    E. None of the above

（2）What's the role of divorce in the development of depression?

    A. Reason
    B. Result
    C. Causative factor
    D. Cause
    E. Precipitating factor

（3）What kind of factors caused the development of depression in this lady?

    A.　Social-psychological factors     B.　Immunological factors

    C.　Nutrition imbalance     D.　Congenital factors

    E.　Biological agent

**Answers**

**Case-based multiple choice questions（single answer）**

    **1.** BCAED；**2.** CCEAA；**3.** DDE；**4.** EDCC；**5.** CEA

（赵　颖）

# Chapter 2　Fluid and Electrolyte Imbalance

## ◇ Water and Sodium Imbalance

## Case-based multiple choice questions（single answer）

**1. A 2-yr-old boy had high fever, vomiting, and diarrhea due to rotavirus infection. He did not eat and only drank small amount of glucose water.**

（1）What kind of fluid imbalance is most likely to occur in this boy?

    A.　Hypertonic dehydration     B.　Hypotonic dehydration

    C.　Isotonic dehydration     D.　Water intoxication

    E.　Sodium intoxication

（2）Which one of the following fluid changes is likely to occur in this boy?

    A.　Decreased ICF     B.　Decreased ECF

    C.　No changes in plasma     D.　No changes in ICF

    E.　None of the above

（3）Which one of the following signs is crucial for diagnosis of fluid imbalance in this boy?

    A.　Facial flushing     B.　Shortness of breath

    C.　Thirst and oliguria     D.　Sunken eyes and poor skin turgor

    E.　Lower limb swelling

（4）Which one of the following dangerous diseases is most likely to occur in this boy?

    A.　Shock     B.　Heart failure

    C.　Renal failure     D.　Hepatic failure

    E.　Internal hemorrhage

（5）Which one of the following solutions should be chosen by a doctor to correct this potential fluid imbalance?

        A. 5% glucose solution         B. 2.5% glucose solution

        C. 0.9% NaCl solution         D. 0.5% NaCl solution

        E. Pure water

**2. A mid-aged healthy man works as a courier. He forgot to bring his water bottle and felt thirsty after sweating a lot in summer.**

（1）What kind of fluid imbalance is most likely to occur in this man?

        A. Hypertonic dehydration         B. Hypotonic dehydration

        C. Isotonic dehydration         D. Hyperkalemia

        E. Metabolic acidosis

（2）Which one of the following fluid changes is likely to occur in this man?

        A. Decreased ICF         B. Decreased ECF

        C. No changes in plasma         D. No changes in ICF

        E. None of the above

（3）Which one of the following signs is crucial for diagnosis of fluid imbalance in this man?

        A. Facial flushing         B. Shortness of breath

        C. Oliguria         D. Sunken eyes and poor skin turgor

        E. Lower limb swelling

（4）Which one of the following laboratory values is most likely to come from this man?

        A. Plasma $[Na^+]$ 160 mmol/L         B. Plasma $[K^+]$ 5.8 mmol/L

        C. HR 120 beats/min         D. BP 100/70 mmHg

        E. Undetectable urine sodium

（5）What should a doctor do to correct this potential fluid imbalance?

        A. Only give an infusion with 5% glucose solution

        B. Only give an infusion with 2.5% glucose solution

        C. Only give an infusion with 0.9% NaCl solution

        D. Only give an infusion with 0.5% NaCl solution

        E. Oral rehydration therapy with glucose, sodium, and potassium

**3. A 3.5-week-old boy had a clear sign of dehydration despite normal feeding. Based on the results of blood and urine analysis, he was diagnosed with renal tubular acidosis with hyperkalemia.**

（1）Which one of the following pathological conditions is NOT possible to occur in this baby?

        A. Metabolic acidosis         B. Hyperchloremia

        C. Hypotonic dehydration         D. Hypertonic dehydration

        E. Hyperkalemia

（2）Which one of the following laboratory values is NOT possible to come from this baby?

    A. [$Na^+$]151 mmol/L

    B. [$Na^+$]139 mmol/L

    C. [$Na^+$]130 mmol/L

    D. Osmotic pressure 295 mmol/L

    E. Osmotic pressure 285 mmol/L

（3）Which one of the following mechanisms may be involved in the development of dehydration in this baby?

    A. Insufficient intake

    B. Skin water loss

    C. Reduced water and sodium reabsorption in the distal convoluted tubule and collecting duct

    D. Reduced water and sodium reabsorption in the proximal convoluted tubule

    E. Altered fluid distribution *in vivo*

（4）Which one of the following molecules may decrease during the development of dehydration in the baby?

    A. Aldosterone

    B. Noradrenalin

    C. Renin

    D. Angiotensin

    E. ADH

**4. A 5-yr-old boy with nausea, vomiting, and fatigue was sent to hospital. 10 days ago, he had a respiratory tract infection. Urinalysis showed the presence of red blood cells and protein. He was diagnosed with acute glomerulonephritis.**

（1）If he has the edema, where may the edema develop first?

    A. Eyelids or face

    B. Upper limbs

    C. Lung

    D. Legs

    E. Abdomen

（2）If he has the edema, which one of the following changes is involved in the development of edema?

    A. Increased capillary hydrostatic pressure

    B. Increased capillary permeability

    C. Reduced lymphatic reflux

    D. Reduced plasma colloid osmotic pressure

    E. None of the above

（3）Which one of the following mechanisms is involved in the development of edema in this boy?

    A. Reduced renal blood flow

    B. Decreased glomerular filtration rate

    C. Increased water and sodium reabsorption in the proximal tubule

    D. Increased water and sodium reabsorption in the distal tubule

    E. All of the above

（4）If he has the edema, which one of the following statements is NOT correct?

    A. This edema fluid maybe a transduate   B. The boy may have a frank edema

C. The boy may have a pitting edema    D. Anasarca may develop in this boy

E. None of the above

**5. A mid-aged woman with progressive tremor and stupor was sent to hospital. She took antibiotics and analgesics, and drank a lot of water due to urinary tract infection. She vomited several times and showed slurred speech.**

(1) Which one of the following fluid imbalances may have occurred in this patient?

A. Hypertonic dehydration          B. Hypotonic dehydration

C. Isotonic dehydration            D. Water intoxication

E. Sodium intoxication

(2) Which one of the following fluid changes may occur in this patient?

A. Increased ICF                   B. Decreased ECF

C. Decreased plasma                D. No changes in ICF

E. Decreased ICF

(3) What caused the patient to have stupor, vomiting, and slurred speech?

A. Dehydration of brain cells      B. Decreased spinal fluid pressure

C. Decreased intracranial pressure D. Cerebral edema

E. None of the above

(4) Which one of the following mechanisms is NOT involved in the occurrence of stupor, vomiting, and slurred speech in the patients?

A. Insufficient sodium intake      B. Excessive water intake

C. Reduced renal water excretion   D. Hypotonic ECF

E. Hypertonic ECF

(5) Which one of the following dangerous conditions may occur in this patient?

A. Cardiorespiratory arrest        B. Ascites

C. Renal failure                   D. Hepatic failure

E. Internal hemorrhage

(6) Which one of the following drugs is effective for this patient to alleviate her clinical signs?

A. Glucose                         B. NaHCO$_3$

C. Calcium                         D. Mannitol

E. Saline

## Case analysis questions

A 37-yr-old nulligravida known to have polycystic ovarian syndrome and depression was admitted to the hospital for lumbar spine fusion to relieve her back pain secondary to a car accident. Home medications included hydrochlorothiazide, 25 mg/d; duloxetine, 60 mg, twice/d; aripiprazole, 10 mg/d; clonazepam, 0.25 mg/d. Preoperative laboratory values were unremarkable. Surgery was performed under general anesthesia, the procedure was uneventful, and she was maintained on maintenance fluids with 0.45% saline and 5% dextrose solution. On postoperative day 1, the patient was found to be agitated and confused and was reporting intensive thirst. Physical examination showed: T 36.4 ℃, HR 105 beats/min, BP 135/80 mmHg, R 15 breaths/min, SaO₂ 100%. Mucous membranes were dry. Cardiac examination findings were unremarkable except for tachycardia. Lungs were clear to auscultation. Abdomen was soft and extremities were without edema. The surgical incision was cleanly opposed without erythema or fluctuance. Serum sodium concentration was elevated to 153 mmol/L. Urine output was not recorded, but urinalysis showed a urine specific gravity of 1.005 and urine osmolality of 129 mOsm/kg. The patient was i. v. injected with 4 μg of desmopressin. However copious urine output continued and urine osmolality was 155 mOsm/kg at 2 hours after treatment. She was diagnosed as nephrogenic diabetes insipidus (DI).

Questions:

(1) What kind of fluid imbalances did this patient have? What's the pathogenesis?

(2) What caused this patient to be agitated and confused with intensive thirsty?

(3) What are the mechanisms underlying the changes of heart rate and blood pressure in this patient?

(4) What should a doctor do with this patient?

## Answers

**Case-based multiple choice questions (single answer)**

1. BBDAC; 2. AACAE; 3. DACA; 4. ADEE; 5. DADEAD

**Case analysis questions**

(1) What kind of fluid imbalances did this patient have? What's the pathogenesis?

Based on [Na⁺] > 145 mmol and her diagnosis, this patient must have hypertonic dehydration due to nephrogenic DI that cause the loss of water more than sodium.

(2) What caused this patient to be agitated and confused with intensive thirsty?

Dehydration of brain cells led to the occurrence of agitation and confusion, while intensive thirst was the consequence of plasma osmolarity elevation that acts on the osmoreceptors in the hypothalamus.

(3) What are the mechanisms underlying the changes of heart rate and blood pressure in this patient?

Massive fluid loss decreases the effective blood volume and subsequent activation of sympathetic system via baroreceptors and volume receptors results in the increase of heart rate. The elevation of blood pressure is attributed to the increase of angiotensin Ⅱ after RAAS activation.

(4) What should a doctor do with this patient?

First of all, the hypertonic condition should be corrected by i. v. infusion of 5% glucose. Oral administration can replace infusion when the patient regains consciousness. Thereafter, DI should be treated according to the underlying cause.

# ◇ Potassium Imbalance

## Case-based multiple choice questions (single answer)

**1. A 60-yr-old man with vomiting and heart palpitation was admitted to hospital. Blood tests revealed: [Na$^+$] 138 mmol/L, [K$^+$] 2.9 mmol/L, [Mg$^{2+}$] 0.95 mmol/L.**

(1) What kind of electrolyte imbalance did this patient have?

    A. Hyperkalemia                 B. Hypokalemia

    C. Hypomagnesemia            D. Hyponatremia

    E. Hypermagnesemia

(2) What caused the development of the electrolyte imbalance in this patient?

    A. Sodium loss from the digestive tract

    B. Magnesium loss from the digestive tract

    C. Sodium and water loss from the digestive tract

    D. Excessive excretion of sodium and water via urine

    E. Potassium loss from the digestive tract

(3) Which one of the following cardiac changes may occur in this patient?

    A. Cardiac excitability ↓, automaticity ↑

    B. Cardiac conductivity ↑, automaticity ↑

    C. Cardiac excitability ↓, conductivity ↑

    D. Cardiac excitability ↓, automaticity ↓

    E. Cardiac automaticity ↑, conductivity ↓

(4) Which one of the following ECG changes is typical for this patient?

    A. Shortened QT interval          B. ST segment elevation

    C. Peaked T wave               D. Prominent U wave

    E. Shortened PR interval

(5) Which one of the following muscular changes may occur in this patient?

    A. Excitability ↑                 B. Excitability ↓

    C. Contractility ↑               D. Contractility ↓

    E. No changes

(6) Which one of the following disorders is most likely to occur in this patient?

    A. Metabolic acidosis            B. Hypoglycemia

    C. Metabolic alkalosis           D. Oliguria

    E. Paradoxical alkaline urine

(7) Which one of the following treatments is a safe and effective way to correct the electrolyte imbalance of this patient?

    A. Intravenous infusion of normal saline

B. Intravenous infusion to replenish potassium

C. Oral supplement with potassium

D. Oral supplement with normal saline

E. Oral supplement with magnesium

**2. A 30-yr-old woman with leg swelling and anuria was rescued after 10 hours of being trapped under rubble due to earthquake. Blood tests showed: [Na$^+$] 136 mmol/L, [K$^+$] 6.6 mmol/L, [Cl$^-$] 95 mmol/L。**

(1) What kind of electrolyte imbalance did this patient have?

A. Hyperkalemia

B. Hypokalemia

C. Hyperchloremia

D. Hyponatremia

E. Hypernatremia

(2) What caused the development of the electrolyte imbalance in this patient?

A. Hypoxia

B. Dehydration

C. Decreased glomerular filtration

D. Increased glomerular filtration

E. Mineralocorticoid deficiency

(3) Which one of the following ECG changes may occur in this patient?

A. Prolonged QT interval

B. Peaked T wave

C. Depressed ST segment

D. Prominent U wave

E. Flattened T wave

(4) Which one of the following cardiac changes may occur in this patient?

A. Cardiac excitability ↓ , automaticity ↑

B. Cardiac conductivity ↑ , automaticity ↑

C. Cardiac excitability ↓ , conductivity ↑

D. Cardiac conductivity ↓ , automaticity ↑

E. Cardiac automaticity ↓ , conductivity ↓

(5) Which one of the following changes is NOT possible to occur in this patient?

A. Arrhythmias

B. Paradoxical alkaline urine

C. Weak limbs

D. Hyperactive deep tendon reflexes

E. Metabolic acidosis

(6) Which one of the following dangerous conditions may occur in this patient?

A. Cardiac arrest

B. Paradoxical alkaline urine

C. Weak limbs

D. Hypoactive deep tendon reflexes

E. Metabolic acidosis

(7) Once this patient shows the cardiac dysfunction, which one of the following treatments should NOT be chosen by a doctor?

A. Intravenouse infusion of insulin with glucose

B. Intravenouse infusion of sodium bicarbonate

C. Intravenouse infusion with calcium reagents

    D. Intravenouse infusion of potassium chloride

    E. Hemodialysis

## Case analysis questions

### • Case 1

A 30-yr-old woman who had juvenile-onset diabetes was scheduled for transplantation of a kidney from a living donor. Problems included hypertension and diabetic nephropathy with chronic renal failure, treated by hemodialysis. Her most recent dialysis had been performed 2 days prior to operation. Diabetic management had been difficult preoperatively, and blood glucose varied between 60 – 600 mg/dL. Blood glucose was 64 mg/dL at midnight, 8 hours prior to operation. Arterial blood-gas analysis 1 day prior to operation revealed pH 7.45, $PaCO_2$ 32 mmHg.

At 5 a. m. on the day of operation, blood glucose was 129 mg/dL, [$Na^+$] 128 mEq/L, [$K^+$] 5.2 mEq/L, [$Cl^-$] 94 mEq/L. Premedication included diazepam (p. o. 10 mg) and methylprednisolone (i. v. 750 mg). Insulin was not given. 5% dextrose in half-normal saline solution was i. v. given and an electrocardiogram (ECG) revealed sinus rhythm with normal QRS and T waves during anaesthesia. Blood glucose was 150 mg/dL at 1 hour and increased to 250 mg/dL at 4 hours after infusion. Insulin was not administrated during this time. Blood pressure varied between 120/80 mmHg and 180/100 mmHg. 5 hours after induction, during surgical closure, widening of the QRS and peaking of the T waves was observed on the ECG. Approximately 3 min later, cardiac arrest occurred. Blood analysis revealed [$K^+$] 7.9 mEq/L, $PaCO_2$ 37 mmHg, pH 7.21. The patient was successfully resuscitated with external cardiac massage, ventilation with 100% oxygen, and intravenous administration of sodium bicarbonate, insulin, calcium chloride, lidocaine and 50% glucose. Blood analysis after resuscitation revealed: [$K^+$] 6.8 mEq/L, $PaCO_2$ 34 mmHg, pH 7.31. 1 hour later, the patient awakened, and blood analysis revealed: [$K^+$] 6.1 mEq/L, $PaCO_2$ 34 mmHg, pH 7.41.

Questions:

(1) What caused the elevation of blood glucose in this patient during operation?

(2) What caused ECG changes and cardiac arrest during renal transplantation?

(3) What pathological states did this patient develop during transplantation? What are the underlying mechanisms?

(4) What cardiac alterations were caused by the electrolyte imbalance in this patient? What are the underlying mechanisms?

(5) Please explain why the doctor treated the patient with sodium bicarbonate, insulin, calcium chloride after the onset of cardiac arrest.

### • Case 2

A 35-yr-old man was admitted to the hospital with myalgias and generalized weakness. 2 weeks before, he had abdominal pain, decreased oral intake, nausea, and vomiting. He denied diarrhea. 1 week before admission, he developed muscle weakness that worsened until he was unable to get out of bed without assistance. His medical history was unremarkable. His only reported medication was over-the-counter ibuprofen for chronic back pain, 2.4 g to 3.2 g daily for several months. He denied alchohol or solvent abuse. On physical examination, he was alert and oriented. His vital signs were normal. He was unable to raise his upper or lower extremities against gravity and had decreased deep tendon reflexes with intact superficial sensations. The rest of his examination findings were unremarkable. Initial laboratory workup showed normal blood cell counts, [$Na^+$] of 142 mEq/L, [$K^+$] of 1.8 mEq/L, metabolic acidosis, and no autoimmune diseases. Urine studies showed: 466 mEq of sodium, 112 mEq of potassium, and 2.25 g of creatinine in 24-hour urine collection with pH 7.0. He was diagnosed as reversible type Ⅰ renal tubular acidosis (RTA), likely from ibuprofen use, because all his manifestations and laboratory analysis were greatly improved after stopping treatment with ibuprofen.

Questions:

(1) What kind of electrolyte imbalance did this patient develop?

(2) What is the relationship between the electrolyte imbalance and type Ⅰ RTA in this patient?

(3) What are the mechanisms underlying muscle weakness in this patient?

(4) If the patient takes an ECG test, what are the potential changes and underlying mechanisms?

(5) What should a doctor do after analysis of blood test results?

## Answers

**Case-based multiple choice questions (single answer)**

**1.** BEEDBCC; **2.** ACBEDAD

**Case analysis questions**

**Case 1**

(1) What caused the elevation of blood glucose in this patient during operation?

This patient had type I diabetes and thus cannot produce insulin. In the absence of insulin infusion prior to operation, continuous administration of 5% dextrose in half-normal saline solution caused the increase of blood glucose.

(2) What caused ECG changes and cardiac arrest during renal transplantation?

Hyperkalemia (above 5.5 mEq/L) caused typical ECG changes include widening of QRS and peaking of T waves.

(3) What pathological states did this patient develop during transplantation? What are the underlying mechanisms?

Hyperkalemia and metabolic acidosis was determined according to the serum $K^+$ (7.9 mEq/L) and pH (7.21). Insulin deficiency and glycemia stimulate the outflow of intracellular $K^+$. The exchange of $H^+$ and $K^+$ through cell membrane in metabolic acidosis also contributed to the rise of plasma $K^+$ levels. Metabolic acidosis may be caused by chronic renal failure, diabetic ketoacidosis or lactic acidosis.

(4) What cardiac alterations were caused by the electrolyte imbalance in this patient? What are the

underlying mechanisms?

This patient had acute severe hyperkalemia during operation. So the excitability of cardiomyocytes was significantly reduced due to depolarization block. The automaticity of heart was also reduced due to the slow influx of $Na^+$ at phase 4 of repolarization. The conductivity of heart was blocked by inactivation of voltage-dependent $Na^+$ channels during depolarization. The reduced calcium influx at the plateau phase of the cardiac action lowered the contractility of cardiomyocytes.

(5) Please explain why the doctor treated the patient with sodium bicarbonate, insulin, calcium chloride after the onset of cardiac arrest.

Sodium bicarbonate was used to correct acidosis. Insulin reduced the blood glucose and plasma $K^+$ by induction of $K^+$ movement into cells. Calcium influx helped to recover the excitability of cardiomyocytes and increased the contractility.

**Case 2**

(1) What kind of electrolyte imbalance did this patient develop?

According to the serum levels of potassium (1.8 mEq/L < 3.5 mEq/L), this patient had hypokalemia.

(2) What is the relationship between the electrolyte imbalance and type Ⅰ RTA in this patient?

The impaired renal excretion of $H^+$ from distal tubules in type Ⅰ RTA stimulates the exchange of $K^+$ and $Na^+$ and subsequently increases excretion of urinary potassium. In line, the amount of potassium in 24-hour urine collection was 112 mEq, much more than the normal value of 30 mEq.

(3) What are the mechanisms underlying muscle weakness in this patient?

In hypokalemia, the concentration of potassium in ECF drops, leading to the increase of transmembane gradient and electrical charge. Therefore, the membrane potential of muscle cells becomes hyperpolarized and less reactive to stimuli.

(4) If the patient takes an ECG test, what are the potential changes and underlying mechanisms?

① ST depression due to the acceleration of $Ca^{2+}$ influx at Phase 2.

② T wave flattening due to the slow efflux of $K^+$ at Phase 4.

③ Prominent U waves due to the slow efflux of $K^+$ at Phase 4 and prolonged repolarization.

(5) What should a doctor do after analysis of blood test results?

The doctor should treat the patient with oral potassium supplements and monitor his serum levels of potassium and ECG changes.

# ◇ **Magnesium Imbalance**

## **Case-based multiple choice questions (single answer)**

1. **A girl with severe diarrhea was admitted to hospital. Blood test showed: [ $Na^+$ ] 142 mmol/L, [ $K^+$ ] 3.3 mmol/L, [ $Mg^{2+}$ ] 0.25 mmol/L, [ $Ca^{2+}$ ] 2.28 mmol/L.**

(1) What kind of electrolyte imbalance did this patient have?

    A. Hyponatremia and hyperkalemia      B. Hyponatremia and hypokalemia

    C. Hypokalemia and hypocalcemia      D. Hypomagnesemia and hypokalemia

    E. Hypokalemia and hypercalcemia

（2）Which one of the following cardiac changes may occur in this patient?

    A. Cardiac excitability ↓ , automaticity ↑

    B. Cardiac conductivity ↑ , automaticity ↑

    C. Cardiac excitability ↓ , conductivity ↑

    D. Cardiac excitability ↑ , automaticity ↑

    E. Cardiac automaticity ↓ , conductivity ↓

（3）Which one of the following changes may occur in this patient?

    A. Reduced muscular irritability      B. Hypertension

    C. Anorexia                         D. Bradycardia

    E. Drowsiness

（4）Which one of the following treatments should be chosen to correct the electrolyte imbalance in this patient?

    A. Supplement with potassium and sodium

    B. Supplement with sodium and magnesium

    C. Supplement with magnesium and potassium

    D. Supplement with potassium and calcium

    E. Supplement with calcium and magnesium

**2. A mid-aged woman with myxedema was diagnosed with hypothyroidism.**

（1）Which one of the following laboratory values is most likely to come from this patient?

    A. $[K^+]$ 3.3 mmol/L           B. $[Na^+]$ 155 mmol/L

    C. $[Ca^{2+}]$ 1.85 mmol/L      D. $[Mg^{2+}]$ 0.55 mmol/L

    E. $[Mg^{2+}]$ 3.25 mmol/L

（2）Which one of the following changes is most likely to occur in this patient?

    A. Increased neuromuscular excitability    B. Decreased arterial pressure

    C. Polyuria                         D. Tachycardia

    E. Irritability/anxiety

## Case analysis questions

A 69-yr-old woman was admitted to the hospital with a 3-day history of headache and confusion. She had suffered from non-insulin dependent diabetes, rheumatoid arthritis, and migraine. There was no history of epileptic fits or transient ischemic attacks. She was taking glibenclamide, prednisolone, and frusemide.

On the day of admission she suffered at least 12 episodes of involuntary head and eye turning (mainly to the left), with associated periods of absence lasting up to 2 minutes. Her husband confirmed that these attacks had started only 2 days earlier. Investigations showed: blood glucose 14.7 mmol/L, haemoglobin A1c (HbA1c) 18.3% (normal 5% – 8%), [Ca] 2.25 mmol/L (normal 2.2 – 2.62 mmol/L), [Pi] 1.03 mmol/L, [K⁺] 3.8 mEq/L. Plasma urea, sodium, and bicarbonate concentrations were normal, as were cardiac enzyme activities. A computed tomogram of the brain was normal, an electroencephalogram (EEG) showed epileptic activity in the right hemisphere.

Despite control of her blood glucose concentration with an insulin infusion (a loading dose of 1 g in the first 24 hours followed by 30 mg daily), she continued to fit with phenytoin, an antiepileptic drug. 48 hours later, her serum magnesium concentration was 0. 29 mmol/L. Magnesium sulphate 3 g was infused and her fits had become less frequent within 12 hours. They had stopped altogether after a further infusion of 2 g magnesium sulphate. Thereafter, her neurological signs resolved completely and her serum magnesium concentrations had become stable at 0. 63 mmol/L.

Questions:

(1) What caused this patient to develop confusion?

(2) Why did this patient develop hypomagnesemia?

(3) What are the cause and pathogenesis of epilepsy in this patient?

(4) If hypomagnesemia was not corrected properly, what metabolic changes may occur in this patient? What are the underlying mechanisms?

## Answers

**Case-based multiple choice questions (single answer)**

**1**. DDBC; **2**. EB

**Case analysis questions**

(1) What caused this patient to develop confusion?

The patient had confusion due to type Ⅱ diabetes and hypomagnesemia.

(2) Why did this patient develop hypomagnesemia?

Diabetes associated hypertonic glycosuria may promote the renal excretion of magnesium; frusemide reduced the renal reabsorption of magnesium in the thick ascending limb. To control the blood glucose concentration, insulin infusion may promote the influx of magnesium into cells. All of these led to the development of hypomagnesemia in this patient.

(3) What are the cause and pathogenesis of epilepsy in this patient?

The development of epilepsy in this patient is due to hypomagnesemia and associated activation of central nervous system. The underlying mechanisms may include:

① Hypomagnesemia leads to the reduced antagonistic action of magnesium on the N-methyl-D-aspartate (NMDA).

② Hypomagnesemia reduces the production of cAMP and the activity of $Na^+$-$K^+$-ATPase.

(4) If hypomagnesemia was not corrected properly, what metabolic changes may occur in this patient? What are the underlying mechanisms?

① Arrythmias due to the increase of cardiac excitability and automaticity, or myocardial potassium insufficiency caused by reduced activity of $Na^+$-$K^+$-ATPase.

② Hypertension due to peripheral vasoconstriction.

③ Coronary heart disease (CHD) due to abnormal cardiac metabolism and coronary spasm.

④ Hypokalemia due to reduced activities of $Na^+$-$K^+$-ATPase and subsequently decreased reabsorption of potassium in the thick ascending limb.

⑤ Hypocalcemia due to the reduced secretion and action of PTH.

## ◇ Calcium and Phosphate Imbalance

### Case-based multiple choice questions (single answer)

**1. A baby was kept indoors since born and his hair became sparse.**

(1) Which one of the following blood test results is most likely to come from this baby?

    A. $[K^+]$ 6.3 mmol/L              B. $[Na^+]$ 155 mmol/L

    C. $[Ca^{2+}]$ 0.8 mmol/L           D. $[Ca^{2+}]$ 1.35 mmol/L

    E. $[Mg^{2+}]$ 3.25 mmol/L

(2) Which one of the following changes is NOT possible to occur in this baby?

    A. Muscle spasm                 B. Hapalonychia

    C. Pectus carinatum             D. Bowlegs

    E. Craniosynostosis

(3) Which one of the following ECG changes is typical for this patient?

    A. Prolonged QT interval         B. Peaked T wave

    C. Shortened ST segment        D. Prominent U wave

    E. ST segment elevation

(4) Which one of the following cardiac changes is likely to occur in this patient?

    A. Cardiac excitability ↓ , automaticity ↑

    B. Cardiac excitability ↓ , contractility ↑

    C. Cardiac excitability ↓ , conductivity ↑

    D. Cardiac excitability ↑ , conductivity ↑

    E. Cardiac excitability ↑ , conductivity ↓

**2. A mid-aged man was diagnosed with chronic lymphocytic leukemia with bone metastasis.**

(1) Which one of the following blood test results is most likely to come from this patient?

    A. $[K^+]$ 3.3 mmol/L              B. $[Na^+]$ 155 mmol/L

    C. $[Ca^{2+}]$ 1.85 mmol/L          D. $[Ca^{2+}]$ 0.6 mmol/L

    E. $[Mg^{2+}]$ 3.25 mmol/L

(2) Which one of the following changes is most likely to occur in this patient?

    A. Increased neuromuscular excitability   B. Ectopic calcification

    C. Muscle spasm                 D. Hyperactive deep tendon reflexes

    E. Irritability/anxiety

(3) Which one of the following ECG changes is most likely to occur in this patient?

    A. Shortened QT interval        B. Peaked T wave

    C. Depressed ST segment       D. Prominent U wave

    E. Inverted T wave

(4) Which one of the following cardiac changes is likely to occur in this patient?

    A. Cardiac excitability ↓, conductivity ↓

    B. Cardiac conductivity ↑, automaticity ↑

    C. Cardiac excitability ↓, conductivity ↑

    D. Cardiac excitability ↑, automaticity ↑

    E. Cardiac automaticity ↓, conductivity ↑

**3. A mid-aged man was diagnosed with acute alcoholism with respiratory alkalosis.**

(1) Which one of the following blood test results is most likely to come from this patient?

    A. $[Na^+]$ 130 mmol/L         B. $[Na^+]$ 155 mmol/L

    C. $[K^+]$ 3.25 mmol/L         D. $[Pi]$ 0.5 mmol/L

    E. $[Pi]$ 1.85 mmol/L

(2) Which one of the following changes is NOT possible in this patient?

    A. Myasthenia         B. Wadding gait

    C. Muscle spasm         D. Ostealgia

    E. Irritability/anxiety

**4. A 5-yr-old boy was diagnosed with Vitamin D intoxication.**

(1) Which one of the following blood test results is most likely to come from this patient?

    A. $[Na^+]$ 130 mmol/L         B. $[Na^+]$ 155 mmol/L

    C. $[K^+]$ 3.25 mmol/L         D. $[Pi]$ 0.5 mmol/L

    E. $[Pi]$ 2.05 mmol/L

(2) Which one of the following changes is NOT likely to occur in this patient?

    A. Increased neuromuscular excitability     B. Ectopic calcification

    C. Muscle spasm         D. Atrioventricular block

    E. Pectus carinatum

## Case analysis questions

A 3-yr-old boy was seen by his pediatrician because of an upper respiratory infection of a week's duration and decreased urination for 1 day. Because of constipation, he was given a single pediatric size Fleet enema with minimal return of fluid in the first minutes. Over the next 2 to 3 hours, this boy had 3 voluminous stools and 3 emeses. He became lethargic and pale. Physical examination revealed: T 38 ℃, pulse 144 beats/min, R 16 breaths/min, BP 96/68 mmHg, BW 8.4 kg. Mucous membrane was dry and skin turgor poor. Deep tendon reflexes were brisk and muscle tone was increased. Blood analysis showed: hemoglobin (Hb) 13.4 mg/dL, hematocrit 40%, serum $[Na^+]$ 152 mEq/L, $[K^+]$ 3.4 mEq/L, $[Cl^-]$ 108 mEq/L, $[Ca^{2+}]$ 0.58 mmol/L, $[Pi]$ 6.78 mmol/L, blood urea nitrogen (BUN) 3.93 mmol/L. He improved after administration of intravenous fluids for 12 hours.

    Questions:

(1) What kind of fluid and electrolytic imbalance is likely to have occurred in this patient?

What are the underlying mechanisms?

(2) What caused the increase of muscle tone in this patient?

(3) If the patient took ECG test, what could be abnormal?

(4) Why did the doctor treat the patient with intravenous fluid infusion?

## Answers

**Case-based multiple choice questions (single answer)**

**1.** CEAD; **2.** CBAA; **3.** DC; **4.** ED

**Case analysis questions**

(1) What kind of fluid and electrolytic imbalance is likely to have occurred in this patient? What are the underlying mechanisms?

① Dehydration occurred due to 3 emeses within 2 to 3 hours.

② Hyperphosphatemia ($[Pi]$ 6.78 mmol/L > 1.9 mmol/L) developed due to the application of Fleet and dehydration.

③ Hypocalcemia ($[Ca^{2+}]$ 0.58 mmol/L < 1 mmol/L) was caused by hyperphosphatemia.

(2) What caused the increase of muscle tone in this patient?

That is the consequence of increased neuromuscular excitability in hypocalcemia.

(3) If the patient took ECG test, what could be abnormal?

Upon hypocalcemia, the cardiac excitability and conductivity increases because of the acceleration of $Na^+$ influx. However, the plateau prolongs due to the reduction of $Ca^{2+}$ influx at Phase 2. Therefore, his ECG may show ST & QT prolongation, flattened or inverted T waves.

(4) Why did the doctor treat the patient with intravenous fluid infusion?

Fluid supplement reduces the plasma levels of phosphate and promotes its excretion. Correction of hyperphosphatemia helps the production of $1,25-(OH)_2 D_3$ and the reabsorption of calcium, thereby elevating the plasma levels of calcium.

(赵丽梅　赵　颖)

# Chapter 3　Acid-base Disturbance

## Case-based multiple choice questions (single answer)

**1. A 61-yr-old man suffered from kidney failure. His blood gas analysis showed: pH 7.28, $PaCO_2$ 30 mmHg, and $[HCO_3^-]$ 14 mmol/L.**

(1) Which one of the following acid-base disturbances is most likely to occur in this patient?

A. Metabolic acidosis　　　　　　B. Respiratory acidosis

C. Metabolic alkalosis　　　　　　D. Respiratory alkalosis

E. None of the above

（2）Which one of the following compensations was mainly induced in this patient?

    A. Extracellular buffers             B. Bone compensation

    C. Intracellular and extracellular ion exchange

    D. Respiratory compensation        E. Kidney compensation

（3）Which one of the following bases is the most important buffer for the acid-base balance in this patient?

    A. $Na_2HPO_4$                 B. K-Hb

    C. $NaHCO_3$                 D. $HbO_2$

    E. $Pro^-$

（4）Which one of the following changes in plasma levels of potassium is correct for this patient?

    A. Decrease                 B. Increase

    C. No change               D. Decrease and then increase

    E. Increase and then decrease

（5）Which one of the following changes in the blood acid-base parameters may occur in this patient?

    A. AB increases            B. SB increases

    C. BB increases           D. AB < SB

    E. AB > SB

（6）Which one of the following changes is NOT likely to occur in this patient?

    A. Increased plasma $[K^+]$

    B. Increased plasma $[Ca^{2+}]$

    C. Increased plasma levels of epinephrine

    D. Enhanced oxidative phosphorylation in the brain

    E. Increased glutamic acid decarboxylase activity in the brain

（7）Which one of the following changes is NOT likely to occur in this patient?

    A. Cardiac arrhythmias

    B. Reduced myocardial contractility

    C. Decreased epinephrine secretion

    D. Impaired metabolism of the central nervous system

    E. Decreased vascular responses to catecholamines

（8）Which one of the following drugs should be taken first for this patient?

    A. Sodium bicarbonate        B. Sodium citrate

    C. Tris(hydroxymethyl)aminomethane    D. Sodium lactate

    E. Disodium hydrogen phosphate

**2. A 6-yr-old boy was admitted to hospital due to drowning when he played with his friends by the river on a hot day. On admission his blood gas analysis revealed: pH 7.1, PaCO$_2$ 76 mmHg, [HCO$_3^-$]28 mmol/L.**

(1) Which one of the following acid-base disturbances is most likely to have occurred in this patient?

    A. Metabolic acidosis　　　　　　　　B. Acute respiratory acidosis

    C. Chronic respiratory acidosis

    D. Metabolic acidosis complicated with respiratory acidosis

    E. None of the above

(2) Which one of the following compensations was mainly induced in this patient?

    A. Phosphate buffer system　　　　　　B. Bicarbonate buffer system

    C. Nonbicarbonate buffer system　　　　D. Protein buffer system

    E. Renal regulation

(3) Which one of the following manifestations could NOT develop in this patient?

    A. Prerenal renal failure　　　　　　　B. Cardiac arrhythmia

    C. Hyperkalemia　　　　　　　　　　D. Decreased blood pressure

    E. Persistent headache

(4) Which one of the following changes is NOT likely to occur in this patient?

    A. Increased plasma [K$^+$]　　　　　　B. Normal plasma [Ca$^{2+}$]

    C. Normal plasma [Na$^+$]　　　　　　D. Increased plasma [Cl$^-$]

    E. Cerebral vasodilation

**3. A 68-yr-old woman with a bad cold was hospitalized due to a rapid fall of air temperature. She had suffered pulmonary heart disease for 25 years. On admission her blood gas analysis showed: pH 7.33, PaCO$_2$ 70 mmHg, [HCO$_3^-$]36 mmol/L.**

(1) What kind of acid-base disturbance did this patient have?

    A. Metabolic acidosis　　　　　　　　B. Metabolic alkalosis

    C. Acute respiratory acidosis　　　　　D. Chronic respiratory acidosis

    E. Respiratory alkalosis

(2) Which one of the following mechanisms is involved in the development of the acid-base disturbance in this patient?

    A. Hysteria　　　　　　　　　　　　B. Airway obstruction induced CO$_2$ retention

    C. Endocrine disorder　　　　　　　　D. Renal insufficiency

    E. Heart failure

(3) Which one of the following compensations was mainly induced in this patient?

    A. Phosphate buffer system　　　　　　B. Bicarbonate buffer system

    C. Non-bicarbonate buffer system　　　　D. Protein buffer system

    E. Renal regulation

（4）Which one of the following changes may occur in this patient?

    A. AB decreased
        B. SB decreased

    C. BB increased
        D. AB < SB

    E. The negative value of BE increased

（5）Which one of the following water-electrolyte imbalances may occur in this patient due to the acid-base disturbance?

    A. Hyperkalemia
        B. Hypercalcemia

    C. Hypophosphatemia
        D. Hyperchloremia

    E. Generalized edema

（6）Which one of the following enzymatic changes in the central nervous system may have occurred in this patient?

    A. Carbonic anhydrase activity ↓

    B. Glutamic acid decarboxylase activity ↓

    C. Glutaminase activity ↓

    D. γ-aminobutyric acid aminotransferase activity ↓

    E. Biological oxidase activity ↑

（7）Which one of the following treatments is NOT appropriate?

    A. Effective ventilation
        B. Antibiotics to control infection

    C. Low-concentration oxygen therapy
        D. Removing mucus

    E. Oral potassium chloride supplementation

**4. A 12-yr-old boy with fever, cough and shortness of breath was admitted to the fever clinic. His blood pressure was 110/75 mmHg, respiratory rate was 28 breaths/min, and moist rales were heard over the lungs. The results of laboratory examinations showed: $[K^+]$ 4.5 mmol/L, $[Na^+]$ 134 mmol/L, $[Cl^-]$ 106 mmol/L, pH 7.51, $PaCO_2$ 30 mmHg, $[HCO_3^-]$ 20.3 mmol/L.**

（1）Which one of the following acid-base disturbances is most likely to have occurred in this patient?

    A. Metabolic acidosis
        B. Respiratory acidosis

    C. Metabolic alkalosis
        D. Respiratory alkalosis

    E. None of the above

（2）Which one of the following mechanisms is involved in the development of acid-base disturbance in the patient?

    A. Excessive excretion of volatile acids
    B. A decrease of fixed acids

    C. Decreased insulin secretion
    D. A decrease of fatty acids

    E. Pulmonary infection

(3) Which of the following may induce one type of acid-base disturbance different from that in this patient?

      A. High-flow mechanical ventilation      B. Massive stock blood transfusions

      C. Hyperthyroidism      D. Hysteria

      E. Excessive intake of ammonium salts

(4) Which one of the following complications is NOT commonly associated with the acid-base disturbance in this patient?

      A. Hypokalemia      B. Convulsion

      C. Hyperphosphatemia      D. Hypoxia

      E. Disorders of consciousness

(5) Which one of the following changes may occur in this patient?

      A. AB increased      B. SB increased

      C. BB increased      D. AB > SB

      E. AB < SB

(6) Which one of the following treatments is NOT appropriate?

      A. Cooling down      B. Inhalation of carbon dioxide

      C. Application of antibiotics      D. High-concentration oxygen theapy

      E. Fluid infusion

**5. A 60-yr-old woman was admitted to the hospital due to recurrent vomiting. She was diagnosed with pyloric obstruction. Her blood gas analysis showed: pH 7. 5, $PaCO_2$ 48 mmHg, $[HCO_3^-]$ 36 mmol/L.**

(1) Which one of the following acid-base disturbances is most likely to have occurred in this patient?

      A. Metabolic acidosis      B. Respiratory acidosis

      C. Metabolic alkalosis      D. Respiratory alkalosis

      E. Mixed acid-base disturbance

(2) Which of the following may induce one type of acid-base disturbance different from that in this patient?

      A. Pneumonia      B. Application of diuretics (furosemide)

      C. Adrenocortical hyperplasia      D. Hypokalemia

      E. Hepatic failure

(3) Which one of the following mechanisms is NOT involved in the development of the acid-base disturbance in this patient?

      A. Loss of $H^+$      B. Loss of $Na^+$

      C. Loss of $K^+$      D. Massive loss of ECF

      E. Loss of $Cl^-$

（4）Which one of the following statements is NOT correct about the compensatory regulation in this patient?

    A. Respiratory compensation is quite fast

    B. Blood buffer capacity is limited

    C. Renal compensation is quite fast

    D. Renal compensation is quite slow

    E. Respiration is depressed

（5）Which of the following is the main functional buffer system in this patient?

    A. $HCO_3^-/H_2CO_3$           B. $Hb^-/HHb$

    C. $Pr/HPr$               D. $HbO_2^-/HHbO_2$

    E. $HPO_4^{2-}/H_2PO_4^-$

（6）Which one of the following enzymatic changes is associated with the decrease of central inhibitory mediators in this patient?

    A. Glutamic acid decarboxylase activity ↓

    B. γ-aminobutyric acid aminotransferase activity ↓

    C. Carbonic anhydrase activity ↑

    D. Glutaminase activity ↑

    E. Pyruvate dehydrogenase activity ↓

（7）Which one of the following alterations may occur in this patient?

    A. $K^+$ influx, and $K^+$-$Na^+$ exchange at proximal convoluted tubule ↓

    B. $K^+$ influx, and $H^+$-$Na^+$ exchange at proximal convoluted tubule ↑

    C. $K^+$ influx, and $H^+$-$Na^+$ exchange at proximal convoluted tubule ↓

    D. $K^+$ efflux, and $H^+$-$Na^+$ exchange at proximal convoluted tubule ↑

    E. $K^+$ efflux, and $H^+$-$Na^+$ exchange at proximal convoluted tubule ↓

（8）If the patient developed tetany later, which one of the following changes is most likely to cause it?

    A. $[K^+]$ ↓              B. $[Cl^-]$ ↓

    C. $[Na^+]$ ↓            D. $[Ca^{2+}]$ ↓

    E. $[Mg^{2+}]$ ↓

（9）Which one of the following treatments is NOT appropriate?

    A. Thiazide diuretics         B. Normal saline (p. o.)

    C. Potassium chloride        D. Fasting, gastrointestinal decompression

    E. Fluid infusion

**6. A 46-yr-old woman was admitted to hospital because of fever. She had diabetes for more than 10 years. Her physical examinations showed: T 39 ℃, and hyperpnea with a rate of 28 breaths/min. Laboratory analysis revealed that her blood glucose of 10. 1 mmol/L, [Na$^+$] 160 mmol/L, [Cl$^-$] 104 mmol/L, pH 7.38, PaCO$_2$ 24 mmHg, [HCO$_3^-$] 13 mmol/L, and glycouria (+++).**

(1) Which one of the following acid-base disturbances is most likely to have occurred in this patient?

　　　A. Metabolic acidosis　　　　　　B. Metabolic alkalosis

　　　C. Respiratory acidosis　　　　　　D. Respiratory alkalosis

　　　E. Metabolic acidosis complicated with respiratory alkalosis

(2) Which one of the following changes is NOT involved in the development of the acid-base disturbance in this patient?

　　　A. Increased generation of volatile acids

　　　B. Increased generation of lactic acid

　　　C. Increased production of β-hydroxybutyric acid

　　　D. Increased production of acetoacetic acid

　　　E. Enhanced lipolysis

(3) Which one of the following changes is associated with the acid-base disturbance in this patient?

　　　A. Increased plasma $[Cl^-]$　　　　B. Decreased plasma $[Cl^-]$

　　　C. Normal AG　　　　　　　　　D. Increased AG

　　　E. AB > SB

**7. An elderly man was admitted to hospital due to recurrent vomiting, oliguria, and weakness in the last 2 days. He had chronic obstructive pulmonary disease (COPD). His physical examinations showed: BP 118/68 mmHg, R 10 breaths/min, and severe dehydration. Laboratory analysis revealed: $[K^+]$ 2.8 mmol/L, $[Na^+]$ 147 mmol/L, $[Cl^-]$ 95 mmol/L; pH 7.48, $PaCO_2$ 52 mmHg, $[HCO_3^-]$ 38 mmol/L.**

(1) Which one of the following acid-base disturbances is most likely to occur in this patient?

　　　A. Metabolic acidosis　　　　　　B. Metabolic alkalosis

　　　C. Respiratory acidosis　　　　　　D. Respiratory alkalosis

　　　E. Respiratory acidosis complicated with metabolic alkalosis

(2) Which one of the following mechanisms is involved in the development of the acid-base disturbance in this patient?

　　　A. Vomiting　　　　　　　　　　B. Hypokalemia

　　　C. Hypochloridemia　　　　　　　D. Chronic obstructive pulmonary disease

　　　E. All of the above

(3) Which one of the following water-electrolyte imbalances did NOT occur in this patient?

　　　A. Hypokalemia　　　　　　　　　B. Hypernatronemia

　　　C. Hypotonic dehydration　　　　　D. Hypochloridemia

　　　E. Hypertonic dehydration

(4) Which one of the following complications is NOT likely to occur in this patient even when he was not treated in time?

　　　A. Gastrointestinal hemorrhage　　　B. Hepatic encephalopathy

C. Pulmonary encephalopathy          D. Arrhythmia

E. Subarachnoid hemorrhage

(5) Which one of the following treatments is NOT appropriate?

A. Glucose infusion               B. Normal saline infusion

C. Potasssium chloride infusion    D. High-flow oxygen delivery

E. All of the above

## Case analysis questions

- **Case 1**

A 38-yr-old male was admitted to hospital due to recurrent vomiting, intermittent diarrhea, and oliguria in the last 2 weeks. Laboratory analysis showed: pH 7. 54, $PaCO_2$ 6. 8 kPa (52 mmHg), BB 65 mmol/L, BE$^+$12 mmol/L, SB 40 mmol/L, plasma [ K$^+$ ] 3. 1 mmol/L, $\triangle$[ HCO$_3^-$ ]16 mmol/L.

Questions:

(1) What kind of acid-base disturbance did this patient have? Is this disorder in the stage of compensation or decompensation? Why?

(2) What acid-base parameters are changed due to the primary disease in this patient? What acid-base parameters are changed due to the compensation in this patient? What caused the changes of theses parameters?

(3) Why did this patient develop hypokalemia? What is the role of hypokalemia in the development of the acid-base disturbance in this patient?

- **Case 2**

A 55-yr-old female was admitted to the emergency room with 1 day history of abdominal pain in the right lower quadrant and around the colostomy site and markedly reduced oral intake, dry-heaving and shortness of breath. Her past medical history was significant for type I diabetes, diastolic heart failure, chronic pancreatitis and gastroparesis. Her surgical history consisted of having an appendicectomy, cholecystectomy, a whipple procedure, J-tube placement, and a diverting colostomy. The patient noted that she needed to empty her ileostomy bag more frequently over the past several days. She was compliant with taking her insulin, but had not taken it that day. On physical examination, she was normotensive with a heart rate of 87 with tachypnea, normal pulse ox and normothermia. However, she was ill appearing and cachectic. She had dry mucus membranes and had pain over abdomen diffusely without rebound or guarding. Suddenly, she started to be confused. Blood analysis showed that serum glucose of 594 mg/dL, [ Na$^+$ ] 124 mmol/L, [ K$^+$ ] 5. 1 mmol/L, [ Mg$^{2+}$ ] 0. 9 mmol/L, [ Ca$^{2+}$ ] 0. 7 mmol/L, [ Pi] 6. 8 mg/dL (normal 3. 0 – 4. 5 mg/dL), [ Cl$^-$ ] 68 mmol/L, pH 7. 85, $PaCO_2$ 21 mmHg, $PO_2$ 99 mmHg, [ HCO$_3^-$ ] 33 mmol/L, lactate 4. 3 mmol/L (normal 0. 5 – 1. 7 mmol/L), BUN 44 mg/dL, creatinine 3. 9 mg/dL. Liver function test, urinalysis, coagulation profile were unremarkable.

Questions:

(1) What type of acid-base disturbance did this patient have?

(2) What is the pathogenesis of the acid-base disturbance in this patient?

(3) What other functional metabolic changes may have occurred in this patient? What are the underlying mechanisms?

## Answers

### Case-based multiple choice questions (single answer)

1. ADCBDDCA; 2. BCAD; 3. DBECADE; 4. DABCED; 5. CABCAACDA; 6. EAD; 7. EECBE

### Case analysis questions

#### Case 1

(1) What kind of acid-base disturbance did this patient have? Is this disorder in the stage of compensation or decompensation? Why?

This patient had metabolic alkalosis:

① His blood pH (7.54) indicates alkalosis.

② A simple or mixed acid-base disturbance can occur in this patient based on the elevation of both plasma [$HCO_3^-$] and $PaCO_2$.

③ His primary complaints of vomiting and diarrhea could lead to an increase of plasma [$HCO_3^-$].

④ Primary changes of plasma [$HCO_3^-$] induce compensatory hypoventilation. According to the expected compensation [$PaCO_2 = 40 + (0.7 \triangle HCO_3^- \pm 5) = 40 + (0.7 \times 16 \pm 5) = 51.2 \pm 5$], the actual $PaCO_2$ is still within the range of $51.2 \pm 5$, indicating he had a simple metabolic alkalosis.

This patient had decompensated metabolic alkalosis because his blood pH (7.54) is out of the normal range (7.35 − 7.45).

(2) What acid-base parameters are changed due to the primary disease in this patient? What acid-base parameters are changed due to the compensation in this patient? What caused the changes of theses parameters?

The primary changes included elevation of SB and BB as well as the positive value of BE, which were the consequences of massive gastric acid loss and a subsequent increase of [$HCO_3^-$] *in vivo*. Increased $PaCO_2$ was a secondary change due to the impaired respiration and a subsequent decrease of $CO_2$ expiration during the development of metabolic alkalosis.

(3) Why did this patient develop hypokalemia? What was the role of hypokalemia in the development of the acid-base disturbance in this patient?

The pathogenesis of hypokalemia in this patient included:

① Potassium loss from the digestive tract due to vomiting and diarrhea.

② Massive digestive fluid loss can lead to the activation of RAAS and the subsequent release of aldosterone promotes the renal excretion of potassium.

③ $H^+$-$K^+$ exchange in alkalosis stimulated the influx of $K^+$ into cells.

④ A decrease of $H^+$ in the renal tubular epithelial cells reduced $H^+$-$Na^+$ exchange and subsequently enhanced $K^+$-$Na^+$ exchange, thereby leading to massive $K^+$ excretion into urine.

Hypokalemia played an important role in the development of metabolic alkalosis:

① A decrease of $K^+$ in extracellular fluids stimulated $H^+$-$K^+$ exchange and the influx of $H^+$ into cells.

② A decrease of $K^+$ in renal tubular epithelial cells reduced $K^+$-$Na^+$ exchange and subsequently stimulated

$H^+$-$Na^+$ exchange. Increased excretion of $H^+$ from tubular epithelial cells promoted the reabsorption of $HCO_3^-$.

**Case 2**

(1) What type of acid-base disturbance did this patient have?

① According to the Henderson equation, $[H^+] = 24 \times (PaCO_2)/[HCO_3^-] = 24 \times 21/33 = 15.3$, the corresponding pH is 7.81 that is close to 7.85. Thus, the blood gas results in the case are reliable.

② Based on the blood pH (7.85 > 7.45), it is a decompensated alkalosis. The patient had short of breath and a decrease of $PaCO_2$, indicating the development of acute respiratory alkalosis, while elevated plasma $[HCO_3^-]$ maybe due to metabolic alkalosis according to increased frequency of emptying the ileostomy bag. The changes of plasma $[HCO_3^-]$ and $PaCO_2$ are opposite and no compensations result in a decompensated alkalosis.

③ $AG = [Na^+] - ([Cl^-] + [HCO_3^-]) = 124 - (68 + 33) = 23$. Based on $AG > 16$, it is deduced that this patient also had metabolic acidosis.

Therefore, the patient had a triple acid-base disturbance of respiratory alkalosis, metabolic alkalosis, and metabolic acidosis.

(2) What is the pathogenesis of the acid-base disturbance in this patient?

① Respiratory alkalosis: shortness of breath in the patient causes hyperventilation and excessive $CO_2$ excretion, leading to a primary decrease in $PaCO_2$.

② Metabolic alkalosis: the increased frequency of emptying the ileostomy bag suggests the development of diarrhea in this patient. Diarrhea can lead to severe hypokalemia through a gastrointestinal loss of potassium as well as aldosterone-induced renal excretion of potassium. Increased renal excretion is the consequence of decreased effective circulating volume and subsequent RAAS activation. Hypokalemia stimulates the influx of $H^+$ into cells by $H^+$-$K^+$ exchange, while the impaired $K^+$-$Na^+$ exchange in distal tubules increases the excretion of $H^+$ by $H^+$-$Na^+$ exchange. In addition, hypochloremia not only reduces the secretion of $HCO_3^-$ but also increases the excretion of $H^+$ in distal tubule. The subsequent increase of $HCO_3^-$ reabsorption also leads to a primary elevation of $[HCO_3^-]$.

③ Metabolic acidosis: the patient had diabetes mellitus with abnormal glucose metabolism and elevated plasma levels of lactate indicate the accumulation of lactic acid. Moreover, a leftward shift in the hemoglobin oxygen dissociation curve in alkalosis leads to tissue hypoxia and subsequently enhances anaerobic glycolysis and lactic acid production. Therefore, this patient also had a metabolic acidosis with increased AG.

(3) What other functional metabolic changes may have occurred in this patient? What are the underlying mechanisms?

Alkalosis increases the catabolism of the central inhibitory transmitter GABA and induces the subsequent excitation of central nervous system, while leftward shift of the hemoglobin oxygen dissociation curve in alkalosis may lead to cerebral hypoxia. This patient may thus have irritability, confusion, and impaired consciousness. Alkalosis-associated tissue hypoxia may trigger ischemia and hypoxia of gastric mucosa and thereby lead to gastrointestinal hemorrhage. In addition, pH elevation reduces the plasma levels of $Ca^{2+}$ to induce neuromuscular stress, hyperactive tendon reflex, and tetany.

(郑　栋　赵丽梅)

# Chapter 4   Fever

## Case-based multiple choice questions (single answer)

1. A 33-yr-old female was hospitalized due to lobar pneumonia in the third trimester of pregnancy. She had a history of myocarditis. On admission, her BT was 39 ℃ and tended to increase, and HR was 120 beats/min.

(1) Which of the following is most likely to cause fever in this patient?

A. Infection
B. Endocrine metabolic disorder
C. Anaphylaxis
D. Central disturbance of thermoregulation
E. Connective tissue disease

(2) Which of the following is the role of the pneumococcus in the development of fever in this patient?

A. Endogenous pyrogen
B. TNF
C. Antigen-antibody complexes
D. Exogenous pyrogen
E. Leukocyte pyrogen

(3) Which of the following is the feature of thermometabolism in this patient if her BT continued to rise?

A. Heat dissipation > heat production
B. Heat dissipation dysfunction
C. Heat production = heat dissipation
D. Heat production dysfunction
E. Heat production > heat dissipation

(4) Which one of the following was most likely to occur in this patient according to BT?

A. Irregular fever
B. Remittent fever
C. Continued fever
D. Intermittent fever
E. Rheumatic fever

(5) The patient should receive infusion in time to prevent dehydration. Which one of the following contaminations should be noticed to prevent infusion-associated secondary infection?

A. Anaphylaxis
B. Endotoxin contamination
C. Exotoxin contamination
D. Mycoplasma contamination
E. Virus contamination

**2.** A 2-yr-old boy was admitted to hospital after 3-day coughing and 1-day fever with 2 episodes of convulsion. His highest BT was 39.1 ℃ before admission. During convulsion, he had rolling of the eyes back, clenching of the teeth, blue lips, skeletal muscle contraction and rigidity, and loss of consciousness. His parents reported that he was delivered smoothing as a full-term newborn, and developed normally with average intelligence and physical strength. After a series of examinations after admission, he was diagnosed with febrile seizure.

（1）Which of the following is the pathogenesis of febrile seizure in this boy?

A. Excited cerebral cortex and subcortical center

B. Congenital temperature center diseases

C. Dysfunctional thermoregulation

D. Immature central nervous system

E. Inhibited cerebral cortex and subcortical center

（2）Which one of the following disorders might develop immediately if this patient was not given any treatment?

A. Hypotonic dehydration　　　　　B. Respiratory acidosis

C. Renal fluid retention　　　　　　D. Hypertonic dehydration

E. Isotonic dehydration

（3）Which one of the following metabolic changes was NOT likely to occur in this patient?

A. Decreased vitamin consumption　　B. Increased glycogenolysis

C. Increased lipolysis　　　　　　　　D. Negative nitrogen balance

E. Increased metabolic rate

（4）Which one of the following antipyretic drugs can be used to this boy?

A. Deoxycorticosterone　　　　　　B. Diphenhydramine

C. Theophylline　　　　　　　　　　D. cAMP

E. Ibuprofen

**3.** A 79-yr-old man was admitted to hospital due to fever of unknown origin for 1 month. He reported that his BT stayed at about 38 ℃ and was not affected by antipyretic drugs. After admission, his BT rose to 39.1 ℃, and he failed to respond to an anti-inflammatory treatment. PET/CT combined with bone marrow biopsy analysis were performed and he was diagnosed with non-Hodgkin's lymphoma.

（1）Which one of the following cells is the main producer of endogenous pyrogens in this patient?

A. Monocytes　　　　　　　　　　B. Macrophages

C. Tumor cells　　　　　　　　　　D. Stellate cells

E. Endothelial cells

（2）Which one of the following substances is an endogenous pyrogen?

A. PGE　　　　　　　　　　　　　B. MIP-1

C. LPS　　　　　　　　　　　　　D. AVP

E. MAN

（3）Which one of the following treatments can effectively lower the patient's BT?

A. Sodium salicylate

B. Glucocorticoid

C. Nicotinic acid

D. Ice blanket

E. Theophylline

## Case analysis questions

- **Case 1**

A 70-yr-old woman with fever was admitted to the hospital. She caught a cold 2 days ago and then had headache, cough, and fever with poor appetite. She could only eat a small amount of porridge per meal. On admission, physical examinations showed BT of 39 ℃, HR of 80 beats/min, BP of 128/80 mmHg and scattered rales over the left lower lung. She was too weak to walk and transferred to the in-patient department by a wheelchair. She denied any previous medical history.

Questions:

（1）What other examinations should be included for diagnosis and treatment?

（2）What are the causes for fever in this patient? Please briefly describe the involved mechanisms.

（3）Why did this patient have poor appetite?

- **Case 2**

A 68-yr-old man was admitted to hospital because of severe cough and chest pain. He was married and had been retired for a few years. He complained of fever and a cough productive of mucoid sputum for 5 days. He was a smoker and had a 15-yr history of hypertension. Administration of ibuprofen slightly lowered his BT. However, the BT gradually increased to 39 ℃ the next day.

Physical examinations: T 39.5 ℃, P 100 beats/min, R 29 breaths/min, BP 160/82 mmHg.

Lab tests: WBC $12 \times 10^9/L$, neutrophil 75%.

Chest X-ray showed increased bilateral bronchrovascular makings and prominent effusion in the left pleural space.

He was thus preliminarily diagnosed with upper respiratory tract infection with high fever.

Questions:

（1）Should the antipyretics be administrated to this patient timely? Why?

（2）What cardiovascular changes may have occurred in this patient?

（3）What are the metabolic changes in this patient?

（4）What other pathological processes may occur in this patient?

（5）What are potential nursing interventions for this patient?

## Answers

**Case-based multiple choice questions (single answer)**

　　**1**. ADECB; **2**. DDAE; **3**. CBD

**Case analysis questions**

　　**Case 1**

　　(1) What other examinations should be included for diagnosis and treatment?

Blood cell analysis (WBC count and classification, neutrophil counts), urine examination, chest X-ray examination, and sputum culture should be included to determine the pathogen and pulmonary inflammation.

　　(2) What are the causes for fever in this patient? Please briefly describe the involved mechanisms.

Invasion of pyrogenic activator induces massive production of endogenous pyrogens (EP) and subsequent signal transmission to the CNS elevates the set-point of temperature, thereby leading to fever.

　　(3) Why did this patient have poor appetite?

Poor appetite may be due to decreased secretion of digestive juice and reduced activities of various digestive enzymes.

　　**Case 2**

　　(1) Should the antipyretics be administrated to this patient timely? Why?

The patient did need the timely administration of antipyretics due to his BT of 39 ℃ and a history of hypertension. On one hand, high fever for an extended period of time can be dangerous and life-threatening. On the other hand, fever may induce heart failure in hypertensive patients by increase of heart load.

　　(2) What cardiovascular changes may have occurred in this patient?

Elevated blood temperature stimulates sinoatrial node to increase heart rate, while increased plasma levels of LPS and hypothalamic levels of PGE after infection activates sympathetic-adrenal medulla system to speed up heart rate. The heart rate has a direct effect on the cardiac output. However, cardiac output tends to fall when heart rate surpasses 180 beats/min. Moreover, long term complications of hypertension and smoking greatly impair the functions of cardiovascular systems. Upon high fever, aggravation of myocardial overload may induce heart failure in this patient.

　　(3) What are the metabolic changes in this patient?

Increased metabolic demands in high fever enhance the catabolism, which is reflected in the following aspects:

　　① Glucose metabolism: increased glycogen decomposition, elevated blood glucose, and decreased glycogen reservation.

　　② Protein metabolism: increased catabolism, a negative nitrogen balance and elevated blood urea nitrogen.

　　③ Fat metabolism: enhanced fat decomposition was induced by low appetite and insufficient carbohydrate intake. Massive fat decomposition and incomplete oxidation increase the generation of ketone bodies.

　　④ Water, electrolyte and vitamin metabolisms: dehydration was induced by a large loss of water, and vitamin deficiency caused by limited food intake and increased consumption.

　　(4) What other pathological processes may occur in this patient?

　　① Hypertonic dehydration may occur due to the increased water loss via sweat, urine and insensible evaporation from the skin and respiratory tract.

　　② Metabolic acidosis may occur due to the increased generation of lactic acid and ketone bodies.

③ Hyperkalemia may occur due to enhanced catabolism and subsequently increased release of intracellular potassium into the blood.

(5) What are potential nursing interventions for this patient?

① Treatment of underlying diseases.

② Physical cooling includes head ice packs, rubbing alcohol or warm water bath.

③ Administration of antipyretics such as acetaminophen and ibuprofen, etc. to lower body temperature according to the doctor's advices.

④ Drinking more water and taking high calorie liquid/semiliquid diet, and correction of water and electrolyte imbalance by fluid therapy if necessary.

(孙丽娜)

# Chapter 5   Stress

## Case-based multiple choice questions (single answer)

1. A 32-yr-old male chef was sent to the Emergency Department due to a severe cooking oil burn. Physical examinations showed: unconsciousness, T 36.3 ℃, P 143 beats/min, R 36 breaths/min, BP 82/68 mmHg. 4 hours later, the patient awoke with stable vital signs. However, he had 3 episodes of black (tar) watery diarrhea accompanied with abdominal distension in 2 days. His stool occult blood test was strongly positive. He denied any history of stomach diseases.

(1) Which one of the following diseases is most likely to have occurred in this patient?

    A. Essential hypertension         B. Atherosclerosis

    C. Stress ulcer                 D. Bronchial asthma

    E. Coronary heart disease

(2) Which one of the following changes is NOT likely to occur in this patient?

    A. Increased heart rate          B. Increased myocardial contractility

    C. Increased cardiac output      D. Skeletal muscle vasodilation

    E. Renal vasodilation

(3) Which one of the following hormones is most likely to decrease in the patient?

    A. β-endorphin             B. Insulin

    C. Glucagon               D. ADH

    E. Prolactin

（4）Which one of the following mechanisms is NOT involved in the development of symptoms in this patient?

    A. Gastric ischemia

    B. Bile reflux

    C. Increased secretion of gastric mucin

    D. Back-diffusion of $H^+$ into the mucosa

    E. Acidosis

（5）Which one of the following proteins did NOT rapidly change in this patient?

    A. C-reactive protein

    B. Hemopexin

    C. Heat shock protein

    D. Ceruloplasmin

    E. Fibrinogen

**2. A 60-yr-old man was sent to the local hospital because of chest pain aggravated by emotional excitement. He had a 10-year history of hypertension and complained of chest tightness and palpitation for 1 year. On admission, his BP was 160/100 mmHg. The bedside ECG results showed ST segment depression and T wave inversion. He was diagnosed with non-ST segment elevation myocardial infarction.**

（1）Which one of the following mechanisms is mainly involved in the induction of myocardial infarction by emotional excitement in this patient?

    A. Activation of sympathetic-adrenal medulla system

    B. Concentric cardiac hypertrophy

    C. Elevated plasma levels of cholesterol, increased blood viscosity

    D. Activation of renin-angiotensin-aldosterone system（RAAS）

    E. Renal vasoconstriction, water and sodium retention

（2）Which one of the following endocrine glands is most likely to have response in this patient?

    A. Thyroid glands

    B. Adrenal glands

    C. Parathyroid glands

    D. Gonads

    E. Pancreas

（3）Which one of the following cardiovascular changes did this patient have before the onset of myocardial infarction?

    A. Increased ventricular fibrillation threshold

    B. Decreased coronary blood flow

    C. Decreased heart rate and cardiac output

    D. Increased cardiac output and blood pressure

    E. Decreased peripheral resistance

（4）Which one of the following changes is most likely to have occurred in this patient?

    A. Decreased levels of adrenaline

    B. Decreased levels of glucagon

    C. Decreased levels of insulin

    D. Decreased levels of endorphin

    E. Decreased levels of norepinephrine

（5）Which one of the following is the potential mechanism of oliguria in this patient?

    A. Activation of sympathetic-adrenal medulla system

    B. Inhibition of renin-angiotensin-aldosterone system

    C. Increased secretion of atrial natriuretic peptide (ANP)

    D. Activation of hypothalamus-pituitary-adrenal cortex system

    E. Decreased secretion of antidiuretic hormone (ADH)

**3. A 17-yr-old male student at junior 3rd year was hospitalized for psychological treatment due to extreme depression and attempted suicide. He complained of inexplicable depression with loss of interest in daily activities as well as pains and hopelessness over the past year.**

（1）Which one of the metabolic changes may occur in this patient?

    A. Polyuria

    B. Hypoglycemia

    C. Increased plasma levels of free fatty acids

    D. Low blood coagulation

    E. Decreased heart rate

（2）Which one of the following hematological changes may occur in this patient?

    A. Decreased leukocyte count

    B. Reduced levels of coagulation factor Ⅷ

    C. Decreased levels of complement component 3 (C3)

    D. Decreased levels of fibrinogen

    E. Decreased number of red blood cells

（3）Which one of the following digestive changes may occur in this patient?

    A. Decreased secretion of gastric acid    B. Increased gastric blood flow

    C. Decreased secretion of pepsin    D. Gastric mucosal erosion

    E. Increased gastric mucosal repair

（4）Which one of the following renal changes may occur in this patient?

    A. Increased urine output    B. Low urine specific gravity

    C. Proteinuria    D. Decreased glomerular filtration rate

    E. Decreased renal tubular $H^+$ secretion

## Case analysis questions

- **Case 1**

A 50-yr-old man was admitted to hospital for hematemesis and tarry stools. 3 days ago, he was involved in a life-threatening accident in which his boat was overturned and he almost drowned. Afterward he was too agitated to sleep for the following 3 days. He denied any history of stomach diseases. Admission physical examinations showed: T 37.5 ℃, HR 125 beats/min, BP 135/80 mmHg. Laboratory analysis revealed: mild anemia, WBC of $1.5 \times 10^9/L$, normal gastrin, GLU of 10 mmol/L (normal 3. 9 – 6. 0 mmol/L). An esophagogastroduodenoscopy demonstrated an open gastric ulcer with an exposed vessel.

Questions：

(1) Why did this patient have tarry stools? What's the pathogenesis?

(2) What changes of neuroendocrine system may occur in this patient?

- **Case 2**

A 17-yr-old female high-school student accompanied by her mother was admitted to hospital. She complained of nervousness, insomnia, and mind blanking during exams. Her mother indicated that this girl had an excellent academic performance and a cheerful personality since childhood. However, with the increasing study pressure and high self-demanding after admission to a key middle school, she became more diligent and aimed to get into a prestigious university. In order to improve her scores, she had no time for all her hobbies. Even so, as the college entrance examination ( CEE ) was approaching, she gradually had nervousness, insomnia, weight loss, irritability and preferred to be alone most of the time with declining academic performance. Moreover, she had a " stomachache" just before each exam, but no abnormality was found upon examination in the hospital.

After communication with the psychologist, she adjusted her learning goals and made a reasonable allocation of leisure time, study and rest. All her symptoms gradually disappeared in half a year.

Questions：

(1) Why did this patient have abnormal physical and psychological manifestations?

(2) Please discuss the potential mechanisms of neuroendocrine changes in this patient.

(3) Please discuss the pathogenesis of "stomachache" in this patient before each exam.

## Answers

**Case-based multiple choice questions ( single answer)**

1. CEBCC；2. ABDCA；3. CEDD

**Case analysis questions**

**Case 1**

(1) Why did this patient have tarry stools? What's the pathogenesis?

This patient suffered stress ulcer as the psychophysical stress he experienced the life-threatening boat accident was so enormous that he was extremely agitated and could hardly sleep. Gastric erosion and bleeding leads to the formation of tarry stools.

The pathogenesis of stress ulcer includes：

① Decreased mucosal blood flow and ischemia：strong activation of locus ceruleus-norepinephrine ( LC-NE) system induced mucosal ischemia is the basic cause for gastric erosions, ulcer and bleeding.

② Breakdown of normal mucosal defense abilities：mucosal ischemia decreases the production of ATP and impairs the production of bicarbonate and mucus. The back-diffusion of $H^+$ into mucosa is increased and causes more lesions.

③ Bile juice reflux or free radicals may also been involved in the ischemic mucosal injury.

（2）What changes of neuroendocrine system may occur in this patient?

① Activation of LSAM system: stress induced activation of LSAM system produces significant cognitive and emotional effects, including excitement, alertness, nervousness and anxiety. Also, activation of LSAM system leads to a rapid increase in plasma levels of epinephrine and norepinephrine.

② Activation of HPAC system: during the stress, the hypothalamus produces corticotrophin-releasing hormone (CRH) acts on other areas within the brain where it suppresses appetite, increases anxiety, and improves memory and selective attention. Also, CRH stimulates pituitary gland to secrete adrenocorticotropin hormone (ACTH), then stimulates the adrenal glands to make and release glucocorticoid into blood. CRH also stimulates the release of endorphins from hypothalamus and pituitary.

③ Activation of RAAS: increased plasma levels of aldosterone, BP elevation, oliguria, and blood volume maintenance are the consequences of RAAS activation.

**Case 2**

（1）Why did this patient have abnormal physical and psychological manifestations?

This girl had a lot of physical and psychological symptoms, including nervousness, insomnia, weight loss, irritability, and mind blanking during exams. That is due to excessive psychological stress induced by study pressure and high self-demanding.

（2）Please discuss the potential mechanisms of neuroendocrine changes in this patient.

① Excitation of sympathetic-adrenal-medulla system: overactivation of NE neurons in locus-ceruleus and subsequent overproduction of NE →patients had bad emotions, such as anxiety and fear.

② Excitation of hypothalamic pituitary adrenocortical system→ overactivation of paraventricular nucleus (PVN) to release CRH→excessive CRH caused general adaptation disorder, such as anxiety, depression, learning and memory ability, anorexia, etc.

（3）Please discuss the pathogenesis of "stomachache" in this patient before each exam.

The stomachache may be a sign of a functional gastrointestinal disease without morphological and biochemical abnormalities. That is due to the neuroendocrine dysfunction induced by the long-term mental stress, excessive anxiety and depression.

（孙丽娜）

# Chapter 6　Hypoxia

## Case-based multiple choice questions（single answer）

**1. A female patient had a test on her blood oxygen levels. It showed $PaO_2$ value was 98 mmHg, $CO_2$ max was 13 mL/dL, $CaO_2$ was 15 mL/dL, and $C(a\text{-}v)O_2$ was 3 mL/dL.**

（1）Which one of the following disorders is most likely to have occurred in this patient?

　　A. Asthma　　　　　　　　　　B. Anemia

    C. Vitamin $B_1$ deficiency      D. Carbon monoxide poisoning

    E. Myocardial hypertrophy

（2）Which one of the mechanisms is crucial for the development of hypoxia in this patient?

    A. Increased capillary mean $PaO_2$      B. Decreased $CaO_2$

    C. Increased $CO_2$ max      D. Decreased $PaO_2$

    E. Decreased tissue blood flow

（3）Which one of the following metabolic changes may develop in this patient?

    A. Metabolic alkalosis      B. Decreased intracellular $[Na^+]$

    C. Enhanced aerobic oxidation      D. Enhanced glycolysis

    E. Enhanced oxygen consumption

（4）Which one of the following cellular changes may occur response to hypoxia in the patient?

    A. Increased lysosomal membrane permeability

    B. Outflow of intracellular $[K^+]$

    C. Decrease of intracellular $[Na^+]$

    D. Increased amount of mitochondria

    E. Decreased capillary density

**2. A 18-yr-old boy traveled to Tibet with his classmates after the college entrance examination (CEE). When they reached the altitudes over 4,000 meters, he was so excited that he could not help jumping around. Due to hyperventilation, he showed general numbness and limb twitching, followed by fainting. He recovered after treatment in the local hospital.**

（1）Which type of hypoxia is most likely to have occurred in this patient?

    A. Hemic hypoxia      B. Ischemic hypoxia

    C. Hypoxic hypoxia      D. Histogenous hypoxia

    E. Congestive hypoxia

（2）Which one of the following cardiovascular compensatory responses is NOT likely to develop in this patient?

    A. Increased HR      B. Increased myocardial contractility

    C. Cardiac and cerebral vasodilation      D. Increased venous return

    E. Pulmonary vasodilation

（3）Which one of the following mechanisms is NOT involved in the development of fainting in this patient?

    A. Insufficient ATP production in brain cells

    B. Dehydration of brain cells

    C. Increased cerebral microvascular permeability

    D. Decreased nerve cell membrane potential

    E. Nerve cell destruction

（4）Which one of the following changes might occur in this patient?

    A. Excited sympathetic system, decreased cardiac output

    B. Dehydration of brain cells, clear mental symptoms

    C. Increased myocardial contractility, adenosine production, and contraction of coronary arteries

    D. Pulmonary vasoconstriction, increased pulmonary artery pressure

    E. Increased EPO synthesis and significantly elevated levels of RBC and Hb

**3. A resident patient Li had a blood gas analysis and the results showed: $PaO_2$ 85 mmHg, $PvO_2$ 60 mmHg, $CO_2$max 10.8 mL/dL, $SaO_2$ 97%, and $C(a\text{-}v)O_2$ 2.8 mL/dL.**

（1）Which one of the following statements is NOT true about blood oxygen parameters in the patient?

    A. $CO_2$max depends on Hb concentration and Hb oxygen affinity

    B. $SaO_2$ is independent of Hb concentration

    C. $PaO_2$ depends on the inspired $PO_2$

    D. $CO_2$ refers to the actual volume of $O_2$ carried in each 100 mL blood

    E. Normal $C(a\text{-}v)O_2$ is 5 mL/dL

（2）Which type of hypoxia did this patient have?

    A. Hypotonic hypoxia                B. Hemic hypoxia

    C. Circulatory hypoxia             D. Histogenous hypoxia

    E. Mixed hypoxia

（3）If hypoxia was not corrected timely, which one of the following ion changes might occur in this patient?

    A. Increased intracellular $[Na^+]$       B. Decreased extracellular $[K^+]$

    C. Decreased intracellular $[Ca^{2+}]$     D. Decreased extracellular $[H^+]$

    E. Decreased intracellular $[H^+]$

（4）Which one of the following statements is correct about the metabolic changes in this patient?

    A. Significantly increased respiration and pulmonary ventilation

    B. Cerebral vasoconstriction

    C. Blood transfusion should be given immediately

    D. Cherry-red discoloration of the skin and mucous membranes

    E. The patient improved significantly after hyperbaric oxygen treatment

**4. A 6-month-old baby was admitted to hospital due to shortness of breath and cyanosis after crying. She was finally diagnosed as congenital heart disease (tetralogy of Fallot).**

（1）Which one of the following changes caused cyanosis in this baby?

    A. An increase of hemoglobin        B. An increase of carboxyhemoglobin

    C. An increase of methemoglobin     D. An increase of deoxyhemoglobin

    E. An increase of cyanohemoglobin

（2）Which kind of hypoxia caused the cyanosis in this baby?

    A. Hypoxic hypoxia

    B. Hemic hypoxia

    C. Circulatory hypoxia

    D. Histogenous hypoxia

    E. Mixed hypoxia

（3）Which one of the following mechanisms is involved in the development of hypoxia in this baby?

    A. Decreased inspired $PO_2$

    B. Decreased Hb count

    C. Systemic circulatory dysfunction

    D. Mitochondrial injury

    E. Venous admixture

（4）Which one of the following changes in blood oxygen levels was NOT likely to occur in this baby?

    A. Decreased $PaO_2$

    B. Decreased $SaO_2$

    C. Decreased $CaO_2$ max

    D. Decreased $CaO_2$

    E. Decreased $C(a\text{-}v)O_2$

（5）Which one of the following treatments is NOT right for this patient?

    A. Calmness

    B. Lying flat

    C. Oxygen inhalation

    D. Palliative surgery

    E. Prostaglandin therapy

**5. A 22-yr-old female was sent to the emergency room because of a severe pain in the left upper abdomen after a traffic accident. Admission physical examinations showed paleness, BP 80/40 mmHg, P 125 beats/min, and R 26 breaths/min. Abdominal CT demonstrated rupture of spleen and massive bleeding in abdominal cavity. She was diagnosed with spleen rupture and hemorrhagic shock.**

（1）Which kind of hypoxia is most likely to occur in this patient?

    A. Hypoxic hypoxia

    B. Hemic hypoxia

    C. Circulatory hypoxia

    D. Histogenous hypoxia

    E. All of the above

（2）Which one of the following blood oxygen levels may change in this patient?

    A. Decreased $PaO_2$

    B. Decreased $SaO_2$

    C. Decreased $CaO_2$ max

    D. Decreased $CaO_2$

    E. Increased $C(a\text{-}v)O_2$

（3）Which one of the following descriptions is NOT correct about hypoxia in this patient?

    A. Normal external respiratory function without the decrease of $PaO_2$ and $SaO_2$

    B. Ischemia hypoxia in peripheral tissues

    C. No cyanosis due to reduced cellular oxygen uptake

    D. A right shift of the oxygen-Hb dissociation curve after tissue hypoxia.

    E. Unchanged quantity and quality of Hb in this patient

（4）Which kind of hypoxia may occur after massive transfusion in this patient?

　　A. Hypotonic and hemic hypoxia　　　B. Hemic and circulatory hypoxia

　　C. Circulatory and hypotonic hypoxia　　D. Histogenous and hypotonic hypoxia

　　E. Histogenous and hemic hypoxia

**6. A 6-yr-old boy was sent to the emergency room by his parents because of headache and weakness after eating a pot of pork stew with pickled vegetable at dinner. The patient looked blue and showed obvious cyanosis. After blood analysis, he was diagnosed with nitrite poisoning.**

（1）Which one of the following hypoxia is most likely to have occurred in this patient?

　　A. Hypoxic hypoxia　　　　　　　B. Hemic hypoxia

　　C. Circulatory hypoxia　　　　　　D. Histogenous hypoxia

　　E. All of the above

（2）Which one of the following changes caused cyanosis in this patient?

　　A. An increase of hemoglobin　　　B. An increase of carboxyhemoglobin

　　C. An increase of methemoglobin　　D. An increase of deoxyhemoglobin

　　E. An increase of cyanohemoglobin

（3）Which one of the following changes about blood oxygen levels is NOT likely to occur in this patient?

　　A. Decreased $PaO_2$　　　　　　　B. Decreased $SaO_2$

　　C. Decreased $CaO_2 max$　　　　　D. Decreased $CaO_2$

　　E. Decreased $C(a\text{-}v)O_2$

（4）Which one of the following treatments is essential for this patient?

　　A. Toxin removal by emetics and gastric lavage

　　B. Increase of $PaO_2$ by the oxygen therapy

　　C. Treatment of methemoglobinemia

　　D. Toxin removal by drinking water and fluid infusion

　　E. None of the above

## Case analysis questions

- **Case 1**

A 67-yr-old woman was admitted to hospital because of cough with copious phlegm, worsening dyspnea for 3 days. She started to have recurrent cough with expectoration 15 years ago, and developed progressive worsening dyspnea. She complained to get cold 2 days ago, followed by fever, chills, cough with thick sputum, wheezing, and difficult breathing when lying down at night.

Physical examinations demonstrated blue lips and fingernails, T 39.0 ℃, P 120 beats/min, R 28 breaths/min, a slight barrel chest and widening of the intercostal spaces, bilateral rough breath sounds with rhonchi, decreased breath sounds in the right lower lungs on auscultation.

Arterial blood gas analysis showed: pH 7. 14, $PaO_2$ 50 mmHg, $PaCO_2$ 80 mmHg, decreased values of AB, SB and BB, AG 18 mmol/L, $[K^+]$ 6. 6 mmol/L, $[Na^+]$ 140 mmol/L, $[Cl^-]$ 92 mmol/L.

She was preliminarily diagnosed with chronic obstructive pulmonary disease (COPD), and greatly improved after oxygen therapy.

Questions:

(1) What type of hypoxia did this patient have? Please describe the alterations of blood oxygen levels and the typical manifestations of hypoxia in this patient.

(2) What are the significance and principles of oxygen therapy for this patient?

(3) What type of acid-base disturbance did this patient have? What are the causes and pathogenesis?

- **Case 2**

A 12-yr-old male patient named Zhang in a coma was sent to hospital by his family. 1 hour ago, he was found lying down unconsciously in the bathroom. On admission, the patient showed convulsed limbs and gatism, and received urinary catheterization, fluid infusion and oxygen therapy.

Diagnosis: severe carbon monoxide poisoning.

He regained consciousness and physical examinations showed: T 36. 5 ℃, P 110 beats/min, BP 110/62 mmHg and $SaO_2$ 100%. Hyperbaric oxygen therapy was performed to prevent/alleviate brain edema, and nutritional therapy helps the patient in recovery.

Questions:

(1) What type of hypoxia did this patient have? Please describe the alterations of blood oxygen levels and the typical manifestations of hypoxia in this patient.

(2) Why did this patient receive hyperbaric oxygen therapy (HOT)?

(3) Please analyze the reason why the patient is easy to have brain edema.

## Answers

**Case-based multiple choice questions (single answer)**

1. BBDD; **2.** CEBD; **3.** CEAC; **4.** DAECB; **5.** CECB; **6.** BCAC

**Case analysis questions**

**Case 1**

(1) What type of hypoxia did this patient have? Please describe the alterations of blood oxygen levels and the typical manifestations of hypoxia in this patient.

Airway obstruction in chronic obstructive pulmonary disease (COPD) significantly reduces the alveolar ventilation, thereby leading to low $PaO_2$ and hypotonic hypoxia. This patient showed cyanosis as the increased level of deoxyhemoglobin in capillary exceed 5 g/dL. The characteristics of blood oxygen levels include decreased $PaO_2$ (50 mmHg < 100 mmHg), $CO_2$ and $SaO_2$, increased $CO_2$max, and no acute changes of $C(a\text{-}v)O_2$.

（2）What are the significance and principles of oxygen therapy for the patient?

Oxygen therapy has multiple effects on patients with hypotonic hypoxia, including the increase of $PaO_2$ and $SaO_2$ by elevating alveolar $PO_2$, reduction of tissue injury, restoration of organ functions, as well as the decrease of the right ventricular load by alleviating hypoxic pulmonary hypertension.

Different oxygen concentration and delivery methods should be chosen according to the diseases treated and blood oxygen levels. In principle, delivered oxygen concentrations should be low enough to rapidly raise $PaO_2$ to 60 mmHg or $SpO_2$ to 90%.

（3）What type of acid-base disturbance did this patient have? What are the causes and pathogenesis?

According to the underlying disease (COPD), decreased $PaO_2$, increased $PaCO_2$, decreased AB, SB and BB, and a significant decrease of pH, it can be preliminarily concluded that the patient had respiratory acidosis complicated with metabolic acidosis. Despite AG > 16, decreased AB, SB and BB together with normal plasma levels of $Cl^-$ indicate the absence of metabolic alkalosis. Sustained low levels of $PaO_2$ due to long-term hypotonic hypoxia increase anaerobic glycolysis for accumulations of acidic substances, thereby resulting in the increase of AG and the decrease of AB, SB and BB. COPD impairs pulmonary ventilation and elimination of $CO_2$ and thereby increases $PaCO_2$.

**Case 2**

（1）What type of hypoxia did this patient have? Please describe the alterations of blood oxygen levels and the typical manifestations of hypoxia in this patient.

The patient had hemic hypoxia as increased HbCO reduces the ability of blood to carry oxygen. The analysis of blood oxygen levels may show decreased $CO_2$ max, $CaO_2$, and $C(a\text{-}v)$ $O_2$, despite normal $PaO_2$ and $SaO_2$. Increased plasma levels of HbCO results in cherry-red discoloration of the skin and mucous membranes.

（2）Why did this patient receive hyperbaric oxygen therapy (HOT)?

Despite no effects on functions of the respiratory system in patients with hemic hypoxia, HOT can improve the tissue hypoxia and reduce cell damage, especially brain cell damage, through increasing the blood oxygen binding capacity and brain oxygen content. Moreover, HOT can accelerate the metabolism of the body and the elimination of carbon monoxide.

（3）Please analyze the reason why the patient is easy to have brain edema.

① Hypoxia causes cerebral vasodilation and increases cerebral blood flow, thereby resulting in fluid leakage and brain edema.

② Hypoxia suppresses energy metabolism in cells and subsequent ATP deficiency impairs sodium pump, thereby leading to water and sodium retention in brain cells.

③ Hypoxia damages the cerebral endothelial cells to increase endothelial permeability, thereby resulting in brain edema.

（孙丽娜）

# Chapter 7　Shock

## Case-based multiple choice questions (single answer)

**1. An 8-yr-old boy presented with an itchy rash, palpitation, dizziness, cyanosis, and dyspnea 1 hour after vaccination.**

(1) Which one of pathological processes may have occurred in this boy?

    A. Septic shock
    B. Hypovolemic shock

    C. Cardiogenic shock
    D. Neurogenic shock

    E. Anaphylactic shock

(2) Which one of the following drugs should be given to this boy when the type of shock was determined?

    A. Vasoconstrictors
    B. Adrenocortical hormones

    C. Vasodilators and fluid infusion
    D. Correction of acidosis

    E. Antibiotics

(3) Which one of the following changes in blood pressure did this boy have?

    A. Increased systolic pressure
    B. Increased diastolic pressure

    C. Significantly decreased BP
    D. No significant change

    E. Decreased pulse pressure

(4) Which one of the following alterations is crucial for the onset of shock in this boy?

    A. Decreased blood volume

    B. Cardiac pump dysfunction

    C. Increased capacity of the vascular bed

    D. Increased capacity of the vascular bed + decreased blood volume

    E. Cardiac pump dysfunction + increased capacity of the vascular bed

**2. A 65-yr-old man with 15 years of coronary heart disease, suddenly developed chest pain, chest tightness, tachypnea during sleep in the early morning. He complained of weakness, sweating, palpitations, and cold extremities with blood pressure of 60/40 mmHg.**

(1) What type of shock did this patient have?

    A. Septic shock
    B. Hemorrhagic shock

    C. Traumatic shock
    D. Cardiogenic shock

    E. Anaphylactic shock

（2）Which one of the following acid-base disturbance may have occurred in this patient?

    A.  Metabolic acidosis and respiratory alkalosis

    B.  Respiratory acidosis

    C.  Metabolic alkalosis

    D.  Metabolic alkalosis and respiratory acidosis

    E.  Metabolic alkalosis and respiratory alkalosis

（3）Which one of the following alterations is crucial for the onset of shock in this patient?

    A.  Decreased blood volume           B.  Cardiac pump dysfunction

    C.  Increased vascular bed volume      D.  Increased blood volume

    E.  Peripheral vasoconstriction

（4）Which one of the following mechanisms is involved in the decrease of blood pressure in this patient?

    A.  Decreased blood volume           B.  Increased vascular bed volume

    C.  Decreased cardiac output          D.  Pulmonary circulation stasis

    E.  Peripheral vasoconstriction

**3. A 31-yr-old woman with postpartum hemorrhage had confusion, cyanosis, petechiae and purpura on the skin. She had a 24-hour urine output of 280 mL. Her blood pressure was 80/55 mmHg, and slightly recovered after treatment with vasoconstrictors.**

（1）Which stage of shock was this patient at?

    A.  Microcirculatory ischemic hypoxia stage

    B.  Microcirculatory stagnant hypoxia stage

    C.  Microcirculatory failure stage

    D.  Compensatory stage

    E.  Refractory stage

（2）Which one of the following microcirculatory alterations is most likely to occur in this patient?

    A.  Inflow ↓ , outflow ↑ , inflow < outflow, ischemic hypoxia

    B.  Inflow ↓ , outflow ↓ , inflow < outflow, ischemic hypoxia

    C.  Inflow ↑ , outflow ↓ , inflow > outflow, stagnant hypoxia

    D.  No inflow, no outflow, blood hypercoagulation, and no blood supply

    E.  Disseminated intravascular coagulation

（3）Which one of the following changes in vascular resistance is most likely to occur in this patients?

    A.  Increased precapillary resistance and postcapillary resistance

    B.  Decreased precapillary resistance and postcapillary resistance

    C.  Higher precapillary resistance than postcapillary resistance

    D.  Higher postcapillary resistance than precapillary resistance

    E.  Increased precapillary resistance and decreased postcapillary resistance

（4）Which one of the following mechanisms is involved in the development of cyanosis and purpura in this patient?

    A. Skin vasoconstriction

    B. Blood stasis in skin with increased plasma levels of deoxyhemoglobin

    C. Decreased plasma levels of deoxyhemoglobin

    D. Capillary plasma extravasation

    E. Significantly decreased blood pressure

## Case analysis questions

### • Case 1

A 45-yr-old woman was brought to the Emergency Deparment one night by her family because of bleeding for the whole day. She presented with pallor, cold sweats, wet and cold extremities, anxiety, accelerated and deepened breathing, and oliguria. On that morning, she noticed bright red blood in her stool. She thought it was hemorrhoids and continued her regular daily activities. On admission physical examinations, her BP was 105/85 mmHg, and HR was 100 beats/min.

The patient was infused with saline, and blood crossmatching was taken for blood transfusion. Colonoscopy showed that the bleeding from a hernia in colon was spontaneously stopped. Due to massive blood loss, the patient was hospitalized and 400 mL of blood was transfused. In the next morning, she improved without cold sweats. Her skin color, breathing, BP and HR turned to normal.

Questions:

（1）Did the patient have shock? Please analyze the etiology and type of shock in this patient.

（2）What are stages of shock? Which stage was this patient at when admitted to hospital? What are the characteristics of microcirculatory perfusion at this stage?

（3）Why did the arterial BP not drop significantly in this patient with bleeding for a whole day?

（4）Why did the patient show pallor, cold sweats, and oliguria?

### • Case 2

An 18-yr-old man was admitted to hospital with fever and rash on extremities. On admission, the physical examinations showed: T 39.5 ℃, HR 120 beats/min, and BP 90/40 mmHg. The arterial blood gas analysis showed: pH 7.30, $[HCO_3^-]$ 16 mmol/L, $PaCO_2$ 26 mmHg, and elevated lactate (3.5 mmol/L). The chest radiograph showed bilateral interstitial and alveolar pulmonary infiltrates. Staining of cerebrospinal fluid smear suggested the presence of Gram-negative cocci, *Neisseria meningitidis* was found to grow in later cultures of blood and cerebrospinal fluid samples. After hospitalization, the patient was treated with intravenous fluids, broad-spectrum antibiotics, and dopamine. The dose of dopamine and normal saline infusion was increased, and epinephrine was given to correct persistent hypotension and oliguria. The patient's mean arterial pressure and urine output gradually increased. He improved with the decreased arterial levels of lactate 12 hours later.

Questions:

(1) Did the patient have shock? Please analyze the etiology, type, and primum movens of shock in this patient.

(2) What are the mechanisms underlying the increase of pulse pressure in this patient?

(3) Based on the blood gas analysis, please analyze the type of acid-base disturbance that this patient had.

(4) What are the mechanisms underlying the elevation of lactate in this patient?

## Answers

### Case-based multiple choice questions (single answer)

1. EACD; 2. DABC; 3. BCDB

### Case analysis questions

#### Case 1

(1) Did the patient have shock? Please analyze the etiology and type of shock in this patient.

The patient showed early manifestations of shock due to blood loss including pallor, cold sweat, wet and cold extremities, anxiety, deepened and accelerated respiration, slightly lowered blood pressure, reduced pulse pressure, accelerated heart rate, reduced urine output, and the patient's symptoms disappeared after being treated with blood and fluid transfusion after admission, so it can be judged that the patient developed shock. The etiology of the patient was decreased blood volume due to persistent bleeding from a hernia in colon. According to etiology, she had hemorrhagic shock. According to primum movens, she was experiencing hypovolemic shock.

(2) What are stages of shock? Which stage was this patient at when admitted to hospital? What are the characteristics of microcirculatory perfusion at this stage?

There are three stages of shock: microcirculatory ischemic hypoxia stage (compensatory stage), microcirculatory stagnant hypoxia stage (decompensatory stage) and microcirculatory failure stage (refractory stage). The patient's symptoms and signs were consistent with the clinical manifestations of the compensatory stage. She didn't have purpura and cyanosis. Her blood pressure didn't drop significantly and she was conscious. So the patient was at the compensatory stage of shock. The characteristics of microcirculatory perfusion at the compensatory stage of shock include less inflow, less outflow, inflow < outflow, and ischemic hypoxia.

(3) Why did the arterial BP not drop significantly in this patient with bleeding for a whole day?

The patient was at the compensatory stage of shock. The decrease of blood volume after bleeding induced activation of sympathetic system and increased release of vasoconstrictors, thereby leading to:

① Contraction of volume vessels and blood storage organs such as liver and spleen to increase the venous return through "auto-blood transfusion".

② Higher precapillary versus postcapillary vasoconstriction to reduce capillary hydrostatic pressure and subsequently increased venous return through "auto-fluid infusion".

③ Contraction of resistance vessels to increase peripheral resistance.

④ Activation of β-receptors in cardiomyocytes to increase heart rate, myocardial contractility, and cardiac output. Increased venous return, peripheral resistance, and cardiac output contributed to the maintenance of arterial blood pressure.

(4) Why did the patient show pallor, cold sweats, and oliguria?

Blood loss induced activation of the sympathetic adrenomedullary system and the renin-angiotensin-aldosterone system (RAAS), leading to peripheral vasoconstriction, with more significant responses in skin and kidney. Skin ischemia led to pallor and cold extremities, while decreased blood perfusion of kidneys reduced the urine output. In addition, sympathetic activation stimulated sweat gland secretion cold sweat.

**Case 2**

(1) Did the patient have shock? Please analyze the etiology, type, and primum movens of shock in this patient.

This patient was in shock as he had hypotension, oliguria, acidosis, and other signs of reduced effective circulating blood volume and tissue blood hypoperfusion. He had septic shock as evidenced by fever and the growth of *Neisseria meningitidis* in his blood and cerebrospinal fluid cultures. The primum movens of septic shock involve:

① Cytokines and vasoactive substances increased capillary permeability, resulting in plasma extravasation and reduced blood volume.

② Vasoactive substances caused vasodilation and increased the peripheral vascular bed volume.

③ Bacterial toxins and inflammatory mediators can directly damage cardiomyocytes and lead to cardiac dysfunction.

(2) What are the mechanisms underlying the increase of pulse pressure in this patient?

Septic shock activates the sympathetic adrenomedullary system and enhances myocardial contractility via β-receptors, thereby maintaining systolic BP. Meanwhile, massive production of inflammatory mediators and vasodilators reduces peripheral resistance and diastolic BP more significantly. Therefore, the pulse pressure that is the difference between systolic and diastolic BP increases.

(3) Based on the blood gas analysis, please analyze the type of acid-base disturbance that this patient had.

This patient had metabolic acidosis due to septic shock with altered blood gas analysis including pH 7.30, the decreased levels of $HCO_3^-$, and increased plasma levels of lactate. According to the predicted compensatory formula for metabolic acidosis, predicted $PaCO_2 = 1.5 \times [HCO_3^-] + 8 \pm 2 = 32 \pm 2$. However, the actual $PaCO_2$ of this patient (26 mmHg) is out of this range, indicating that the development of respiratory alkalosis. Therefore, he had a mixed disorder with metabolic acidosis and respiratory alkalosis.

(4) What are the mechanisms underlying the elevation of lactate in this patient?

In shock, ischemia and hypoxia stimulate anaerobic glycolysis and increase production of lactic acid, while impaired hepatic and renal functions decrease the metabolism and elimination of lactic acid, respectively.

(赵丽梅)

# Chapter 8　Disturbances of Hemostasis

## Case based multiple choice questions (single answer)

1. A 56-yr-old man complained of cough and chest pain for 5 days and yellow purulent sputum for 3 days. Physical examination showed: T 39 ℃, HR 96 beats/min, R 24 breaths/ min, BP 129/85 mmHg, noisy breathing sound, moist rales from the right lower lobe of lung, and large ecchymotic lesions on both lower limbs. Laboratory examination revealed: WBC $22 \times 10^9$/L, Hb 94 g/L (normal 120 – 160 g/L), PLT $100 \times 10^9$/L. APTT 48. 2 s (control 30.2 s), PT 19.5 s(control 14.2 s), TT 35.6 s (control 12.8 s), Fg 1.6 g/L (normal 1.8 – 4.5 g/L). X-ray showed thickened lung markings on both sides and patchy shadow in the right lower lobe of lung.

(1) If the doctor wants to make sure whether this patient has DIC, which one of the following laboratory values is required?

　　A. Circulating WBC count

　　C. Plasma levels of D-dimer

　　E. APTT

　　B. Results of platelet function tests

　　D. Platelet count

(2) If the patient was diagnosed with DIC, which one of the following blood coagulation states is likely to occur in the development of DIC?

　　A. Hypercoagulability

　　B. Hypocoagulability

　　C. Hypercoagulability followed by hypocoagulability

　　D. Hypocoagulability followed by hypercoagulability

　　E. No obvious changes

(3) If the patient was diagnosed with DIC, which one of the following statements is NOT correct?

　　A. Pulmonary infection is the cause of DIC

　　B. Large ecchymotic lesions on both lower limbs indicate local bleeding

　　C. The decrease of PLT is involved in the formation of ecchymosis in this patient

　　D. The coagulation tests showed the reduction of coagulation factors in this patient

　　E. The decrease of Fg had no contribution to the formation of ecchymosis

(4) If the patient was diagnosed with DIC, which one of the following emergent treatments should NOT be included?

　　A. Anti-shock therapy

B. Anti-infection therapy

C. Infusion of fresh frozen plasma

D. Administration of low molecular weight heparin

E. Supplement with coagulation factors

**2. A 49-yr-old female with blurred consciousness was admitted to hospital. She complained of high fever and chills for 1 week and oliguria for 3 days. Physical examination showed: T 39. 6 ℃, HR 129 beats/min, R 28 breaths/min, BP 79/55 mmHg. She had multiple scattered petechiae and ecchymosis in the skin. Laboratory examination revealed: WBC 27 × 10^9/L, Hb 88 g/L, PT 21 s(control 13.5 s), Fg 1.4 g/L (normal 1.8 − 4.5 g/L), DD > 1.0 mg/L (control < 0.5 mg/L). Peripheral blood smear showed schistocytes. The growth of *Escherichia coli* was detected in blood culture. Intracranial subarachnoid hemorrhage was detected by MRI. Thus, she was diagnosed as *Escherichia coli* septicemia complicated with DIC.**

(1) Which one of the following diseases is the cause of DIC in this patient?

A. Malignant tumor
B. Obstetric accident

C. Metabolic diseases
D. Major surgical trauma

E. Infectious diseases

(2) Which one of the following manifestations is NOT due to DIC in this patient?

A. Shivering, high fever
B. Oliguria

C. Anemia
D. Ecchymosis

E. Confusion

(3) Which one of the following mechanisms is NOT involved in the bleeding of this patient?

A. Coagulation disorders

B. Fibrinolytic system activation

C. Formation of fibrin degradation products

D. Myelosuppression

E. Microvascular injury

(4) Which one of the following changes is associated with schistocytes in this patient with DIC?

A. Anemia
B. Bleeding

C. Shock
D. Renal failure

E. Sheehan syndrome

(5) Which one of the following is NOT true about schistocytes on peripheral blood smear of this patient?

A. Schistocytes are circulating red blood cell fragments

B. Schistocytes are of similar shape

C. Schistocytes are fragile

D. The filaments of fibrin in the microvessels lead to the formation of schistocytes

E. Schistocytes indicate that anemia in this patient is due to hemolysis

**3.** A 37-yr-old woman at 39 weeks' gestation who was experiencing irregular contractions of the uterus for 1 hour was admitted to the hospital. She had given birth to a healthy baby girl 5 years ago. At admission, the patient's HR was 70 beats/min, BP was 110/80 mmHg, respiratory rate was 18 breaths/min, and oxygen saturation was 98% on room air. Laboratory examination showed unremarkable results from platelet, hemoglobin, routine coagulation, liver and renal functions tests and normal D-dimer, and fibrin degradation products. The fetal heart rate was 150 beats/min. Within 4 hours after admission, the patient experienced a spontaneous rupture of the membranes. The amniotic fluid was clear and the cervix was dilated 10 cm. After 10 minutes, the patient complained of dyspnea, dysphoria and exhibited cyanosis of her lips. Her BP dropped to 98/60 mmHg, HR increased to 120 beats/min. The fetal heart rate dropped to 70 beats/min. Alive, 3 150 g female infant was immediately delivered by forceps and subsequently transferred to the neonatal intensive care unit (ICU). Approximately 20 minutes until the expulsion of the placenta, completing the delivery, at this time, large amounts of unclotted blood flowed from her vagina. Her blood loss was 2 100 mL, her BP dropped to 40/20 mmHg, and her HR was 156 beats/min. She was unconsciousness and exhibited pale lips and extreme dyspnea. She was thus transferred to ICU and received intravenous transfusions of red blood cell suspensions, fresh frozen plasma, hemostatic drugs, large amounts of colloidal and crystalline solutions. She was placed on a ventilator, and hemofiltration and various support measures were carried out. Laboratory analysis revealed: Hb 54 g/L, PLT $67 \times 10^9$/L, APTT > 180 s(control 30.2 s), PT 40 s(control 14.2 s), DD > 20 μg/mL, FDP > 120 μg/mL. She was diagnosed as amniotic fluid embolism complicated with DIC.

(1) What type of DIC did this patient have?

A. Acute compensated DIC

B. Acute decompensated DIC

C. Acute overcompensated DIC

D. Acute consumptive hypocoagulable DIC

E. Acute hyperfibrinolytic DIC

(2) Which one of the following mechanisms is essential for the development of DIC in this patient?

A. The release tissue factor releases activates and initiates coagulation

B. Endotoxin damages endothelial cells

C. Leukocytes are massive damaged

D. Platelet primary activation occurs

E. Primary acute hemolysis occurs

(3) Which one of the following factors is involved in the development of DIC in this

patient?

    A. Impaired functions of mono/macrophages

    B. Severe impairment of hepatic functions

    C. Blood hypercoagulable state

    D. Microcirculation dysfunction

    E. None of the above

(4) Which one of the following mechanisms is involved in the development of dyspnea in this patient?

    A. Pulmonary embolism leads to restrictive ventilation defect

    B. Pulmonary embolism leads to obstructive ventilation defect

    C. Pulmonary infarction leads to alveolar hypoventilation

    D. During pregnancy, cardiac preload increased

    E. During pregnancy, cardiac afterload increased

(5) Which one of the following statements on the pathogenesis of shock in this patient is NOT correct?

    A. The formation of microthrombosis in DIC blocks microvessels, thereby leading to a decrease of venous return in this patient

    B. Massive bleeding led to decreased blood volume in this patient

    C. Vasoactive substances produced in DIC dilate blood vessels lowered the peripheral resistance

    D. Anemia in DIC did not affect the development of shock in this patient

    E. Microvascular injury is an important mechanism underlying the development of shock in patients with DIC

## Case analysis questions

A 36-yr-old man was referred to hospital. He complained of sore throat for 3 weeks, aggravated in recent 1 week. He had cough with blood-tinged sputum and a high fever of 39 ℃, and exhibited hemorrhage from the nose and under the skin. In the previous hospital, laboratory tests showed: Hb 94 g/L, WBC $2.4 \times 10^9$/L, PLT $38 \times 10^9$/L. He had no hematuria or hematochezia, but less food intake and poor sleep. He was previously healthy and had no history of liver and kidney diseases and tuberculosis. Admission physical examination revealed: T 37.8 ℃, R 20 breaths/min, HR 88 beats/min, BP 120/80 mmHg, scattered bleeding points on the skin and subcutaneous ecchymosis, no big superficial lymph nodes, no yellow sclera, pharyngeal congestion (+), Grade Ⅰ tonsil enlargement with no secretion, no big thyroid, slight tenderness of the sternum, normal cardiac boundary, regular rate and rhythm without murmur, a few moist rales in the right lower lung, flat and soft abdomen, no enlarged liver and spleen. Laboratory examination showed: Hb 90 g/L (normal 120 ~ 160 g/L), WBC 2.8 × $10^9$/L, classification revealed 12% primordial granules, 28% early and young granules, 8%

middle and young granules, 8% lobulated granules, 40% lymphoid granules, 4% monocytes, PLT $30 \times 10^9$/L (normal $100 \times 10^9 - 300 \times 10^9$/L). Bone marrow hyperplasia was extremely active with promyelocyte 91% and erythroid 1.5%, one megakaryocyte/film, and peroxidase activities were strongly positive. Coagulation tests showed: PT 19.9 s (control 15.3 s), fibrinogen 1.5 g/L (normal 1.8 – 4.5 g/L), FDP 180 μg/mL (control 5 μg/mL), and the plasma protamine paracoagulation (3P) test was positive. The results of the fecal occult blood test and urine analysis were unremarkable. Chest X-ray revealed a cloud in the right lower lung. The patient was diagnosed as acute promyelocytic leukemia and pulmonary infection complicated with DIC.

Questions:

(1) What's the diagnostic basis for DIC in this patient?

(2) What are the stages and types of DIC? What stage and type of DIC did this patient have?

(3) According to the pathogenesis of DIC, what are emerging manifestations in this patient and underlying mechanisms?

(4) Please analyze the mechanisms underlying the development of DIC in this patient.

(5) What molecules are detectable in the 3P test? How important is the 3P test in the diagnosis of DIC?

## Answers

**Case-based multiple choice questions (single answer)**

1. CCED; 2. EADAB; 3. BACCD

**Case analysis questions**

(1) What's the diagnostic basis for DIC in this patient?

The patient suffered from promyelocytic leukemia and pulmonary infection, both of which are the main causes of DIC. The physical examination showed bleeding in many parts of the body, typical signs of DIC. The laboratory examination showed prolonged PT, decreased fibrinogen, increased FDP and positive 3P test, indicating the impairment of coagulation and the activation of fibrinolytic system in DIC.

(2) What are the stages and types of DIC? What stage and type of DIC did this patient have?

The typical course of DIC can be divided into three stages: hypercoagulable, hypocoagulable, and secondary hyperfibrinolysis stages. According to the disease onset speed, DIC can be categorized into acute, subacute and chronic types, while the compensation state is used to distinguish compensated, decompensated and overcompensated DIC. In this case, the occurrence of DIC took a few days, so it is subacute. The massive formation of FDP indicates the secondary hyperfibrinolysis, while decompensated DIC is associated with thrombocytopenia in the patient.

(3) According to the pathogenesis of DIC, what are emerging manifestations in this patient and underlying mechanisms?

The patient may deteriorate rapidly, present with massive hemorrhage, shock and multiple organ dysfunction.

① Massive hemorrhage is the result of excess fibrinolytic activity in DIC.

② Shock: multiple microvascular thrombosis reduces the venous return; extensive bleeding reduces the blood volume; myocardial injury reduces cardiac output; the activation of kinin, complement and fibrinolytic system produces vasoactive substances, such as kinin, histamine and complement components, which increase vascular permeability, promote vasodilation, reduce peripheral resistance and subsequent venous return; FDP increases the vasodilative effects of histamine and kinin, and further promotes microvascular dilation.

③ MODS: microvascular thrombosis blocks organ microcirculation, resulting in ischemia and necrosis and subsequently promoting the development of shock and multiple organ dysfunctions (i. e. kidney, gastrointestine and heart).

(4) Please analyze the mechanisms underlying the development of DIC in this patient.

First, malignant tumor and infection caused tissue damage, and the release of tissue factors initiated the coagulation. Second, malignant tumor and infection damaged vascular endothelium and induced dysfunctions of coagulation and anticoagulation. In addition, the massive death of blood cells and activation of platelets may also contribute to the development of DIC in this patient with leukemia.

(5) What molecules are detectable in the 3P test? How important is the 3P test in the diagnosis of DIC?

Fibrinogen degradation products (FDP) were examined by the plasma protamine paracoagulation (3P) test. In DIC, secondary hyperfibrinolysis leads to the production of FDP by plasmin. These fragments can form soluble complexes with fibrin monomers. Protamine can separate fibrin monomers and FDP, and fibrin monomers subsequent form visible white precipitation. The 3P test is useful in identifying DIC as results of 3P test from patients with DIC are positive.

(刘立民　赵丽梅)

# Chapter 9　Ischemia-reperfusion Injury

## Case-based multiple choice questions (single answer)

**1. A 74-yr-old woman with left limb weakness and unclear speech for 1 hour was admitted to hospital. Cranial MRI showed acute patchy infarcts in her right frontal and temporal lobes and she was diagnosed with cerebral infarction. She improved after conservative intra-arterial thrombolytic therapy. Shortly afterwards, her family found her unconsciousness and some vomituses on the pillow, and paralysis of the left side of body. Emergent cranial CT showed multiple hyperdense hemorrhage foci in both frontal and temporal lobe and the sum of volumes was 40 mL.**

(1) Which one of the following disorders caused severe intracerebral hemorrhage in this woman with cerebral infarction after treatment with the conservative intra-arterial thrombolytic therapy?

A. Cerebral ischemia　　　　　　　B. Cerebral artery thrombosis

C. Reperfusion　　　　　　　　　　D. Reperfusion of cerebral artery thrombosis

  E. Cerebral ischemia-reperfusion injury

（2）Which one of the following mechanisms is NOT directly related to the aggravation of a preexisting injury after thrombolysis in this patient?

  A. Increased excitatory amino acids

  B. Increased free radicals

  C. Over activation of inflammatory response

  D. Calcium overload

  E. Astrocyte proliferation

（3）Which one of the following changes may occur in the brain of this woman during the aggravation of a preexisting injury?

  A. cAMP ↑ and cGMP ↑      B. cAMP ↓ and cGMP ↓

  C. cAMP ↑ and cGMP ↓      D. cAMP ↓ and cGMP ↑

  E. Both cAMP and cGMP were normal

**2. A 53-yr-old man with severe chest pain for half an hour was admitted to hospital. Based on ECG and laboratory analysis, he was diagnosed with ST segment elevation myocardial infarction. He improved after the percutaneous coronary intervention. 10 minutes later, ECG monitoring demonstrated tachycardia.**

（1）Which one of the following caused tachycardia in this patient after interventional therapy?

  A. Decreased cardiac output

  B. Increased ventricular end diastolic pressure

  C. Decreased myocardial contractility

  D. Cardiac ischemia-reperfusion injury

  E. Myocardial stunning

（2）Which one of the following arrhythmias is most likely to have occurred in this patient?

  A. Atrial arrhythmia       B. Atrioventricular block

  C. Atrioventricular junction block    D. Ventricular arrhythmia

  E. Atrial fibrillation

（3）What is the definition of the reversible myocardial systolic and diastolic dysfunction in this patient after treatment?

  A. Decreased cardiac output

  B. Decreased ventricular end diastolic pressure

  C. Decreased peak systolic pressure

  D. The maximum rate of change in the ventricle decreased

  E. Myocardial stunning

**3.** A 71-yr-old man felt a slight abdominal pain and obstipation, with pallid and frigid extremities at 12 hours before death in a nursing home. He had hypertension but no history of abdominal disorders or abdominal surgery. He did not receive any medical examination or medications meanwhile. 4 hours before the death, his extremities were extremely frigid and showed severe pallor. His systolic blood pressure was 76 mmHg. An intravenous drip injection of saline was started. Several hours later, the victim was found in cardiopulmonary arrest, and was confirmed dead after resuscitation attempts. At autopsy, a mesenteric hematoma and hemoperitoneum was observed with approximately 1,000 mL of blood in the abdominal cavity. The peripheral branch of inferior mesenteric artery near the hematoma ruptured. The sigmoid colon and the mesentery were twisted and the condition was determined to be a sigmoid volvulus that was observed to be loosened. The victim was speculated to die from hemorrhagic shock caused by intestinal ischemia-reperfusion injury.

(1) Which one of the following statements is true about the ischemia-reperfusion injury in this patient?

    A. Ischemia-reperfusion injury is mainly caused by ischemia

    B. Ischemia-reperfusion injury aggravates ischemic injury

    C. Ischemia-reperfusion injury is irreversible

    D. The ischemic time for intestinal reperfusion injury is similar to that for heart and brain

    E. The development of reperfusion injury is not related to the concentrations of electrolytes in reperfusion fluid

(2) Which one of the following factors regulates the development of intestinal ischemia-reperfusion injury in this patient?

    A. Ischemic time               B. The pressure of blood for reperfusion

    C. pH of blood for reperfusion     D. All of factors above

    E. None of factors above

(3) Which one of the following mechanisms is crucial for this patient to get pale and cold limbs before his death?

    A. Pain stress leads to the activation of sympathetic system

    B. Pain stress leads to the increased release of glucocorticoids

    C. RAAS activates due to the abdominal hemorrhage

    D. Cardiac output decreases and sympathetic system activates in hemorrhagic shock

    E. None of the above is correct

(4) Which one of the following metabolic changes may cause cardiac arrest in this patient with hemorrhagic shock?

    A. Hyperkalemia            B. Hypokalemia

    C. Respiratory alkalosis     D. Decreased catabolism

    E. None of the above

## Case analysis questions

- **Case 1**

A 50-yr-old man was admitted to hospital due to persistent and severe chest pain for 5 hours. He had an oppressive pain radiating to the left arm, sweating and nausea. Physical examination showed sinus rhythm, HR 110 beats/min, BP 75/50 mmHg. The patient was confused and short of breath. Laboratory analysis revealed that serum creatine phosphokinase (CK) was 1,660 U/L (normal < 198 U/L), creatine phosphokinase isoenzyme was 35 U/L (normal < 16 U/L), and serum malondialdehyde increased as well. ECG showed ST segment elevation in leads $V_1 - V_6$. Left ventricular ejection fraction (LVEF) was 31%. Chest X-ray demonstrated severe pulmonary edema. He was diagnosed as myocardial infarction and treated with i. v. infusion of furosemide (diuretic) and tissue plasminogen activator (tPA, thrombolytic). However, BP was still 80/50 mmHg. Coronary angiography showed a complete occlusion of the left main coronary artery. His symptoms of dyspnea and pain disappeared after balloon angioplasty, BP and LVEF rise to 100/70 mmHg and 38%, respectively. This was followed by transient ventricular tachycardia.

Questions:

(1) What type of shock did this patient have? Please briefly describe its pathogenesis.

(2) Please briefly describe mechanisms involved in the development of dyspnea and pulmonary edema in this patient.

(3) Why did this patient develop ventricular tachycardia after reperfusion of clogged coronary artery, despite the improvement of BP and LVEF? Please analyze the underlying mechanisms.

(4) What should a doctor do to prevent ischemia-reperfusion injury during reperfusion of coronary arteries after myocardial infarction?

- **Case 2**

A 25-yr-old man was admitted to the intensive care unit (ICU) after accidental CO poisoning at home. Before admission, he was resuscitated twice because of cardiac arrest. Upon admission he was unconscious, with inefficiently spontaneous breathing and hypotension. Mechanical ventilation was started along with fluids and inotropic catecholamines. His carboxyhemoglobin (CO-Hb) was 48.7%. After 1 hour of ventilation with 100% oxygen it decreased to 12.1% with a further decline to 1.2% after 5 hours. Urine output was > 250 mL/h; excessive diuresis was alleviated by vasopressin administration. Serum creatinine levels were < 1.0 mg/dL. Brain death was declared by a medical commission, and his kidneys were harvested for transplantation.

One recipient was a 46-yr-old man with end-stage renal disease owing to chronic glomerulonephritis, who had been previously treated with continuous peritoneal dialysis for 20 months. Kidney transplantation was started using the standard approach with typical sites for vascular anastomoses. Arterial anastomosis was complicated by dissection of the external iliac artery owing to extensive atherosclerosis. A segment of external iliac artery was replaced with a dacron prosthesis to which the renal artery of the graft was implanted, and the total kidney ischemia time increased to 100 minutes. Strikingly, ischemia-reperfusion injury did not occur and the kidney regained its normal tension and color, and immediately resumed urine production. In the post-transplant course, his serum creatinine declined steadily. He was discharged on the 10th day after surgery.

Questions:

(1) Please discuss the factors that affect the development of ischemia-reperfusion injury after renal transplantation.

(2) Please discuss the mechanisms of ischemia-reperfusion injury after renal transplantation.

(3) Please analyze why this patient did not have ischemia-reperfusion injury after renal transplantation.

## Answers

**Case-based multiple choice questions (single answer)**

1. EEC; **2.** DDE; **3.** BDDA

**Case analysis questions**

**Case 1**

(1) What type of shock did this patient have? Please briefly describe its pathogenesis.

This patient had cardiogenic shock. Its pathogenesis is as follows. Myocardial infarction → cardiac dysfunction→decreased output→decreased pulse pressure→cardiogenic shock.

(2) Please briefly describe mechanisms involved in the development of dyspnea and pulmonary edema in this patient.

Left heart failure→increased left ventricular end diastolic volume/pressure→increased left atrial pressure→ impaired pulmonary venous return → pulmonary congestion → increased capillary pressure/permeability → pulmonary edema→dyspnea.

(3) Why did this patient develop ventricular tachycardia after reperfusion of clogged coronary artery, despite the improvement of BP and LVEF? Please analyze the underlying mechanisms.

The ventricular tachycardia that this patient developed is reperfusion arrhythmia, which is related to myocardial ischemia-reperfusion injury. The mechanism of reperfusion arrhythmia is related to heterogeneities in action potential durations, delayed after depolarization, and altered electrophysiological characteristics of injured myocardium.

(4) What should a doctor do to prevent ischemia-reperfusion injury during reperfusion of coronary arteries after myocardial infarction?

The development of reperfusion injury is mainly related to the severity and duration of the ischemic insult, electrolyte abnormalities, and rate of reperfusion blood flow. The strategies for prevention and treatment include control of the initial reperfusion, improvement of myocardial metabolism, elimination of free radicals, reduction of calcium load and leukocyte activation.

**Case 2**

（1）Please discuss the factors that affect the development of ischemia-reperfusion injury after renal transplantation.

Ischemia-reperfusion injury is a frequent event in kidney transplantation. The occurrence of ischemia-reperfusion injury was related with warm ischemia time and conditions of reperfusion including the pressure, temperature, pH and electrolyte concentrations. In this case, the duration of warm ischemia was >60 minutes. Despite no organic necrosis, this transplanted kidney may be more susceptible to ischemia-reperfusion injury. In order to reduce reperfusion injury in transplantation, the speed, pressure, temperature, pH of reperfusion fluids as well as concentrations of sodium and calcium should be properly controlled, while an appropriate increase of potassium and magnesium in reperfusion fluid is beneficial.

（2）Please discuss the mechanisms of ischemia-reperfusion injury after renal transplantation.

So far, it is considered that the increase of free radicals, calcium overload and over-activation of the inflammatory responses are the main mechanisms of ischemia-reperfusion injury. The increase of free radicals leads to membrane lipid peroxidation, protein denaturalization and enzyme inhibition, DNA damage. Calcium overload plays an essential role in the disturbance of energy metabolism, the damage of cell membrane and structural proteins, and the aggravation of acidosis. Inflammation-associated microvascular and cellular injury are also involved in the development of ischemia-reperfusion.

（3）Please analyze why this patient did not have ischemia-reperfusion injury after renal transplantation.

In this case, CO poisoning could induce the hypoxia and ischemia in donor kidney. This preconditioning might activate the endogenous protective mechanisms. Moreover, the surprisingly unexpected outcome is most likely due to the protective effects of CO on renal ischemia-reperfusion injury. It was reported that inhalation of CO and low levels of endogenous CO alleviating the ischemia-reperfusion injury in vital organs（i. e. heart, liver, kidney, lung and intestine）of experimental animals. Small quantities of CO are remarkably cytoprotective, anti-apoptosis, and anti-inflammatory.

（刘立民　赵丽梅）

# Chapter 10　Cardiac Insufficiency

## Case-based multiple choice questions（single answer）

**1. A 59-yr-old man had a night attack of suffocation during sleep and was forced to sit up with violent coughing. Pink foamy sputum was coughed up.**

（1）Which one of the following disorders did this patient have?

    A. Left heart failure　　　　　　B. Right heart failure

    C. Compensated cardiac insufficiency　D. Septic shock

    E. Anaphylactic shock

（2）Which one of the following mechanisms is NOT involved in the development of dyspnea in this patient?

    A. Increased blood volume via reabsorption of edema fluids from lower extremities when lying down

    B. Aggravation of pulmonary stasis due to increased venous return when lying down

    C. Reduced alveolar ventilation due to an upward shift of the diaphragm when lying down

    D. Vagal inhibition and small bronchial dilatation during sleep

    E. Only severe hypoxemia and ventilation dysfunction can wake up the patient as the sensitivity of the central nervous system was reduced during sleep

（3）Which one of the following results is likely to come from this patient?

    A. HR 50 beats/min         B. pH 7.59

    C. BP 120/80 mmHg       D. Circumoral cyanosis

    E. $PaO_2$ 100 mmHg

（4）Which one of the following disorders is NOT likely to occur in this patient?

    A. Hypertension          B. Coronary artery disease

    C. Pulmonary valve insufficiency     D. Aortic stenosis

    E. Mitral stenosis

**2. A 62-yr-old woman with palpitation and dyspnea was admitted to hospital. She had had aortic stenosis for 12 years. She complained of palpitation and dyspnea after climbing stairs or doing housework in the last 6 months. Physical examinations showed no hepatosplenomegaly or leg edema. Echocardiography revealed left ventricular hypertrophy with a left ventricular ejection fraction of 53%.**

（1）Which one of the following is the main cause of heart failure in this patient?

    A. Left heart volume overload     B. Right heart volume overload

    C. Left heart pressure overload     D. Right heart pressure overload

    E. Reduced myocardial contractility

（2）Which one of the following statements is correct about the mechanisms of dyspnea on exertion in this patient?

    A. Reduced oxygen demand during physical activity

    B. Increased left ventricular filling during physical activity

    C. Reduced venous return during physical activity

    D. Aggravation of pulmonary stasis and edema during physical activity

    E. Respiratory muscle paralysis due to physical exertion

（3）Which one of the following changes is NOT likely to occur in this patient?

    A. Increased blood volume       B. Decreased renal blood flow

    C. Decreased number of red blood cells   D. Increased heart rate

    E. Ventricular remodeling

（4）What type of heart failure did this patient have according to left ventricular ejection fraction?

  A. Heart failure with increased ejection fraction

  B. Heart failure with preserved ejection fraction

  C. Heart failure with mild-range of ejection fraction

  D. Heart failure with decreased ejection fraction

  E. Low-output heart failure

（5）Which one of the following is NOT the significance of left ventricular hypertrophy in this patient?

  A. Increased contractility per unit weight of myocardium

  B. Ventricular wall thickening and tension reduction

  C. Reduction of myocardial oxygen consumption

  D. Reduction of cardiac load

  E. Maintenance of cardiac output

**3. A 56-yr-old man was admitted to the Emergency Department with shortness of breath and syncope. He had a prostatectomy 5 days ago and stayed in bed after it. Echocardiography showed normal left ventricular ejection fraction, elevated right ventricular systolic pressure, moderate right ventricular dilatation, and decreased right ventricular function. Chest CT revealed extensive bilateral pulmonary embolism, and acute deep vein thrombosis was detected in the left leg by a venous duplex scan.**

（1）Which one of the following is the main cause of heart failure in this patient?

  A. Left heart volume overload     B. Right heart volume overload

  C. Left heart pressure overload     D. Right heart pressure overload

  E. Reduced myocardial contractility

（2）Which one of the following signs or symptoms is NOT likely to occur in this patient?

  A. Decreased BP         B. Increased respiratory rate

  C. Coughing up pink foamy sputum    D. Decreased oxygen saturation

  E. Increased central venous pressure

（3）Which one of the following changes is NOT possible to occur in this patient?

  A. Pitting edema in the lower extremities

  B. Jugular engorgement

  C. A positive hepatojugular reflux sign

  D. Hepatosplenomegaly

  E. Decreased pulmonary artery wedge pressure

## Case analysis questions

• **Case 1**

A 68-yr-old man was admitted to hospital with progressive shortness of breath in the last 3 days. He complained of increased dyspnea and weakness during physical activity and relief at rest. He often woke up and coughed severely at night when lying down to sleep. He had to sit up in a comfortable position and coughed up pink sputum. The patient had a 20-yr history of hypertension, a 15-yr history of coronary artery disease, and recently became depressed due to a telecommunication fraud. His father died of myocardial infarction 20 years ago.

On admission examinations showed his body height of 170 cm, BW of 90 kg, R of 24 breaths/min, HR of 112 beats/min, thready pulse, BP of 150/90 mmHg, T of 37 ℃, bilateral swelling of ankles with pits/indents on pressure, elevated jugular venous pressure. On auscultation, his apical impulse was displaced downward to left with audible fourth heart sound and moist rales at the base of the lungs. The edge of liver was palpable 10 cm below the costal margin.

Questions:

(1) What is heart failure? What type of heart failure did this patient have?

(2) What are the manifestations of venous congestion in this patient?

(3) What are the risk factors of heart failure in this patient?

(4) Why did this patient cough up pink frothy sputum?

- **Case 2**

A 63-yr-old woman with shortness of breath was sent to the Emergency Department. She had a cold 2 days ago and the subsequent onset of dyspnea at rest, forgetfulness, mild fatigue, and bilateral leg swelling. She stayed in bed for 2 days because of weakness, fatigue, and shortness of breath. The patient had a 30-yr history of smoking and stopped it 2 years ago due to shortness of breath. 1 year ago, he was hospitalized due to acute exacerbation of chronic obstructive pulmonary disease (COPD) with similar symptoms.

On admission examinations showed T of 38.6 ℃, HR of 120 beats/min, R of 24 breaths/min, BP of 104/54 mmHg, $SaO_2$ of 90%, cardiac index of 1.4 L/(min · m$^2$), left ventricular ejection fraction (LVEF) of 40%, jugular engorgement, and pitting edema in bilateral lower extremities. Arterial blood gas analysis revealed pH of 7.49, $PaCO_2$ of 27.6 mmHg, $PaO_2$ of 53.6 mmHg, [$HCO_3^-$] of 20.6 mmol/L, and $SaO_2$ of 90%. Chest X-ray indicated alveolar edema, pericardial effusion, cardiomegaly, small bilateral pleural effusions, and partial collapse of the left lungs.

Questions:

(1) Please analyze the cardiac alterations in this patient and underlying mechanisms.

(2) Please discuss the role of the cold in the development of heart failure in this patient.

(3) Why did this patient have increased heart rate? What are the effects of increased heart rate on cardiac function?

(4) What are the mechanisms underlying the development of bilateral leg swelling and jugular engorgement in this patient?

# Answers

## Case-based multiple choice questions (single answer)

**1**. ADDC; **2**. CDCBA; **3**. DCE

## Case analysis questions

### Case 1

(1) What is heart failure? What type of heart failure did this patient have?

Heart failure is a condition in which impaired ventricular ejection and/or filling significantly reduce cardiac output and subsequently result in no enough blood to meet the body's needs and a series of clinical syndromes including insufficient organ perfusion and pulmonary and/or systemic congestions. The dyspnea in this patient is a manifestation of left heart failure, while the pitting edema of the lower extremities, liver enlargement and elevated jugular venous pressure are manifestations of right heart failure. Therefore, this patient developed acute whole heart failure.

(2) What are the manifestations of venous congestion in this patient?

Exertional dyspnea, nocturnal paroxysmal dyspnea, and coughing up pink frothy sputum are signs of pulmonary congestion. Pitting edema of the lower limbs, liver enlargement and elevated jugular vein pressure are signs of systemic congestion.

(3) What are the risk factors of heart failure in this patient?

Family medical history, hypertension, coronary artery disease, obesity, and mood swings are risk factors involved in the development of heart failure in this patient.

(4) Why did this patient cough up pink frothy sputum?

Coughing up pink frothy sputum is an indicator of pulmonary edema. Left-sided heart failure reduces cardiac output and increases pulmonary vascular resistance, thereby leading to pulmonary congestions. Increased pulmonary venous and capillary pressure as well as increased capillary permeability induce the plasma extravasation into the interstitium and alveoli, leading to pulmonary edema.

### Case 2

(1) Please analyze the cardiac alterations in this patient and underlying mechanisms.

The patient had reduced cardiac function as evidenced by cardiac index of $< 2.2$ L/(min $\cdot$ m$^2$) and left ventricular ejection fraction of $< 50\%$. This is due to increased right ventricular afterload and hypoxia in COPD and subsequent impaired function of the left heart, while the induction of metabolism in cold aggravates the clinical manifestations of heart failure.

(2) Please discuss the role of the cold in the development of heart failure in this patient.

Fever with the upper respiratory tract infection not only increases the basic metabolic rate and cardiac load, but also accelerates the heart rate to increase myocardial oxygen consumption. Shortened diastolic time also reduces coronary blood perfusion. Moreover, the upper respiratory tract infection elevates pulmonary vascular resistance and increases right heart afterload. In addition, inflammatory mediators and bacterial toxins may also directly impair myocardial function.

(3) Why did this patient have increased heart rate? What are the effects of increased heart rate on cardiac function?

Decreased cardiac output activates the sympathetic system to increase heart rate by β-receptors. Within a certain range, increase in heart rate raises cardiac output and diastolic blood pressure to elevate coronary blood flow, thereby maintaining arterial blood pressure and blood supply to vital organs. However, acceleration of heart rate can increase myocardial oxygen consumption, and significantly shorten the diastolic time when a heart rate is more than 180 beats/min. The subsequent reduction of ventricular blood filling and coronary blood perfusion not only decreases cardiac output but also aggravates myocardial ischemia and hypoxia.

(4) What are the mechanisms underlying the development of bilateral leg swelling and jugular engorgement in this patient?

Right heart failure causes a decrease of right heart output and an increase of right ventricular diastolic pressure that blocks the venous return from the superior and inferior vena cava, thereby resulting in bilateral leg swelling and jugular engorgement.

(赵丽梅)

# Chapter 11　Pulmonary Insufficiency

## Case-based multiple choice questions (single answer)

**1.** A 17-yr-old high school male student was sent to hospital due to a sudden right chest pain with dyspnea for 1 hour after PE class.

Physical examinations: HR 145 beats/min, BP 92/60 mmHg, purple lips, right thoracic distention and tympanic sounds heard over the chest. He was then hospitalized for the treatment of close pneumothorax.

(1) Which one of the following pathological processes might occur in the patient?

  A. Obstructive hypoventilation    B. Restrictive hypoventilation

  C. Diffusion defects       D. Increased dead space

  E. Less pulmonary surfactant

(2) Which one of the following blood oxygen parameters can be used to determine the type of respiratory failure?

  A. $PaO_2$ and $SO_2$       B. $PaCO_2$ and $[HCO_3^-]$

  C. $PaO_2$ and $PaCO_2$     D. $CO_2$ and $[H^+]$

  E. $CO_2max$ and $[HCO_3^-]$

(3) Which one of the following statements is NOT true about the pulmonary and circulatory changes in this patient?

  A. Hypoxia excites cardiovascular center and subsequently increases HR and myocardial contractility

  B. Pneumothorax reduces venous reflux and cardiac output, thereby lowering systolic blood pressure

C. Activation of cardiovascular center helps to maintain the PR and redistribute the blood flow

D. Rapid shallow breathing the patient had is a sign of dyspnea

E. Pulmonary hypoxia and $CO_2$ retention increase the plasma levels of $[H^+]$ and thereby lead to pulmonary vasodilation

（4）Which one of the following acid-base disturbances is likely to occur in this patient?

A. Metabolic acidosis

B. Metabolic alkalosis

C. Respiratory acidosis

D. Respiratory alkalosis

E. Mixed acid-base disturbances

（5）Which one of the following diagnosis or treatments is NOT correct for this patient?

A. Chest X-ray can be used to determine closed pneumothorax

B. The patient may have acute respiratory failure due to closed pneumothorax

C. Pericardiocentesis can help this patient to relieve dyspnea

D. Thoracic puncture to remove air can help this patient to relieve dyspnea

E. Oxygen therapy can alleviate the symptoms of hypoxia

**2. A 65-yr-old man had been suffering from chronic bronchitis for more than 10 years. His symptoms had worsened with obvious dyspnea in the last month. Blood gas analysis revealed: pH 7.2, $PaO_2$ 50 mmHg, $SaO_2$ 80%, $PaCO_2$ 82 mmHg and $[HCO_3^-]$ 36.2 mmol/L.**

（1）Which one of the following changes is essential for the diagnosis of chronic respiratory failure?

A. Dyspnea

B. A medical history of chronic bronchitis

C. $SaO_2 < 90\%$

D. $PaO_2 < 60$ mmHg and $PaCO_2 > 50$ mmHg

E. pH < 7.35

（2）Which one of the following respiratory changes is mainly occur in this patient?

A. Inspiratory dyspnea

B. Expiratory dyspnea

C. Bradypnea

D. Shallow breathing

E. None of the above

（3）Which one of the following mechanisms is mainly involved in the development of chronic respiratory failure in this patient?

A. Diffusion defects

B. Partial alveolar hypoventilation

C. Obstructive hypoventilation

D. Partial alveolar hypoperfusion

E. Arterial-venous shunt

（4）Which one of the following respiratory changes may NOT induce the chronic respiratory failure in this patient?

A. Airway wall thickening and stenosis

B. Bronchospasm

C. Less pulmonary surfactant and decreased surface tension

D. Blocked small airways due to mucus glands and overabundance of goblet cells

E. Small airways compression due to pulmonary hyperplasia and fibrosis

(5) Which one of the following parameters from this patient can effectively assess the airway resistance?

  A. Forced vital capacity (FVC)

  B. Forced expiratory volume in one second (FEV1)

  C. FEV1% (FEV1/FVC × 100%)

  D. Minute ventilation (VE)

  E. Alveolar ventilation per minute(VA)

(6) Which one of the following changes is associated with functional intrapulmonary shunt in this patient?

  A. Total lung $V_A/Q = 0.8$      B. Total lung $V_A/Q < 0.8$

  C. Total lung $V_A/Q > 0.8$      D. Increased $CaO_2$

  E. Decreased $CaCO_2$

(7) Which one of the following acid-base disturbances may occur in this patient according to the blood gas analysis?

  A. Metabolic acidosis       B. Respiratory acidosis

  C. Metabolic alkalosis       D. Respiratory alkalosis

  E. Mixed acid-base disturbances

(8) Which one of the following treatments should NOT be given to this patient?

  A. Prevention and treatment of respiratory infections

  B. Oxygen inhalation, and increase $PaO_2$ to more than 60 mmHg as soon as possible

  C. Increasing ventilation to decrease $PaCO_2$

  D. Correction of acid-base disturbances and electrolyte imbalances

  E. Improvement of the internal environment and protection of the vital organs (i. e. heart and brain)

**3. A 25-yr-old woman was hospitalized for wound debridement due to a left femoral segmental open fracture and a tibia-fibular fracture. At the end of surgery, several pieces of gauze dressing containing epinephrine were placed over the wound area. At arrival in the recovery room, the patient was conscious and physical examination tests showed BP 165/115 mmHg, HR 110 beats/min, and R 20 breaths/min. 1 hour later, BP decreased to 106/74 mmHg, and tachycardia (HR 135 beats/min) was noted. Arterial blood gas analysis showed: pH 7.35, $PaO_2$ 64 mmHg, $SaO_2$ 91.6%, $PaCO_2$ 34 mmHg, $[HCO_3^-]$ 19 mmol/L, Hb 8.9 mg/dL, $[Na^+]$ 131 mmol/L, $[K^+]$ 2.26 mmol/L. 500 mL packed erythrocytes and 20 mEq KCl in 800 mL of Ringer's lactate were infused slowly. HR increased rapidly to 145 beats/min despite treatment, chest auscultation revealed bilateral moist rales, and central venous pressure was 27 cmH$_2$O (normal 3−10 cmH$_2$O) with poor urine output. The patient was given furosemide. Chest radiography, performed 50 minutes later, confirmed the diagnosis of pulmonary edema. 1 hour later, hypotension (82/59 mmHg) and hypoxia ($SpO_2$ <85%) developed with**

**coughing up frothy pink sputum. Tracheal intubation was immediately performed and arterial blood analysis showed: pH 7.09, PaO$_2$ 45 mmHg, SaO$_2$ 63.7%, PaCO$_2$ 52 mmHg, [HCO$_3^-$] 15.6 mmol/L, Hb 12.5 mg/dL, [Na$^+$] 131 mmol/L and [K$^+$] 8.0 mmol/L.**

（1）Which one of the following statements is correct according to the arterial blood analysis results before confirmation of pulmonary edema?

    A. The patient had type I respiratory failure

    B. The patient had type Ⅱ respiratory failure

    C. The patient had acute respiratory failure

    D. The patient had chronic respiratory failure

    E. None of the above

（2）Which type of the following respiratory failure might develop in this patient according to the arterial blood gas analysis results after tracheal intubation?

    A. Type I respiratory failure    B. Type Ⅱ respiratory failure

    C. Acute respiratory failure, type Ⅰ    D. Acute respiratory failure, type Ⅱ

    E. Chronic respiratory failure, type Ⅱ

（3）Which one of the following pathophysiological mechanisms is involved in the development of respiratory failure in this patient?

    A. Restrictive hypoventilation    B. Obstructive hypoventilation

    C. Diffusion defects    D. Ventilation perfusion dismatch

    E. All of the above

（4）Which one of the following respiratory changes is right for the patient before tracheal intubation?

    A. Inspiratory and expiratory dyspnea    B. Only inspiratory dyspnea

    C. Only expiratory dyspnea    D. Shallow breathing

    E. Slow breathing

（5）Which one of the circulatory changes might happen after this patient suffered pulmonary edema?

    A. Increased BP    B. Cardiac arrest

    C. Increased afterload of left heart    D. Decreased afterload of right heart

    E. None of the above

（6）Which one of the following acid-base disturbances did this patient have after tracheal intubation?

    A. Metabolic acidosis    B. Respiratory acidosis

    C. Metabolic alkalosis    D. Respiratory alkalosis

    E. Metabolic acidosis complicated with respiratory acidosis

（7）Which one of the following complications might occur in this patient during treatment?

    A. Acute renal failure    B. Gastrointestinal mucosal bleeding

    C. Brain herniation    D. Multiple organ failure

    E. All of the above

**4.** A 20-yr-old woman was admitted to the emergency room due to mild dyspnea and diffuse right upper abdominal pain. Admission physical examinations showed: T 38. 6 ℃, P 72 beats/min, R 15 breaths/min, BP 98/70 mmHg. Examinations of the heart and lungs were normal. The abdomen was soft with tenderness in the right upper quadrant and the bowel sounds hypoactive. The extremities had no signs of deep venous thrombosis. Over the next 2 hours she developed rebound and guarding in the right upper quadrant of the abdomen. The serum electrolytes, glucose, creatinine, and blood urea nitrogen were normal. Complete blood count, β-human chorionic gonadotropin, and serum thyroxine were unremarkable. An arterial blood gas analysis revealed pH of 7. 42, $PaO_2$ of 65 mmHg, $PaCO_2$ of 31 mmHg. The alveolar arterial oxygen gradient [$P_{(A-a)}O_2$] was 46 mmHg. The chest radiograph was normal, and intestinal obstruction was ruled out by an abdominal ultrasound. With a ventilation perfusion scan and pulmonary angiography, she was diagnosed with a pulmonary embolism.

(1) Which one of the following statements is correct about the respiratory dysfunction in this patient?

    A. The patient had type I respiratory failure

    B. The patient had type Ⅱ respiratory failure

    C. The patient had pulmonary ventilation disorder

    D. The patient had gas exchange disorder

    E. None of the above

(2) According to the arterial blood gas analysis, which one of the following gas exchange disorders is involved in the development of dyspnea in this patient?

    A. Diffusion defect                B. Functional shunt

    C. Dead space ventilation       D. Anatomic shunt

    E. True shunt

(3) Which one of the following is correct on ventilation/perfusion ratio and arterial blood analysis?

    A. Total lung $V_A/Q = 0.8$         B. Total lung $V_A/Q < 0.8$

    C. Total lung $V_A/Q > 0.8$         D. Increased $CaO_2$

    E. Increased $CaCO_2$

(4) Which one of the following cardiovascular changes was induced by pulmonary embolism in the patient?

    A. Increased cardiac output       B. Decreased peripheral resistance

    C. Increased preload of left heart    D. Increased preload of right heart

    E. Increased afterload of right heart

(5) Which one of the following treatments is urgently required for this patient?

    A. Thrombolytic therapy to prevent respiratory failure

    B. Pure oxygen inhalation to increase $PaO_2$

  C. Increasing pulmonary ventilation to reduce $PaCO_2$

  D. Correction of acid-base disturbances and electrolyte imbalances

  E. Improvement of the internal environment and protection of the vital organs ( i. e. heart and brain)

## Case analysis questions

- **Case 1**

A 68-yr-old man was admitted to the hospital because of the serve asthmatic cough, dyspnea and drowsiness. The patient had a 30-yr history of smoking. He complained of cough and expectoration with small amount of white phlegm since 15 years ago and more frequently to get sick in winter. These symptoms were recurring more often and worsening with yellow phlegm, but could be relieved by the treatment. In the recent 3 years, the patient showed palpitation, shortness of breath and bilateral lower limb edema on exertion, and rest alleviated the dyspnea. In the last 10 days asthmatic coughs with dyspnea was worsening, while drowsiness occurred 2 days ago.

Physical examination: T 36.5 ℃, BP 120/80 mmHg, HR 118 beats/min, R 25 breaths/min, blurred consciousness, blue lips, slight shortness of breath, and jugular vein distension. Hyperresonance to percussion, dry and moist rales were heard over bilateral lungs. Weakened cardiechema without obvious enlargement of heart boundary or murmurs was heard on auscultation. The abdomen was flat and soft with tenderness in the right upper quadrant. The liver was palpable below the ribs and shifting dullness was noted. Pitting edema was remarkable on both lower limbs.

After hospitalization, dyspnea was aggravated despite of the treatment with oxygen therapy. Blood gas analysis showed: pH 7.10, $PaO_2$ 70 mmHg, $PaCO_2$ 90 mmHg, and $[HCO_3^-]$ 27.3 mmol/L.

Diagnosis: COPD, pulmonary heart disease (PHD), and pulmonary encephalopathy (PE).

Questions:

(1) What is the pathogenesis of COPD, PHD and PE in this patient?

(2) What are the mechanisms of ascites and bilateral lower limb edema in this patient?

(3) What is the mechanism of unconsciousness in this patient?

(4) Which type of acid-base disturbance did this patient develop?

(5) Why was the dyspnea worsening in this patient after oxygen therapy? What kind of treatment was the first choice for this patient at this moment?

- **Case 2**

A 48-yr-old male patient was admitted to hospital due to fever, cough and dyspnea for 8 days. He had a history of hypertension on therapy. On admission physical examinations showed as follows: BP 131/78 mmHg, HR 88 beats/min, R 30 breaths/min, T 37.7 ℃, $SpO_2$ 77%, rhonchi on bilateral lungs. Chest CT scan showed ground-glass opacity (GGO) and multifocal crazy paving pattern involving both lungs, predominantly in peripheral distribution. Laboratory examinations showed lymphopenia and increased neutrophil count, erythrocyte sedimentation rate, and D-dimer count. Blood gas analysis (BGA) prior to admission showed: pH 7.5, $PaO_2$ 57 mmHg, $PaCO_2$ 29 mmHg, [$HCO_3^-$] 22.4 mmol/L, $SpO_2$ 92.2%. His COVID-19 test was positive. Therefore, he was diagnosed with COVID-19 with type I respiratory failure and acute respiratory distress syndrome (ARDS).

The patient was immediately admitted to ICU and given oxygen via high flow nasal cannula, which corrected the $SpO_2$ into 100%. He also received treatment with a variety of drugs. On day 4 of hospitalization in ICU, the patient developed worsening symptom of dyspnea. Serial BGA showed pH 7.45, $PaO_2$ 69.9 mmHg, $PaCO_2$ 31.9 mmHg, [$HCO_3^-$] 22.1 mmol/L, and $SpO_2$ 95.5%. The patient was intubated and supported with mechanical ventilation. Laboratory examination showed a D-dimer count of 4.49 (N<0.05), on the next day, intravenous heparin was started and continued for 4 days. On day 14 of hospitalization in ICU, the patient suddenly developed right lung hydropneumothorax and atelectasis, revealed by chest X-ray, therefore, insertion of water seal drainage (WSD) and bronchoscopy were done. Bronchoscopy results showed a very thick mucous plug on the left and right main bronchus, and *Acinetobacter baumannii* was found in the culture of the bronchial washing. The chest X-ray after the first bronchoscopy showed the improvement of hydropneumothorax and atelectasis, and serial BGA showed improved oxygenation after 4 days of treatment. On day 18 of hospitalization in ICU, serial laboratory examinations showed overt dissemination intravascular coagulation (DIC). The patient was thus given fresh frozen plasma immediately. Then he gradually improved, and WSD and tracheostomy were removed on day 36. The patient was discharged on day 41 and the last chest X-ray examination revealed massive right lung fibrosis and right pleura thickening. During follow-up on the next 2 weeks, the chest X-ray showed residual but improved massive right lung fibrosis and right pleura thickening.

Questions:

(1) What is the basis for the patient's diagnosis with type I respiratory failure and ARDS on admission?

(2) What is the relationship between COVID-19, type I respiratory failure and ARDS?

(3) What is the pathogenesis of ARDS in this patient?

(4) What blood parameter is required for the diagnosis of DIC in this patient?

(5) Why was the development of DIC related to ARDS in this patient?

(6) What kind of respiratory dysfunction may this patient have according to the chest X-ray results on hospital discharge?

# Answers

**Case-based multiple choice questions (single answer)**

1. BCEEC; **2**. DBBCCBBB; **3**. EDEABEE; **4**. DCCEA

**Case analysis questions**

### Case 1

(1) What is the pathogenesis of COPD, PHD and PE in this patient?

COPD refers to chronic airway obstruction with chronic bronchitis and emphysema. This is confirmed by a chronic history of cough, asthma and dyspnea as well as hyporesonance to percussion and dry and moist rales on auscultation. The pathogenesis of COPD includes:

① Obstructive hypoventilation due to bronchial wall swelling, airway hyperresponsiveness, bronchospasm and bronchial obstruction.

② Restrictive hypoventilation due to respiratory muscle failure.

③ Diffusion defects due to alveolar damage and alveolar membrane thickening.

④ Ventilation-perfusion dismatch due to partial alveolar hypoventilation and hypoperfusion, or pulmonary vasoconstriction and remodeling.

PHD: patients with COPD had systemic congestion due to the right heart failure as evidenced by jugular vein distension, ascites and pitting edema of upper and lower limbs. The pathogenesis of PHD in this patient with COPD includes:

① Alveolar hypoxia and $CO_2$ retention in COPD increase plasma levels of $[H^+]$ and thereby lead to pulmonary vasoconstriction, which gradually stimulates pulmonary vascular remodeling to induce pulmonary hypertension and increased afterload of right heart.

② Hypoxia and acidosis impair systolic and diastolic functions of the heart.

③ Long-term hypoxia induces production of erythropoietin (EPO), and the subsequent elevation of blood viscosity due to polycythemia increases the cardiac load.

④ Abnormal changes of intrathoracic pressure due to pulmonary lesions may impair systolic and diastolic functions of the heart.

PE: PE in COPD is one brain dysfunction due to respiratory failure. Drowsiness is the sign of the neurological-cognitive alterations in this case. The development of PE in COPD is related to cerebral edema and neurological dysfunction caused by hypercapnia, acidosis and hypoxia.

① Acidosis and hypoxia induce cerebral vasodilation and increase the cerebral blood flow. Vascular endothelial injury not only increases the vascular permeability for induction of cerebral interstitial edema, but also leads to intravascular coagulation.

② Reduced ATP production under hypoxia impairs the sodium-potassium pump and thereby leads to cerebral edema.

③ Acidosis promotes the production of inhibitory transmitter GABA and thereby leads to central inhibition.

④ Enhanced phospholipase activity and increased lysosomal hydrolases in response to acidosis lead to nerve tissue damage.

(2) What are the mechanisms of ascites and bilateral lower limb edema in this patient?

Ascites and bilateral lower limb edema are the signs of systemic congestion due to respiratory failure-induced the right heart failure. The pathological changes in lungs cause pulmonary hypertension and increase the afterload of the right heart, thereby leading to heart failure. Reduced venous return results in systemic congestion, while peripheral edema is the consequence of increased capillary hydrostatic pressure.

(3) What is the mechanism of unconsciousness in this patient?

The patient had PE, and unconsciousness is a sign of cerebral edema and neurological dysfunction as hypoxia, hypercapnia and acidosis induce neurovascular injuries.

(4) Which type of acid-base disturbance did this patient develop?

Given pH of 7.10, this patient developed decompensated acidosis. He had respiratory acidosis according to COPD as the underlying disease and increased $PaCO_2$. Because COPD is a chronic disease, according to the expected compensation formula, $\Delta[HCO_3^-] = 0.35 \times \Delta PaCO_2 \pm 3 = 0.35 \times (90 - 40) \pm 3 = 17.5 \pm 3$. However, the actual $\Delta[HCO_3^-]$ was 3.3 mmol/L (27.3 - 24 = 3.3), which is out of the compensation limit. This indicates that this patient also had metabolic acidosis due to hypoxia.

(5) Why was the dyspnea worsening in this patient after oxygen therapy? What kind of treatment was the first choice for this patient at this moment?

This patient had type II respiratory failure. High-concentration and high-flow oxygen therapy could rapidly raise $PaO_2$ to relieve hypoxia. However, hypercapnia with increased $PaCO_2$ may directly depress the respiratory center and thereby lead to the aggravation of dyspnea. The first choice for this patient is thus to improve ventilation and reduce $PaCO_2$.

**Case 2**

(1) What is the basis for the patient's diagnosis with type I respiratory failure and ARDS on admission?

The type I respiratory failure was diagnosed because the value of $PaO_2$ (57 mmHg) is lower than 60 mmHg, while $PaCO_2$ (29 mmHg) is not higher than 50 mmHg. ARDS is an acute respiratory failure due to acute lung injury (ALI). In this case, the patient showed diffused alveolar injury due to COVID-19 infection as evidenced by ground-glass opacity (GGO) and multifocal crazy paving pattern involving both lungs, predominantly in peripheral distribution on chest CT scan.

(2) What is the relationship between COVID-19, type I respiratory failure and ARDS?

In this case, the patient had ARDS because of COVID-19 infection-induced acute lung injury. Injuries of alveolar-capillary membranes and inflammatory mediators increased the permeability of pulmonary capillary endothelial and alveolar epithelial barriers, thereby resulting in osmotic pulmonary edema and hyaline membrane formation, and subsequent diffusion defects. Diffusion defects together with increased pulmonary functional shunt and dead space ventilation lead to the decrease of $PaO_2$ and the development of type I respiratory failure in this patient.

(3) What is the pathogenesis of ARDS in this patient?

① COVID-19 acts on pulmonary capillaries, alveolar epithelial cells and alveolar-capillary membranes, and thereby induces massive pulmonary injuries.

② COVID-19 activates leukocytes, macrophages and platelets, and indirectly causes lung injury.

③ COVID-19 promotes neutrophils to adhere to pulmonary capillary endothelium and subsequent migration into lungs. Neutrophil activation increases the release of cytokines, oxygen free radicals, proteases and other inflammatory mediators and thereby leads to injuries of alveolar epithelial cells and capillary endothelial cells.

④ The release of procoagulant substances due to vascular endothelial and pulmonary injury and neutrophil infiltration induces intravascular coagulation and microthrombus formation, which further aggravate lung injury by reduction of blood flow and increase pulmonary vascular permeability by generation of fibrin degradation products (FDP) and secretion of $TXA_2$.

(4) What blood parameter is required for the diagnosis of DIC in this patient?

DIC is disseminated intravascular coagulation characterized by widespread coagulation and bleeding in the vascular compartment. DIC is initiated by massive release of procoagulants into the blood and subsequent activation of coagulation factors and platelets induced by some pathogenic factors. The increase of intravascular thrombin induces formation of massive thrombus in microcirculation, overconsumption of clotting factors and platelets, as well as secondary activation of fibrinolysis. D-dimer is a fragment of degraded fibrin and reflects the secondary activation of fibrinolysis in responses to thrombosis as no fibrin is present in primary hyperfibrinolysis. ISTH scoring system is used to diagnose DIC in clinical, which includes the parameters of platelet (PLT) count (decrease: 0 – 2), D-dimer (decrease: 0,2,3), prothrombin time (PT) (prolongate: 0 – 2) and fibrinogen ( > 1.0 g/L = 0, < 1.0 g/L = 1), and the diagnose of DIC can be confirmed when the sum of scores is greater than or equal to 5.

(5) Why was the development of DIC related to ARDS in this patient?

ARDS is an important cause of DIC in this patient. COVID-19 induced ALI promotes the development of DIC through the following mechanisms:

① ALI increases the release of tissue factor (TF), which activates exogenous coagulation system (ECS) and initiates the coagulation.

② Vascular endothelial cell injuries not only enhance TF-induced coagulation, but also impair endothelial anticoagulant functions.

③ The destruction of leukocytes releases TF and activates ECS.

④ The exposure of collagen on vascular basement membrane in ALI also activates aggregation of platelets.

(6) What kind of respiratory dysfunction may this patient have according to the chest X-ray results on hospital discharge?

The last chest X-ray examination before discharge revealed massive right fibrosis and right pleura thickening, which may cause respiratory insufficiency through restrictive ventilation, impaired diffusion, functional shunt and dead space ventilation.

(孙晓东　孙丽娜)

# Chapter 12　Hepatic Insufficiency

## Case-based multiple choice questions (single answer)

1. A 56-yr-old male patient was admitted to hospital due to lethargy and confusion for 2 days. He had a 10-year history of cirrhosis. Physical examination showed: P 95 beats/min, R 32 breaths/min. The liver was firm and palpable two fingers below the costal margin. Ascetic fluid was detectable. The patient was preliminarily diagnosed with hepatic encephalopathy (HE).

（1）Which stage of hepatic encephalopathy did this patient have?

  A. Stage Ⅰ         B. Stage Ⅱ

  C. Stage Ⅲ         D. Stage Ⅳ

  E. Stage Ⅴ

（2）Which one of the following statements is NOT true in this patient?

  A. Neuropsychiatric syndrome is secondary to liver cirrhosis in this patient

  B. The patient is in the advanced stages of hepatic encephalopathy

  C. Flapping tremor should be remarkable in this patient

  D. Portal hypertension may occur in this patient

  E. Low plasma levels of albumin are due to insufficient production in this patient

（3）Which one of the following mechanisms is NOT involved in the development of hepatic encephalopathy in this patient?

  A. Impaired ornithine cycle due to liver cirrhosis

  B. Impaired ammonia metabolism due to the decrease of hepatic ATP production

  C. Decreased digestion and absorption

  D. Increased intestinal ammonia production

  E. Increased renal tubular secretion of ammonia

（4）Which one of the following mechanisms is NOT involved in the development of ascites in this patient?

  A. Portal hypertension

  B. Decreased plasma colloid osmotic pressure

  C. Impaired lymphatic circulation

  D. Decreased glomerular filtration rate（GFR）

  E. Decreased plasma levels of aldosterone

（5）Which one of the following acid-base disturbances may develop in this patient?

  A. Metabolic acidosis      B. Respiratory acidosis

  C. Metabolic alkalosis      D. Respiratory alkalosis

  E. None of the above

（6）Which one of the following water and electrolyte disorders may occur in this patient?

  A. Hypokalemia        B. Hypertonic dehydration

  C. Hypotonic dehydration     D. Salt poisoning

  E. None of the above

（7）Which one of the following treatments is NOT appropriate for this patient?

  A. Epsom salt as an osmotic cathartic

  B. Oral administration of lactulose

  C. Administration of alkaline drugs

  D. Administration of levodopa

  E. Oral or intravenous administration of a branched chain amino acid mixture

**2.** A 55-yr-old male patient was sent to hospital due to sudden hematemesis (500 mL). He had a 10-year history of hepatitis B and cirrhosis. Physical examinations showed: anemic signs, BP 90/60 mmHg, HR 90 beats/min. The abdomen was soft, and the liver was firm and palpable 3 cm below the costal margin. The blood analysis showed: Hb 70 g/L, WBC 5.5 × $10^9$/L, and platelet 100 × $10^9$/L. He was preliminarily diagnosed with upper gastrointestinal bleeding (UGIB); chronic hepatitis B and liver cirrhosis.

(1) Which one of the following disorders led to the hematemesis in this patient?

    A. Gastrorrhagia

    B. Hematobilia

    C. Stress ulcer bleeding (SUB)

    D. Bleeding ulcers

    E. Bleeding esophageal varices

(2) If the patient had portal hypertension, which one of the following mechanisms is NOT involved in it?

    A. Splenomegaly

    B. Hepatic fibrosis

    C. Nodular hepatocyte regeneration

    D. Intrahepatic arterioportal shunts

    E. Portal vein compression

(3) If UGIB induces hepatic encephalopathy (HE) in this patient, which one of the following mechanisms is mainly involved in it?

    A. Destruction of BBB

    B. Increased intestinal production of ammonia

    C. Cerebral ischemia and hypoxia

    D. Increased cerebral contents of false neurotransmitters (FNT)

    E. Shock induced by massive blood loss

(4) If UGIB induces HE in this patient, which one of the following factors may promote the development of HE?

    A. Increased brain sensitivity due to hypoxia

    B. increased nitrogen load by Hb proteolysis in the intestine

    C. Increased endogenous nitrogen load due to hepatorenal syndrome

    D. Increased BBB permeability due to abnormal energy metabolism

    E. All of the above

(5) If the patient developed HE, which one of the following mechanisms was NOT involved in it?

    A. Increased ammonia toxicity to brain

    B. Increased ammonia suppression to GABA inhibitory neurotransmission

    C. Increased production of aromatic amino acids by hyperammonemia

    D. Increased false neurotransmitter production by aromatic amino acids

    E. Impaired detoxification of ammonia due to decreased cerebral levels of BCAA

(6) If the patient developed hepatorenal syndrome, which one of the following changes might NOT occur in this patient?

A. Elevated blood urea nitrogen levels

B. Parenchymal renal failure

C. Activation of sympathetic-adrenal medulla system

D. Activation of RAAS

E. Increased levels of ADH

## Case analysis questions

- **Case 1**

A 50-yr-old male pestcide factory worker was taken by ambulance to the Emergency Department due to the sudden onset of hematemesis during eating. He vomited about 1,200 mL of blood with dizziness, heart palpitation and cold sweat. He had a 5-yr history of cirrhosis. He was hospitalized after his vitals were stablized by treatment with blood transfusion and hemostasis. 1 day later, he developed somnipathy, auditory hallucination and incoherent speech. Then he was unconscious and went into a coma. Blood biochemical analysis showed: blood ammonia 140 μg/dL, blood glucose 3.5 mmol/L, and BUN 7.3 mmol/L. He was diagnosed with hepatic encephalopathy.

Questions:

(1) What is hepatic encephalopathy (HE)? What are the clinical manifestations of HE in this patient?

(2) What are the precipitating factors of HE in this patient? What are other precipitating factors?

(3) Please analyze the pathogenesis of hyperammonemia in this patient and toxic effects of hyperammonemia on central nervous system.

(4) What are the treatments for HE?

- **Case 2**

A 35-yr-old male patient was transferred to our hospital after diagnosis of cirrhotic ascites in a local hospital. He was treated with blood transfusion and hemostasis in the local hospital because of 2-day tarry stool and suspected gastrointestinal bleeding. He had a 5-yr history of alcoholic liver disease. Physical examination showed the presence of jaundice, spider angioma on upper chest, and shifting dullness. Laboratory analysis revealed: serum albumin 17 g/L (normal 34 – 47 g/L), total bilirubin (TBIL) 350.6 μmol/L (normal 1.7 – 21 μmol/L), prothrombin time (PT) 14.9 s (normal 8.9 – 10.7 s), BUN 17.5 mmol/L (normal 2.9 – 7.1 mmol/L), serum creatinine (SCr) 185.6 μmol/L (normal 61.9 – 106.1 μmol/L), and no remarkable results of hepatitis serologic test. Abdominal ultrasound showed peritoneal fluid accumulation, liver nodules and splenomegaly, but no sign of renal parenchymal or obstructive lesions. He was diagnosed with alcoholic liver disease, cirrhosis and hepatorenal syndrome. After 8 months of treatment, his plasma levels of BUN and SCr decreased to 5.4 mmol/L and 79.6 μmol/L, respectively.

Questions:

(1) What signs and laboratory test results in this patient are the consequence of hepatic dysfunction?

(2) What is hepatorenal syndrome (HRS)? What are signs of HRS in this patient?

(3) What is the pathogenesis of ascites in this patient?

(4) What is the pathogenesis of HRS in this patient?

(5) Is this patient susceptible to HE? Why?

## Answers

**Case-based multiple choice questions (single answer)**

**1**. BBEEDAC; **2**. EABEBB

**Case analysis questions**

**Case 1**

(1) What is hepatic encephalopathy (HE)? What are the clinical manifestations of HE in this patient?

HE refers to a broad range of neuropsychiatric abnormalities secondary to advanced hepatic insufficiency or portosystemic shunting in the absence of primary brain disorders. The patient had upper gastrointestinal bleeding, probably due to portal hypertension in cirrhosis. Moreover, somnipathy, auditory hallucination, incoherent speech, unconsciousness and a coma that the patient had are the symptoms of neurological disorders.

(2) What are the precipitating factors of HE in this patient? What are other precipitating factors?

Upper gastrointestinal bleeding (UGIB) is the precipitating factor of HE in this patient.

The precipitating factors of HE include: exo/endogenous factors increasing nitrogen load; various factors increasing BBB permeability; various factors increasing neuronal sensitivity to toxins.

(3) Please analyze the pathogenesis of hyperammonemia in this patient and toxic effects of hyperammonemia on central nervous system.

In the current case, the patient had a 5-yr history of cirrhosis. Portal hypertension in cirrhosis causes the development of upper gastrointestinal bleeding and subsequently increases the intestinal production of ammonia, while ornithine cycle defects in the liver impaired clearance of ammonia. Therefore, elevation of blood ammonia levels in this patient was the consequence of increased ammonia production together with decreased ammonia clearance.

Ammonia toxicity to the brain includes: abnormal brain energy metabolism; altered neurotransmitter profiles in the brain; alterations in neuronal membrane.

(4) What are the treatments for HE?

① To eliminate precipitating factors by decreasing nitrogen load, preventing hemorrhage of GI/constipation, correcting water and electrolyte disorders, and administrating analgesics/sedatives with caution.

② To reduce the plasma levels of ammonia by administrating enema and cathartics with magnesium sulfate (p. o.), suppressing activity of intestinal bacteria with neomycin (p. o.), reducing intestinal pH with fructose (p. o.), and taking glutamic acid together with arginine.

③ Others: administration of BCAA-enriched supplements (p. o. or i. v.) to correct amino acid imbalance, and administration of levodopa to promote a transition toward a full consciousness.

④ Liver transplantation to rebuild its metabolic functions.

**Case 2**

（1）What signs and laboratory test results in this patient are the consequence of hepatic dysfunction?

① Jaundice and the elevation of total bilirubin are due to impaired hepatic uptake, transport, esterification and excretion of bilirubin in this patient.

② Spider angioma is due to reduced inactivation of estrogen by the liver in this patient.

③ Decreased plasma levels of serum albumin and prolonged prothrombin time are due to decreased hepatic protein synthesis in this patient.

（2）What is hepatorenal syndrome（HRS）? What are signs of HRS in this patient?

HRS refers to the reversible renal dysfunction or failure secondary to advanced liver cirrhosis or acute severe hepatitis. The following changes in the patient indicate the development of HRS:

① Jaundice, spider angioma, and the elevation of total bilirubin are the signs of hepatic insufficiency, while ascites is a landmark of the progression into the decompensated phase of cirrhosis.

② Increased plasma levels of BUN and SCr indicate the reduction of renal function.

③ No renal parenchymal and obstructive lesions shown by ultrasound indicate that the decrease of renal function is secondary to cirrhotic ascites, probably due to the reduction of the effective circulating blood volume and renal blood supply.

④ The renal dysfunction is reversible as evidenced by a decline in plasma levels of BUN and SCr after treatment.

（3）What is the pathogenesis of ascites in this patient?

① The decrease of plasma colloidal osmotic pressure is due to significantly decreased plasma levels of albumin.

② Portal hypertension as evidenced by splenomegaly is probably due to the compression of portal branches by regenerative nodules in the liver.

③ Sodium and water retention is due to decreased effective circulating blood volume and subsequent activation of sympathetic and RAAS as well as induction of ADH secretion in hepatorenal syndrome.

④ Impaired lymphatic reflux may be caused by compression of the hepatic veins and lymphatic vessels.

（4）What is the pathogenesis of HRS in this patient?

The development of ascites in the patient with chronic liver disease reduces the effective circulating blood volume and renal blood supply, thereby leading to renal failure via the following mechanisms.

① Activation of sympathetic-adrenal medulla system increases the release of catecholamine and subsequent renal vasoconstriction to reduce the renal blood flow and GFR.

② Activation of RAAS increases the release of Angiotensin Ⅱ and subsequent renal vasoconstriction to reduce the renal blood flow and GFR.

③ Enhanced ADH secretion not only induces renal water retention but also increases renal vascular resistance, and thereby decreases renal blood flow and GFR.

（5）Is this patient susceptible to HE? Why?

This patient may develop HE. Renal dysfunction in HRS decreases the renal excretion of urea and thereby increases the levels of ammonia in blood. Diffusion of urea from blood to the intestine increases the production of ammonia by *E. coli* urease. At the same time, hepatic dysfunction in HRS impairs the ornithine cycle and elimination of ammonia. Therefore, hyperammonemia may develop in this patient with HRS and thereby induce HE.

（孙晓东　孙丽娜）

# Chapter 13  Renal Insufficiency

## Case-based multiple choice questions (single answer)

1. A 36-yr-old woman was admitted to hospital with jaundice and oliguria for 2 days. She complained of nausea, vomiting, abdominal cramps, watery diarrhea after consumption of a gall bladder isolated from a carp fish weighing more than 5 kg 6 days ago and had consistent low back pain ever since. On admission physical examination, she was present with yellow discoloration of sclera and skin. Vital signs of heart and lung were stable. The abdomen was soft with tenderness 2 cm below the costal margin. Her BP was 120/80 mmHg. Laboratory examination showed: plasma $[K^+]$ 5.6 mmol/L, glucose 6.7 mmol/L, blood urea nitrogen (BUN) 18.4 mmol/L, serum creatinine 158.6 μmol/L. The results of alanine aminotransferase (ALT) and aspartate aminotransferase (AST) were not remarkable.

(1) Which one of the following diseases did NOT occur in this patient?

    A. ARF                            B. Hepatitis B

    C. Acute gastroenteritis         D. Acute cholecystitis

    E. Hyperkalemia

(2) Which one of the following disorders is involved in the development of oliguria in this patient?

    A. Renal tubular dysfunction due to poisoning

    B. Primary glomerulonephritis

    C. Nephropyelitis

    D. Lumbar muscle degradation

    E. Urolithiasis

(3) Which one of the following pathological states is NOT possible to occur in this patient?

    A. Hematuresis                B. Proteinuria

    C. Acidosis                    D. Edema

    E. Alkalosis

(4) Which one of the following urinalysis results is NOT possible to come from this patient?

    A. Hyponatruria             B. Hyposthenuria

    C. Low specific gravity of urine     D. Proteinuria

    E. Cylindruria

（5）Which one of the following factors is NOT involved in the development of renal disorder in this patient?

    A. Renal tubular epithelial cell injury     B. Reduced renal perfusion pressure

    C. Reduced GFR     D. Impairment of renal ion transporters

    E. Renal brush border injury

**2. A 37-yr-old woman was admitted to hospital due to uncontrolled elevation of blood creatinine. She had dizziness without obvious precipitating factors 2 years ago. Her blood analysis showed blood creatitine of 475 μmol/L and BP of 182/104 mmHg. She was treated in many hospitals thereafter, but her conditions had not obviously improved. Her blood creatinine continued to rise. Recently, she complained of decreased appetite, sour regurgitation, feeling cold, and nocturia 3 – 4 times per night. On admission examinations revealed her blood creatinine of 1,021 μmol/L and the absence of the tendon reflex.**

（1）Which one of the following renal disorders did this patient have?

    A. Compensated chronic renal insufficiency

    B. Chronic renal insufficiency

    C. Compensated acute renal insufficiency

    D. Uremia

    E. Acute renal insufficiency

（2）Which one of the following disorders caused the absence of the tendon reflex in this patient?

    A. Peripheral neuropathy

    B. Hyperphosphatemia

    C. Excessive excretion of growth hormone

    D. Increased protein synthesis

    E. Hyperlipidaemia

（3）Which one of the following changes is involved in the development of sour regurgitation in this patient?

    A. Urea decreases     B. Insulin decreases

    C. PTH decreases     D. Production of ammonium ion decreasses

    E. Gastrin increases

（4）Which one of the following toxins may accumulate in this patient?

    A. Urea     B. Guanidines

    C. PTH     D. Polyamine

    E. All of the above

（5）Which one of the following treatments is NOT proper for this patient?

    A. Nutritional support     B. High-calorie foods full of carbohydrates and fat

    C. High-protein diet     D. Anti-infective therapy

    E. Correction of water-electrolyte disturbances

**3.** A 30-yr-old man with a femur fracture was sent to hospital after a car accident half an hour ago. On admission examinations, his BP was 90/64 mmHg. Laboratory analysis showed: serum creatinine 132 μmol/L, urine specific gravity 1. 021, urine sodium levels < 20 mmol/L, BUN ( blood urea nitrogen) -creatinine ratio 40 : 1, and trace protein in urine.

(1) Which one of the following renal disorders did this patient have?

    A. Functional renal failure　　　　B. Chronic renal insufficiency

    C. Organic renal failure　　　　　D. Uremia

    E. End-stage renal failure

(2) Which one of the following mechanisms is involved in the development of renal dysfunctions in this patient?

    A. Decreased effective circulatory blood volume

    B. Bone fracture

    C. Hyperglycemia

    D. Increased protein synthesis

    E. Hyperlipidaemia

(3) Which of the following might be detected in the microscopic examination of urinary sediment from this patient?

    A. Deformable epithelial cells　　　B. A high number of RBC

    C. White blood cell casts　　　　　D. Granular casts

    E. None of the above

(4) If his levels of serum creatinine increased to 300 μmol/L after blood transfusion, which one of the following urine osmolality values is most likely from this patient?

    A. 550 mM　　　　　　　　　　　B. 700 mM

    C. 330 mM　　　　　　　　　　　D. 500 mM

    E. 600 mM

(5) Which one of the following treatments should be taken first for this patient?

    A. External fixation of fractures　　B. Blood transfusion

    C. Nutritional support　　　　　　D. Anti-infective therapy

    E. Correction of the water-electrolyte disturbances

## Case analysis questions

A 32-yr-old woman was sent to Emergency Department with the chief complaint of anuria for almost 24 hours. She had glomerulonephritis 21 years ago and did not take any regular medicines before. After that, she had recurrent swelling of eyelids ( not affected by gravity). She had frequent urination (more than 10 times per day, 4 – 5 times at night and 2,000 mL/d) since 7 years ago. At that time, her BP was 145/100 mmHg. The blood analysis showed Hb of 40 – 70 g/L and RBC of $1. 3 \times 10^{12}$ – $1. 76 \times 10^{12}$/L. The urinalysis revealed proteinuria ( + ), RBC ( – ), WBC ( – ), epithelial cells 0 – 2/HP ( high power field). In recent 3 years, nocturia had become more frequent. The total volume of urination reached $2,500 - 3,500$ mL/d and its specific gravity was about $1.010$ ($1.015 - 1.025$). Her generalized bone pain became more and more severe, and did not improve after treatments with anti-rheumatics and acupuncture. She complained of oliguria, severe edema, reduced appetite, nausea, vomiting, abdominal pain, generalized pruritus, limb numbness and slight convulsions in recent 15 days. On admission physical examination showed: T 37 ℃, R 20 breaths/min, HR 120 beats/min, BP 150/98 mmHg, RBC $1.49 \times 10^{12}$/L, Hb 47 g/L, WBC $9.6 \times 10^9$/L (normal $4 \times 10^9 - 10 \times 10^9$/L), plasma [Pi] 1.9 mmol/L (normal $0.74 - 1.39$ mmol/L), plasma calcium 1.3 mmol/L (normal $2.25 - 2.75$ mmol/L), serum creatitine 320 μmol/L. The urinalysis revealed: proteinuria (+), RBC $10 - 15$/HP, WBC $0 - 2$/HP, epithelial cell $0 - 2$/HP, granular casts $2 - 3$/HP. A X-ray showed normal lungs and a bit extended border of the heart, as well as cancellous bone loss and bone thinning on both hands. She was diagnosed as chronic renal failure.

Questions:

(1) What are the mechanisms underlying the development of chronic renal failure in this patient? What are the typical manifestations of chronic renal failure in this patient?

(2) Why did this patient have nocturia, diuresis and isosthenuria?

(3) What are the complications of chronic renal failure in this patient? What's the pathogenesis of these complications?

## Answers

**Case-based multiple choice questions (single answer)**

**1**. BAEAB; **2**. DAEEC; **3**. AAECB

**Case analysis questions**

(1) What are the mechanisms underlying the development of chronic renal failure in this patient? What are the typical manifestations of chronic renal failure in this patient?

The patient had "glomerulonephritis" and recurrent swelling for 20 years. That indicates the glomerulonephritis is chronic, which could result in a progressive loss of nephrons. On one hand, the hemodynamic compensations of the remaining nephrons (high perfusion, pressure and filtration) stimulate mesangial cell proliferation and increase extracellular matrix deposition, leading to the glomerular injury, progressive glomerulosclerosis and a vicious circle of nephron loss. On the other hand, the chronic inflammation, hypoxia plus tubular hypermetabolism induce the tubular-interstitial injury, fibrosis and the progressive loss of nephrons. In addition, many other factors such as hypertension, proteinuria and toxin of intoxication, etc. are also related to the progression of CRF. In line, signs and symptoms of chronic renal failure developed over time in this patient: from nocturna (nocturnal > daytime urine volume), diuresis ($ > 2,000$ mL/d), hyposthenuria in early and middle stages to oliguria/anuria, isosthenuria, hematuresis and cylinduria in the late stage. Also this patient had azotemia (serum creatinine 320 μmol/L), hyperphosphatemia ($1.9$ μmol/L $> 1.39$ μmol/L), hypocalcemia ($1.3$ mmol/L $< 2.25$ mmol/L), serious anemia (Hb 47 g/L $< 120$ g/L), hypertension ($150/98$ mmHg $> 140/90$ mmHg), as well as osteodystrophy (cancellous bone loss and bone thinning on both hands).

（2）Why did this patient have nocturia, diuresis and isosthenuria?

Nocturia is an early manifestation of chronic renal failure with similar or even more urine at night as compared to daytime. It develops due to the diminished ability of renal tubules to reabsorb salt and water. Also the glomerular filtration rate（GFR）increases with enhanced venous return and renal blood flow when lying down at night.

Pathogenesis of diuresis includes: massive loss of nephrons increases the renal blood flow and GFR in the remaining nephrons, glomerular hyperfiltration speeds up the flow of tubular fluid and relatively shortens duration of urinary concentration; osmotic diuresis due to the increase of solute in the crude urine; renal medullary damage impairs the formation of the concentration gradient（hyperosmotic environment）and subsequently reduces urinary concentration capacity; reduced water retention due to less responses to ADH in damaged distal convoluted tubule and collecting duct.

Isosthenuria is a late manifestation of chronic renal failure, mainly because of renal inability to concentrate or dilute the urine. The specific gravity of isosthenuria is neither greater nor less than that of protein-free plasma, typically $1.008 - 1.012$.

（3）What are the complications of chronic renal failure in this patient? What's the pathogenesis of these complications?

This patient had renal hypertension, anemia and osteodystrophy. The pathogenesis of these complications is as the following:

① Renal hypertension: the retention of water & sodium and the increase of blood volume lead to "volume-expanded" hypertension. Renal ischemia stimulates the secretion of renin and angiotensin Ⅱ and thereby results in renin-dependent hypertension via the induction of vasoconstriction and peripheral resistance. Moreover, the renal parenchymal damage reduces the secretion of pressure-reducing substances. Reduced generations of kallikrein, plasmakinin and prostaglandin also contribute to the development of renal hypertension. Hypertension in glomerular diseases is primarily volume-dependent. However, it is difficult to separate volume-dependent hypertension from renin-dependent one, as they may occur at the same time. Recent studies indicate that the activation of renal sympathetic nerve may result in refractory hypertension.

② Renal anemia occurs due to the less production of erythropoietin（EPO）. The accumulation of toxic substances（such as methylguandine）inhibits hematopoiesis in bone marrow, damages red blood cells, and induces bleeding via impairment of platelet functions. Some toxins could reduce the intestinal absorption of hematopoeitic raw materials, such as iron and folic acid and hamper their utilization. Aluminum poisoning（or aluminum overload）also inhibits some enzymes essential for hemoglobin synthesis and thereby impairs the functions of red blood cells.

③ Renal osteodystrophy: hyperphosphatemia and hypocalcemia developed in chronic renal failure stimulate the secretion of parathyroid hormone（PTH）and thereby induce the calcium release from bones. As a result, bones are decalcified to be soft. The renal diseases may also reduce the levels of active vitamin $D_3$ to hamper the bone calcification, which worsens secondary hyperparathyroidism and causes a kind of symptoms, including the bone decalcification, soft bones, joint pain and myotenositis, etc. In addition, acidosis and aluminum accumulation may be involved in the development of osteodystrophy.

（郑　栋　赵丽梅）

# Chapter 14    Brain Dysfunction

## Case-based multiple choice questions (single answer)

1. **A 55-yr-old man suddenly felt dizzy with right limb weakness and aphasia 2 hours ago. He had a history of metabolic syndrome and atrial fibrillation. He was diagnosed with ischemic stroke.**

(1) Where are the lesions in the brain of this patient?

    A. Left cerebral hemisphere      B. Right cerebral hemisphere

    C. Occipital lobe      D. Frontal lobe

    E. Temporal lobe

(2) Which one of the following laboratory results is NOT likely to come from this patient?

    A. Glucose 8.98 mmol/L      B. LDL-C 2.7 mmol/L

    C. BP 150/95 mmHg      D. BMI 30

    E. TG 2.7 mmol/L

(3) Which one of the following changes in this patient is the clinical manifestation of cognitive disorders?

    A. Dizzy      B. Limb weakness

    C. Aphasia      D. Hypertension

    E. Atrial fibrillation

(4) Which one of the following statements is NOT true about the pathogenesis of cognitive impairment in this patient?

    A. Cerebral ischemia led to the abnormal energy metabolism of neurons

    B. Cerebral ischemia led to the calcium overload of neurons

    C. Cerebral ischemia led to the excitation of GABAergic neurons

    D. Cerebral ischemia damaged neurons by inflammatory mechanisms

    E. Cerebral ischemia increased the production of oxygen free radicals

(5) Which one of the following treatments is the most important for this patient?

    A. Rapid reperfusion to reduce neuronal damage

    B. Psychotherapy for emotion regulation

    C. Regulation of neurotransmitters to improve neuronal functions

    D. Microenvironment improvement and symptomatic treatment

    E. Conservative drug therapy

**2.** A 63-yr-old female suddenly fell to the ground and became unconscious half an hour ago. Meanwhile, she did not have convulsion, reverse ocular bobbing, foaming at the mouth, or gatism. She had hypertension and diabetes. Physical examination showed BP of 140/85 mmHg, glucose of 25 mmol/L, and results of the cardiopulmonary and abdominal examination were not remarkable. She was still unconsciousness with equal pupils. Pathological reflexes were negative, and withdrawal reflex was normal.

(1) What kind of brain dysfunction did this patient have?

A. Cognitive impairment      B. Disorder of consciousness

C. Psychological disorders      D. Mood disorders

E. Dysmnesia

(2) Which of the following is the arousal level of this patient?

A. Drowsiness      B. Lethargy

C. Coma      D. Confusion

E. Delirium

(3) Which one of the following changes is the most likely cause of fainting for this patient?

A. Abnormal blood pressure

B. Abnormal blood glucose metabolism

C. Electrolyte imbalances

D. Disturbances of neurotransmitter metabolism in brain

E. Cerebral apoplexy

(4) Which one of the following mechanisms is NOT involved in the development of brain dysfunction in this patient?

A. Damaged ARAS

B. Extensive injury and functional inhibition of cerebral cortex

C. Destruction of positive feedback in midbrain-thalamus-cortex circuits

D. Thalamic dysfunction

E. Synaptic dysfunction

(5) Which one of the following treatments is NOT proper for this patient?

A. Regulate neurotransmitters

B. Keep airways clear

C. Find out the cause and the proper treatment

D. Real-time monitor on vital signs and the state of consciousness

E. Reduce the primary and secondary brain injury

**3.** A 68-yr-old woman was present in hospital due to memory loss and getting lost. She did not have hypertension, heart diseases, cerebral hemorrhage or ischemia. However, her symptoms of forgetfulness worsened in the last several years. She lost and forgot things very often. On that morning, she went to buy vegetables, but didn't go back home before her husband found her in the alley near the open market. When he asked her why she didn't go back home, she said, "I didn't recall how I got here, so I can't find the way back home." On admission physical examination showed BP was 130/85 mmHg, and she was alert and oriented, but completely forgot what had happened in the morning. CT showed extensive brain atrophy. She was diagnosed with Alzheimer's disease.

(1) What kind of brain dysfunction did the patient have?

    A. Cognitive disorders        B. Disorder of consciousness

    C. Learning disorders         D. Dementia

    E. Agnosias

(2) Why did this woman have memory loss?

    A. Craniocerebral trauma       B. Brain aging and neuronal loss

    C. Cerebral ischemia          D. Chronic systemic diseases

    E. Mental abnormality

(3) Which one of the following mechanisms is NOT involved in the development of Alzheimer's disease in this woman?

    A. Abnormal protein aggregation in the brain

    B. Abnormal modifications of proteins in the brain

    C. Free-radical damage

    D. Glutamate excitotoxicity

    E. Gene mutations

(4) In addition to brain atrophy, which one of the following abnormalities can lead to the impairment of learning and memory in this patient?

    A. Abnormal expressions of neuromodulators and receptors

    B. Synaptic dysfunction

    C. Neural circuit dysfunction

    D. Decreased protein synthesis and abnormal protein phosphorylation

    E. All of the above

## Case analysis questions

A 70-yr-old man was admitted to hospital due to bradykinesia and hand tremors. He complained of slow movements which started without obvious precipitating factors 8 years ago. At that time, he also had a low-amplitude tremor on left upper limb. The increased amplitude of tremor and decreased sense of smell were ignored by his family. 5 years ago, the tremor also occurred on the right upper limb, which became very obvious at rest and exacerbated by stress. The motor retardation became worse as well. He had taken Madopar 0. 125 g, bid. In the last year, he developed forward/rightward tilt and slower movement, and progressed to be noticeably incapacitated in daily living. His appetite was fine, but sometimes coughing during the eating and drinking. On physical examination, BP was 135/85 mmHg. He was alert and oriented with a "mask-like" face (hypomimia) and rest tremors of both upper limbs. His limbs showed increased muscle tone and normal muscle strength (grade 5), and his alternating hand movement was slow. He was diagnosed as Parkinson disease.

Questions:

(1) How is this patient diagnosed as Parkinson disease (PD)?

(2) What are the mechanisms of brain dysfunction in this patient?

(3) What kind of brain dysfunction did this patient have?

## Answers

**Case-based multiple choice questions (single answer)**

**1**. ABCCA; **2**. BCBEA; **3**. ABDE

**Case analysis questions**

(1) How is this patient diagnosed as Parkinson disease (PD)?

The evidences for diagnosis:

① Rest tremors were worsening over time, progressed from one side to both sides; bradykinesia started with tremors of the left upper limb 8 years ago, the tremor also occurred on the right upper limb and became very obvious at rest and exacerbated by stress, and motor retardation became worsen as well.

② Physical examination showed typical manifestations of PD: masked face, rest tremor and slow movement.

③ Olfactory dysfunction: decreased sense of smell.

(2) What are the mechanisms of brain dysfunction in this patient?

① Abnormal metabolism of dopamine(DA) in brain.

② Genetics of PD.

③ Toxic environments, i. e. long-term exposure to heavy metals and pesticides.

④ Mitonchondrial dysfunction, oxidative stress, glutamate toxicity, inflammation, cell apoptosis, and dysfunction of neurotransmitter transporters.

(3) What kind of brain dysfunction did this patient have?

① Movement dysfunction: rest tremors of upper limbs, increased muscle tone, slow alternating hand movement, and bradykinesia.

② Sensory dysfunction: decreased sense of smell.

(单立冬)

# Chapter 15    Multiple Organ Dysfunction Syndrome

## Case-based multiple choice questions (single answer)

1. A 78-yr-old man was admitted to hospital because of a cough for 2 weeks. CT-guided percutaneous lung biopsy was examined and he was diagnosed with lung cancer. After chemotherapy, he was discharged from the hospital. 3 weeks later, he presented with fever and shortness of breath, followed by jaundice and oliguria. He was thus sent to hospital. On admission physical examination showed: T 38.6 ℃, R 30 breaths/min, BP 140/95 mmHg, HR 125 beats/min.

(1) Which one of the following disorders did this patient have for rehospitalization after chemotherapy discharge?

    A. Infectious shock                  B. Chronic renal dysfunction

    C. Cardiac insufficiency            D. MODS

    E. Hepatic encephalopathy

(2) Which one of the following caused the symptoms in this patient after chemotherapy?

    A. Shortness of breath due to lung cancer    B. Hypoxemia due to lung cancer

    C. Tumor metastasis to various organs     D. Side effects of chemotherapy drugs

    E. Hypoimmunity and severe infection

(3) Which one of the following responses is NOT likely to occur in this patient?

    A. Uncontrolled systemic inflammatory responses caused by SIRS

    B. Stronger pro-inflammatory responses than the anti-inflammatory responses

    C. Stronger anti-inflammatory responses than the pro-inflammatory responses

    D. Bacterial translocation from the intestines

    E. Increased expressions of inflammatory mediators

(4) Which one of the following mechanisms is NOT mainly involved in the development of hepatic injury in this patient?

    A. Liver perfusion is increased and thereby induces hepatic stasis and edema

    B. High hepatic expressions of xanthine oxidase make livers susceptible to ischemia-reperfusion injury

    C. Intestinal bacteria and toxins damage hepatocytes after translocation and transportation into livers

    D. Activation of Kupffer cells leads to the massive production of inflammatory mediators in livers

    E. Toxins damage intrahepatic vascular endothelial cells and induce microthrombosis

**2. A 58-yr-old woman was admitted to hospital with acute right upper abdominal pain and was diagnosed with acute necrotizing pancreatitis upon admission. Thereafter, she quickly deteriorated and developed acute respiratory distress syndrome, and then gradually improved after comprehensive treatment with anti-infection, rehydration, and oxygenation. However, 3 days later, she had high temperature again with dyspnea followed by oliguria, palpitations and leg muscle atrophy, and was diagnosed with MODS.**

（1）Which one of the following disorders is the main cause of MODS in this patient?

    A. Pulmonary infection

    B. Tissue necrosis due to acute necrotizing pancreatitis

    C. Cardiac insufficiency

    D. Renal dysfunction

    E. Hypoimmunity

（2）Which one of the following is the type of MODS in this patient?

    A. Monophase immediate MODS      B. Primary type

    C. One-hit type                 D. Dual-phase delayed MODS

    E. None of the above

（3）Which one of the following metabolic changes is closely associated with leg muscle atrophy?

    A. Hypermetabolism          B. Reduced oxygen consumption

    C. Hyperdynamic circulation     D. Hypodynamic circulation

    E. Reduced basal metabolic rate

（4）Which one of the following is the reason why the patient with MODS is more susceptible to acute pulmonary dysfunction?

    A. Harmful substances accumulate in lungs as all of the mixed venous blood from all of the tissues in the body is pumped out of the right ventricle into the pulmonary circulation

    B. Macrophages rich in lungs are easily activated

    C. Activation of inflammatory cells damages and activates pulmonary vascular endothelial cells

    D. Reactive oxygen species, lysosomal enzymes and inflammatory mediators are easily produced by damaged lungs

    E. All of the above

**3. A 35-yr-old woman was admitted to hospital for hemorrhage after spontaneous delivery. On admission, she was given an anti-shock treatment but her blood pressure remained low. 4 days later, the patient showed a temperature of 39 ℃, leukocytes of 2.0 × 10^10/L, heart rate of 120 beats/min, weak pulse, elevated serum creatinine, and thrombocytopenia, prolonged clotting time, purpura and punctate bleeding spots. However, she had no infectious lesions and no bacteria was grown/detected in her blood culture.**

（1）Which one of the following is the reason why this patient with symptoms of infection had no infectious lesions or detectable bacteria in blood?

　　A. Intestinal endotoxemia　　　　B. Urinary tract infection

　　C. Reproductive system infection　D. Neurological infection

　　E. Respiratory infection

（2）Which one of the following changes is associated with elevated serum creatinine in this patient?

　　A. Oliguria or anuria　　　　　　B. Hyperkalemia

　　C. Elevated blood urea nitrogen　D. Edema

　　E. All of the above

（3）Which one of the following mechanisms is involved in the elevation of serum creatinine in this patient?

　　A. Decreased secretion of aldosterone and antidiuretic hormone

　　B. Renal tubular necrosis

　　C. Decreased renal blood flow

　　D. Sympathetic depression

　　E. Organic injury

（4）Which one of the following pathological states did this patient have?

　　A. Hemorrhagic shock　　　　　　B. Systemic inflammatory response syndrome

　　C. Renal dysfunction　　　　　　 D. DIC

　　E. All of the above

（5）Which one of the following is NOT the principle of treatment for this patient?

　　A. To block the inflammatory responses

　　B. To improve oxygen metabolism and correct hypoxia

　　C. To use anticoagulation therapy

　　D. To prevent and treat the ischemia-reperfusion injury

　　E. To improve the abdominal organ blood perfusion

**Answers**

**Case-based multiple choice questions（single answer）**

1. DECA；2. BDAE；3. AECEC

（赵丽梅）

# Chapter 16    Problem-based Learning

## Case 1: Big trouble from a mild cold

- **Part 1**

Mr. Wang was a 40-yr-old businessman in charge of an advertising company. As a migrant worker, he worked hard for more than a decade to set up his own company from nothing by himself. In Mr. Wang's words, his footprints were everywhere around the world. He traveled on business so frequently that he had poor eating and sleeping habits. He not only depended on a lot of smoking to stay up for making plans, but also had a heavy taste and drank a lot in business dinners. However, Mr. Wang never worried about his health as he thought he was so strong that he seldom went to hospital even when he had headache or fever sometimes. He did not care about minor illness and even postponed his annual medical examination because of his busy work schedule. 3 years ago, his blood pressure was found a bit high, but he did not monitor his blood pressure or get any medication. Since half a year ago, he started to feel tired more easily than before and his appetite was declining. Sometimes he had chest tightness, short of breath and occasional chest pain when he felt exhausted after work, and these symptoms were relieved soon by rest. Moreover, he cannot afford his favorite badminton game and did not take it to heart. 3 days ago, he got a cold with a runny nose. After taking some common cold medicine brought in a drugstore, he started coughing especially at night and had poor urine output and mild leg swelling, despite a significantly reduced runny nose. On that evening, the company had a dinner party. As the boss of the company, he had to drink a lot at the company dinner. When returning home, he felt suffocated like lack of oxygen and did not improve after a long rest. He was thus admitted to hospital.

- **Part 2**

After a brief inquiry of medical history, the attending physician immediately performed a physical examination. His body temperature was 36.5 ℃; heart rate was 115 beats/min; respiratory rate was 30 breaths/min; and blood pressure was 160/105 mmHg. The patient was in a forced position with orthopnea. He had shortness of breath when lying down, which was relieved by sitting upright. He had jugular vein distension and a positive hepatojugular reflux.

Pitting edema was remarkable in his ankles and feet. On auscultation, fine moist rales were heard at the base of lungs. The left heart border extended to the left, and the apex impulse was present about 1 cm lateral to the midclavicular line in the left sixth intercostal space. A soft first heart sound, diastolic gallops (third heart sound), as well as a 2/6 systolic murmur at the cardiac apex can be heard.

## ● Part 3

**Blood routine examination**: RBC $6.4 \times 10^{12}$/L ($4.3 \times 10^{12} - 5.8 \times 10^{12}$/L), WBC $12 \times 10^9$/L ($3.5 \times 10^9 - 9.5 \times 10^9$/L), N 81% (40% − 75%), PLT $230 \times 10^9$/L ($125 \times 10^9 - 350 \times 10^9$/L), Hb 185 g/L (130 − 175 g/L).

**Biochemistry blood test**: TB 28.7 μmol/L (3.5 − 20.5 μmol/L), ALT 80 U/L (4 − 43 U/L), Cr 79 μmol/L (59 − 104 μmol/L), GLU 6.6 mmol/L (3.89 − 6.11 mmol/L), TC 4.5 mmol/L (0 − 5.69 mmol/L), TG 1.2 mmol/L (0.3 − 1.7 mmol/L), LDL-C 3.62 mmol/L (2.07 − 3.36 mmol/L), CK 46 U/L (38 − 172 U/L), troponin (−).

**Urine routine test**: Pro (−).

**Biomarker analysis**: NT-proBNP 5,600 pg/mL (< 300 pg/mL).

**ECG**: sinus tachycardia, HR 110 beats/min, altered ST-T segment (Figure 1).

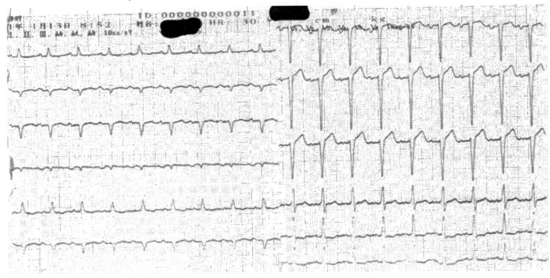

**Figure 1    ECG results**

**Chest X-ray**: enlarged heart, cardiothoracic ratio 0. 66, pulmonary edema (Figure 2).

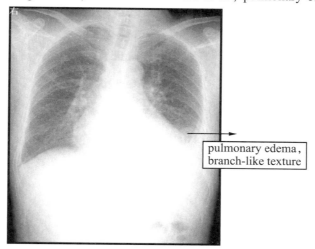

pulmonary edema, branch-like texture

**Figure 2 Chest X-ray results**

**Coronary angiography**: normal right coronary artery (Figure 3A), 40% stenosis in proximal segment of left anterior descending artery (Figure 3B), and 40% stenosis in left circumflex artery (Figure 3C).

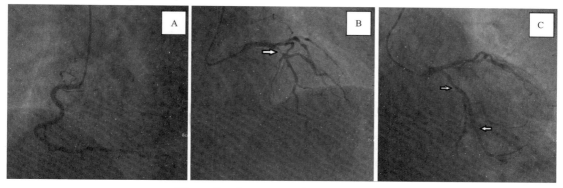

**Figure 3 Coronary angiography results**

**Echocardiography**: enlargement of the whole heart, significantly impaired left ventricular systolic function (left ventricular ejection fraction, LVEF 23. 67%), moderate mitral and tricuspid regurgitation, moderate pulmonary hypertension, aortic valve stiffness, and mild aortic insufficiency.

● **Part 4**

**Diagnosis**:

Dilated cardiomyopathy

Biventricular heart failure

Cardiac function: NYHA Ⅳ

Hypertension, grade 2

Coronary atherosclerosis

**Medication treatment:**

Furosemide injection    20 – 40 mg    three i. v. bolus injection a day,

oral administration when acute symptoms are improved

| | | |
|---|---|---|
| Digoxin | 0. 125 mg | qd |
| Perindopril | 4 mg | qd |
| Spironolactone | 20 mg | qd |

**Medications applied after the coronary angiography:**

| | | |
|---|---|---|
| Atorvastatin | 20 mg | qn |
| Aspirin | 0. 1 g | qd |

**Medication applied at day 4 after the disappearance of edema with stable weight:**

Metoprolol sustained release tablets    11. 875 mg    qd

After 10-day treatment in the hospital, the patient was significantly improved without shortness of breath at rest or when lying down. No rales and lower limb edema were detected, and results of blood and urine routine tests were unremarkable.

**Home medications:**

| | | |
|---|---|---|
| Furosemide | 20 mg | qd |
| Digoxin | 0. 125 mg | qd |
| Perindopril | 4 mg | qd |
| Metoprolol sustained release tablets | 11. 875 mg | qd |
| Spironolactone | 20 mg | qd |
| Atorvastatin | 20 mg | qn |
| Aspirin | 0. 1 g | qd |

Medical advice from the doctor: quit smoking and drinking with low-sodium and fluid-restricted diet, avoid heavy physical activity and catching cold, stay in a good mood.

## • Part 5

After discharge, the patient took the doctor's advice to adjust his lifestyle and gradually improved without lower limb edema. He was able to do some housework and had no shortness of breath.

On the morning of day 10 after discharge, he felt anorexia and nausea. When he read the newspaper in the afternoon, he suddenly had a blurred vision. He told his wife that he saw everything yellow and felt heart palpitations.

The patient was admitted to hospital immediately and had some medical examinations. ECG: HR 120 beats/min, frequent premature ventricular contractions, bigeminy rhythm.

## • Part 6

The physician inquired the medical history and found that he mistakenly took too much digoxin as each tablet contains 0. 25 mg. The blood concentrations of digoxin were 4. 0 ng/mL (0 – 2 ng/mL).

**Diagnosis**: digoxin poisoning.

The physician asked the patient to stop taking digoxin immediately, and gave the patient potassium chloride. Potassium chloride (1. 5 g) in 500 mL normal saline was intravenously infused into the patient. Also the patient orally took potassium chloride sustained release tablet 1. 0 g tid and phenytoin sodium 0. 1 g bid. Blood potassium concentrations and urine volume were monitored meanwhile. Symptoms of the patient disappeared that evening.

Over the next few weeks, digoxin was discontinued, and other medications were continued with gradually increased doses of perindopril and metoprolol. The patient continued to improve and had no symptomatic relapse.

3 months later, Mr. Wang was asymptomatic at rest and on mild exercise. The follow-up medical examination revealed: HR 80 beats/min, BP 110/70 mmHg, LVEF 40%.

**Core learning issues**:

(1) Please analyze the ECG results of the patient in this case using the knowledge on cardiovascular anatomy and functions.

(2) Please analyze the cardiac auscultation results of the patient in this case using the knowledge on cardiovascular anatomy and functions.

(3) Please analyze the echocardiography results of the patient in this case using the knowledge on cardiovascular anatomy and functions.

(4) Please discuss neurohumoral mechanisms underlying the manifestations of the patient in this case, and explain why positive inotropic agents are not the first choice for this patient.

(5) Please analyze the etiology and pathogenesis of heart failure in this patient.

(6) What's atherosclerotic coronary heart diseases (CHD)? What's pathogenesis? What's the relationship of atherosclerotic CHD to heart failure?

(7) What are the pathological changes of hypertension and dilated cardiomyopathy? What are the signs of these disorders?

(8) Please analyze the pharmacological effects of medications used for the patient in this case. What are the mechanisms underlying the therapeutic effects of lipid-lowering drugs and diuretics?

(9) What are the adverse effects of digoxin? How to prevent these adverse effects? Why were potassium chloride and phenytoin sodium given to the patient with digoxin poisoning?

(10) What is the classification of medications for heart failure? What are the representative drugs? What are the pharmacological effects and underlying mechanisms of digoxin, ACE inhibitors and beta blockers?

(盛　瑞　赵丽梅)

# Case 2: Mr. Min, please listen to your doctor!

## • Part 1

Mr. Min was a 56-yr-old man who had recently retired. He was divorced at the age of 40 and lived alone since then. He did not like cooking and always ate out at restaurants. He had been smoking 1 – 2 packs of cigarettes a day for more than 30 years. After retirement, he was crazy about mahjong games and always stayed up playing all night. Mr. Min thought he was in good health and thus forgot/missed the regular physical checkups organized by his original company because of mahjong games. Since July in 2015, Mr. Min noticed foamy urine and slight lower limb swelling. However, he did not go to see the doctor for the fear of disease. 3 months later, he had intermittent fatigue and frequent dizziness. When he attended the family party to celebrate his mother's 82nd birthday, his elder sisters noticed his severe leg swelling and urged him to see the doctor. As he was getting worse and worse, he was finally admitted to hospital.

## • Part 2

On the medical consultation, Mr. Min reported no history of infectious diseases, drug allergy, trauma, and surgery. Also his parents were very healthy.

**Physical examination:** BW 75 kg, H 175 cm, T 36.8 ℃, P 75 beats/min, R 16 breaths/min, BP 145/95 mmHg, facial swelling, no jugular vein distension, normal heart and lung sounds on auscultation, soft abdomen without palpable liver and spleen, no percussion pain in both kidney areas, pitting edema (grade 3, 4 – 6 mm indentation) in lower limbs.

**Blood analysis:** normal blood cell counts, $[K^+]$ 3.76 mmol/L (3.5 – 5.5 mmol/L), $[Na^+]$ 143.5 mmol/L (135 – 145 mmol/L), $[Cl^-]$ 107.9 mmol/L (97 – 107 mmol/L), $[Ca]$ 2.38 mmol/L (2.3 – 2.7 mmol/L), TP 42.5 g/L (65 – 80 g/L), Alb 19.2 g/L (35 – 55 g/L), Glob 23.3 g/L (20 – 35 g/L), Alb/Glob = 0.8 (1 – 2), ALT 15 U/L (0 – 40 U/L), AST 20 U/L (0 – 40 U/L), AST/ALT = 1.33 (1 – 2), T-Bil 12.8 μmol/L (3.42 – 20.5 μmol/L), D-Bil 2.1 μmol/L (0 – 6.8 μmol/L), I-Bil 10.7 μmol/L (0 – 17 μmol/L), TC 8.51 mmol/L (0 – 5.17 mmol/L), TG 1.7 mmol/L (0.5 – 1.7 mmol/L), HDL-C 1.8 mmol/L (1.04 – 1.66 mmol/L), LDL-C 4.74 mmol/L (0 – 3.12 mmol/L), BUN 4.5 mmol/L (1.7 – 8.3 mmol/L), SCr 76.5 μmol/L (60 – 115 μmol/L), BUN/SCr = 58.82 (20 – 100), UA 399 μmol/L (202 – 417 μmol/L), HBsAg (–), Syphilis (–), HIV (–).

**Urinalysis:** specific gravity 1.010 (1.003 – 1.02), pH 6.0 (6.0 – 8.0), RBC (++, 80/μL), WBC (–), protein (+++, ≥3.0 g/L), glucose (–), vitamin C 0.6 mmol/L, Bil (–), ketones (–), URO (–), nitrites (–). After hospitalization, 6.88 g protein in 1.2 L of urine over a 24-hour period.

## • Part 3

**Biomarker analysis**: plasma anti-PLA2R IgG4 (+++).

**Pathological analysis of renal biopsies** (**Figure** 4):

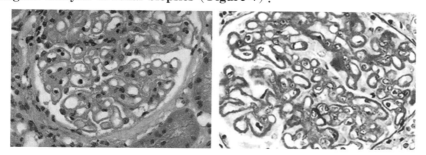

HE stained section          PAS stained section

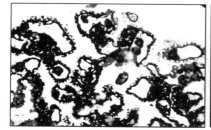   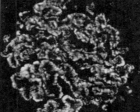   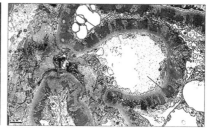

PASM stained section      Immunoflurescence stained section      Electron microscopy section

**Figure 4    Pathological analysis of renal biopsies**

**Light microscopy**:

HE stained section: 2 renal cortical tissues containing 21 glomeruli with no sclerosis and crescent formation, slightly enlarged glomeruli with 80 – 100 cells/glomerulus, 1 – 2 mesangial cells/mesangium, no proliferative cells or mesangial matrix, open capillary loops, obviously diffused thickening and stiffness of the basement membrane. PAS stained section: marked thickening of the basement membrane with subepithelial accumulation of eosinophilic substances. PASM stained section: formation of spikes on the basement membrane.

**Immunofluorescence microscopy**: subepithelial deposits with IgG (+++) and C3 (+++) on the basement membrane.

**Electron microscopy**: subepithelial electron-dense deposits and formation of spikes.

**Diagnosis**: nephrotic syndrome, Stage II membranous nephropathy.

## • Part 4

**Medical treatment and advices**: prednisone 60 mg/(kg · d), p. o. (6 – 8 a. m.); cyclophosphamide 0.6 g/m$^2$, i. v.

Have regular checkups; take adequate rest and sleep; no booze and cigarettes; limit the intake of protein, lipids, sodium, potassium and water; take more healthy carbs.

## ● **Part 5**

Upon his return home, Mr. Min started to take prednisone as prescribed. His tobacco addiction was so high that he could not quit smoking completely. He played mahjong much less than before. But sometimes he still stayed up for it. His food intake continuously increased as he always felt hungry. He ate 3 apples at once, or had 2 bowls of rice and a large bowl of meat (i. e. spareribs) for a meal. Because of heavy taste, he kept drinking water all day long. He had forgotten all the dietary advices from the doctor. 1 month later, Mr. Min noticed reduced urine output, weakness, and shortness of breath after exercise. In the last 2 days, he had barely peeing, marked lower limb swelling, and continuous worsening of dyspnea. He thus went to see a doctor in the hospital.

## ● **Part 6**

**Physical examination**: BW 80 kg, T 37 ℃, R 25 breaths/min, HR 110 beats/min, BP 160/100 mmHg, facial swelling, no conjunctival congestion and edema, centripetal obesity, hyporesonant sounds over lungs without rales or rhonchi, dullness to percussion of the chest, regular heart rhythm without murmur, abdominal distension with shifting dullness, severe pitting edema of lower limbs.

**Blood cell counts**: WBC $6.31 \times 10^9$/L $(3.5 \times 10^9 - 9.5 \times 10^9$/L$)$, Neu 71.9%, Lym 21.9%, HGB 98 g/L $(130 - 175$ g/L$)$, RBC $4.35 \times 10^{12}$/L $(4.3 \times 10^{12} - 5.8 \times 10^{12}$/L$)$, HCT 43.9 $(40 - 50)$, PLT $275 \times 10^9$/L $(125 \times 10^9 - 350 \times 10^9$/L$)$.

**Blood biochemistry test**: $[K^+]$ 3.2 mmol/L $(3.5 - 5.5$ mmol/L$)$, $[Na^+]$ 139 mmol/L $(135 - 145$ mmol/L$)$, $[Ca]$ 1.8 mmol/L $(2.3 - 2.7$ mmol/L$)$, $[HCO_3^-]$ 25 mmol/L $(22 - 29$ mmol/L$)$, glucose 7.2 mmol/L, TP 47 g/L $(65 - 80$ g/L$)$, Alb 20 g/L $(35 - 55$ g/L$)$, ALT 25 U/L $(0 - 40$ U/L$)$, AST 20 U/L $(0 - 40$ U/L$)$, TC 7.13 mmol/L $(0 - 5.17$ mmol/L$)$, TG 1.37 mmol/L $(0.5 - 1.7$ mmol/L$)$, HDL-C 1.8 mmol/L $(1.04 - 1.66$ mmol/L$)$, LDL-C 4.8 mmol/L $(0 - 3.12$ mmol/L$)$, BUN 33 mmol/L $(1.7 - 8.3$ mmol/L$)$, SCr 552 μmol/L $(60 - 115$ μmol/L$)$, UA 652 μmol/L $(202 - 417$ μmol/L$)$, PT 13.30 s $(9 - 14$ s$)$, CT 14 s $(4 - 14$ s$)$, fibinogen 3.8 g/L $(2 - 4$ g/L$)$, FDP 2.07 μg/mL $( <5.0$ μg/mL$)$.

**Urinalysis**: specific gravity 1.020, pH 6.0, RBC $(-)$, WBC $(-)$, protein $(++)$, glucose $(-)$, vitamin C $(+)$, Bil $(-)$, ketones $(-)$, URO $(-)$, nitrites $(-)$, 3.71 g protein in 0.5 L of urine over a 24-hour period.

**ECG**: sinus tachycardia.

**Chest CT**: bilateral pleural effusion with atelectasis of the right lung.

**Abdominal ultrasound**: right kidney 118 mm × 68 mm × 55 mm, left kidney 120 mm ×

70 mm × 52 mm, increased renal cortex echogenicity, normal cortical thickness and renal sinus with the clear corticomedullary junction; unremarkable bile and liver, liquid dark area in the peritoneal cavity.

**Diagnosis**: membranous nephropathy, acute renal injury.

## ● Part 7

**Hospital treatment**:

① Potassium supplement with regular monitoring of blood gas and electrolytes.

② Dialysis for 2 weeks.

③ Prednisone 60 mg/(kg · d), cyclophosphamide 0.6 g/m².

④ Spironolactone 60 mg/d, Norvasc 5 mg/d, Lipitor 10 mg/d.

⑤ Calcium supplement.

During the treatment, Mr. Min gradually improved with increased urine output, well controlled BP, and the alleviation of edema and dyspnea.

On hospital discharge, prednisone (60 mg/d) and cyclophosphamide (0.6 g/m²) were prescribed as a 3-month hormone therapy for membranous nephropathy and prednisone was gradually reduced by 5 mg per week to a dosage of 30 mg/d. In addition, he was required to take medicines including spironolactone 20 mg/d, Norvasc 5 mg/d, Lipitor 10 mg/d as well as calcium supplement. He was advised again to stop smoking, have adequate rest, and control food and water intake.

After this incidence, Mr. Min strictly took medicines as prescribed and went to bed on time. 3 months later, general supportive measures indicated his membranous nephropathy was significantly improved.

**Core learning issues**:

(1) What are the structural characteristics of nephron? Please figure out the pathological changes of renal biopsies in the case and their associations with membranous nephropathy.

(2) What's the functions of kidney? Please analyze the altered renal functions in the patient with acute renal injury.

(3) Please figure out the mechanisms underlying the development of edema in the patient with membranous nephropathy.

(4) Please figure out the mechanisms underlying the development of hyperlipidemia in the patient with membranous nephropathy.

(5) Please figure out therapeutic mechanisms of prednisone and cyclophosphamide for membranous nephropathy, as well as reasons for the control of food and water during the treatment.

(6) What are the physiological and side effects of glucocorticoids?

(7) Please figure out the pathogenesis of acute renal injury developed in the patient with

membranous nephropathy.

（8）Please analyze the types and pathogenesis of electrolyte disorders in the patient with acute renal injury.

（9）Please analyze the pharmacological effects of medicines for this patient and their role in the treatment of acute renal injury.

（10）What kind of antihypertensives and diuretics can be used for patients with renal diseases?

（赵　颖）

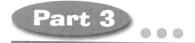

# Experiments: Expansion and Discussion

## Chapter 2　Fluid and Electrolyte Imbalance

### ◇ Water and Sodium Imbalance

**［Course Experiment］: Adrenaline-induced Pulmonary Edema**

(selected from: XIE K M, WANG G Q, JIANG X H, et al. Functional experimental science[M]. Beijing: Higher Education Press, 2014.)

**1. Previous animal studies and reviews on pathogenesis**

➤ AUER J, GATES F L. Experiments on the causation and amelioration of adrenalin pulmonary edema[J]. J Exp Med, 1917,26(2):201－220.

➤ HURLEY J V. Current views on the mechanisms of pulmonary oedema[J]. J Pathol, 1978,125(2):59－79.

**2. Case reports**

➤ ERSOZ N, FINESTONE S C. Adrenaline-induced pulmonary oedema and its treatment: a report of two cases[J]. Br J Anaesth, 1971,43(7):709－712.

➤ CHANG Y J, MIN S K, YOO J Y, et al. Acute pulmonary edema after local infiltration of epinephrine during mastoidectomy: a case report[J]. Korean J Anesthesiol, 2009,56(4):462－465.

Questions:

(1) What small animals except rabbits can be used for induction of pulmonary edema?

(2) Which parameter can be used to determine the development of edema in this experiment?

(3) What kind of fluid is trapped in lungs of mice treated with adrenaline? A transudate or an exudate?

(4) What's the pathogenesis of pulmonary edema in mice treated with overdose of adrenaline? Which parameters in the microcirculation (i. e. capillary/interstitial hydrostatic

pressure/colloid osmotic pressure) are changed for the induction of pulmonary edema?

(5) What are metabolic alterations caused by pulmonary edema in this experiment? What are mechanisms underlying these alterations?

## [Extended Experiments]

### 1. Animal models of inflammatory edema

➤ HORAKOVA Z, BEAVEN M A. Time course of histamine release and edema formation in the rat paw after thermal injury[J]. Eur J Pharmacol, 1974,27(3):305 – 312.

➤ PIETRA G G, SZIDON J P, LEVENTHAL M M, et al. Histamine and interstitial pulmonary edema in the dog[J]. Circ Res, 1971,29(4):323 – 337.

➤ MORRIS C J. Carrageenan-induced paw edema in the rat and mouse[J]. Methods Mol Biol, 2003,225:115 – 121.

### 2. Animal models of lymphedema

➤ FRUEH F S, GOUSOPOULOS E, REZAEIAN F, et al. Animal models in surgical lymphedema research—a systematic review[J]. J Surg Res, 2016,200(1):208 – 220.

➤ SAARISTO A, KARKKAINEN M J, ALITALO K. Insights into the molecular pathogenesis and targeted treatment of lymphedema[J]. Ann N Y Acad Sci, 2002,979: 94 – 110.

### 3. Hyponatremia-induced cerebral edema

➤ OVERGAARD-STEENSEN C, STØDKILDE-JØRGENSEN H, LARSSON A, et al. The frequently used intraperitoneal hyponatraemia model induces hypovolaemic hyponatraemia with possible model-dependent brain sodium loss[J]. Exp Physiol, 2016,101(7):932 – 945.

### 4. Water intoxication-induced cerebral edema

➤ KOZLER P, MARESOVA D, POKORNY J. Cellular brain edema induced by water intoxication in rat experimental model[J]. Neuro Endocrinol Lett, 2018, 39(3): 209 – 218.

Questions:

(1) How does the fluid imbalance develop in different models of edema?

(2) What's the difference between edema and cellular edema?

(3) Which parameters are used to determine the development of all kinds of edema?

(4) What are the manifestations of organ-specific edema?

# ◇ **Potassium Imbalance**

[**Course Experiment**]: **Induction and Treatment of Hyperkalemia-induced Cardiac Dysfunctions in Rabbits**

(selected from: WANG J Z, QIAN R Z. Experimental instructions for pathophysiology[M]. Beijing: People's Medical Publishing House, 2017. )

## 1. Previous animal studies and reviews on pathogenesis

➢ PATERSON D J, BLAKE G J, LEITCH S P, et al. Effects of catecholamines and potassium on cardiovascular performance in the rabbit[J]. J Appl Physiol, 1992, 73(4): 1413 – 1418.

➢ GREENBERG A. Hyperkalemia: treatment options[J]. Semin Nephrol, 1998, 18(1): 46 – 57.

## 2. Case reports

➢ LAMBREW C T, CARVER S T, PETERSON R E, et al. Hypoaldosteronism as a cause of hyperkalemia and syncopal attacks in a patient with complete heart block[J]. Am J Med, 1961, 31:81 – 85.

➢ SAAD S M, YASIN S, JAIN N, et al. Cardiac manifestations in a case of severe hyperkalemia[J]. Cureus, 2021, 13(3):e13641.

Questions:

(1) What parameters can be used to determine the changes of cardiac functions?

(2) What are the mechanisms underlying the pathogenesis of hyperkalemia-induced cardiac dysfunction?

(3) What metabolic changes can be induced by hyperkalemia? What methods and parameters are useful to find out these changes?

## [**Extended Experiments**]

## 1. Type Ⅱ Pseudohypoaldosteronism and Hyperkalemia

➢ LÓPEZ-CAYUQUEO K I, CHAVEZ-CANALES M, PILLOT A, et al. A mouse model of pseudohypoaldosteronism type Ⅱ reveals a novel mechanism of renal tubular acidosis [J]. Kidney Int, 2018, 94(3):514 – 523.

## 2. Crush Syndrome and Hyperkalemia

➢ CLEMENS M S, STULL M C, RALL J M, et al. Extracorporeal filtration of potassium in a swine model of bilateral hindlimb ischemia-reperfusion injury with severe acute hyperkalemia[J]. Mil Med, 2018, 183(11 – 12):e335 – e340.

➢ MURATA I, OOI K, SASAKI H, et al. Characterization of systemic and histologic injury after crush syndrome and intervals of reperfusion in a small animal model[J]. J Trauma, 2011, 70(6):1453 – 1463.

### 3. Digoxin Intoxication and Hyperkalemia

➤ HACK J B, WOODY J H, LEWIS D E, et al. The effect of calcium chloride in treating hyperkalemia due to acute digoxin toxicity in a porcine model[J]. J Toxicol Clin Toxicol, 2004, 42(4): 337 – 342.

### 4. Diabetes associated Hyperkalemia

➤ KIM H J. Mechanisms of hyperkalemia associated with hyporeninemic hypoaldosteronism in streptozotocin-induced diabetic rats[J]. J Korean Med Sci, 1994, 9(2): 107 – 115.

### 5. Aldosterone-induced Hyperkalemia

➤ ORENA S, MAURER T S, SHE L, et al. PF-03882845, a non-steroidal mineralocorticoid receptor antagonist, prevents renal injury with reduced risk of hyperkalemia in an animal model of nephropathy[J]. Front Pharmacol, 2013, 4: 115.

➤ BARRERA-CHIMAL J, GIRERD S, JAISSER F. Mineralocorticoid receptor antagonists and kidney diseases: pathophysiological basis[J]. Kidney Int, 2019, 96(2): 302 – 319.

Questions:

(1) What are the pathogenesis of hyperkalemia in different models shown above?

(2) What mechanisms underlying the development of hyperkalemia are still unknown in different models shown above?

## ◇ Magnesium Imbalance

### [Extended Experiment]: Thiazide-induced Hypomagnesemia in Mice

### 1. Previous animal studies and reviews on pathogenesis

➤ NIJENHUIS T, VALLON V, VAN DER KEMP A W, et al. Enhanced passive $Ca^{2+}$ reabsorption and reduced $Mg^{2+}$ channel abundance explains thiazide-induced hypocalciuria and hypomagnesemia[J]. J Clin Invest, 2005, 115(6): 1651 – 1658.

➤ WHANG R. Magnesium deficiency: pathogenesis, prevalence, and clinical implications [J]. Am J Med, 1987, 82(3A): 24 – 29.

### 2. Case reports

➤ BARNES J N, DREW P J, SKEHAN J D. Diuretic associated hypomagnesaemia[J]. Br Med J (Clin Res Ed), 1983, 286(6359): 146 – 147.

➤ SAAD S M, YASIN S, JAIN N, et al. Cardiac manifestations in a case of severe hyperkalemia[J]. Cureus, 2021, 13(3): e13641.

Questions:

(1) Except diuretics, what methods can be used to induce hypomagnesemia in animals?

(2) What are the mechanisms underlying hypomagnesemia-indueced cardiac dysfunction?

(3) What are functional and metabolic alterations in animal models of hypomagnesemia?

What tests and parameters are required for determination of these changes?

## ◇ **Calcium and Phosphate Imbalance**

### ［Extended Experiment］: Adrenalectomy-induced Hypercalcemia in Rabbits

**1. Previous animal studies and reviews on pathogenesis**

➤ GILDERSLEEVE D L, PEARSON T A, BAGHDIANTZ A, et al. Effect of ACTH, alpha-MSH, and beta-Lipotropin on calcium and phosphorus metabolism in the rabbit ［J］. Endocrinology, 1975,97(6):1593 – 1596.

➤ WALSER M, ROBINSON B H, DUCKETT J W Jr. The hypercalcemia of adrenal insufficiency［J］. J Clin Invest, 1963,42(4):456 – 465.

**2. Case reports**

➤ PEDERSEN K O. Hypercalcaemia in Addison's disease: report on two cases and review of the literature［J］. Acta Med Scand, 1967,181(6):691 – 698.

➤ AGRAWAL S, GOYAL A, AGARWAL S, et al. Hypercalcaemia, adrenal insufficiency and bilateral adrenal histoplasmosis in a middle-aged man: a diagnostic dilemma［J］. BMJ Case Rep, 2019,12(8):e231142.

Questions:

(1) Except adrenalectomy, what methods can be used to induce of hypercalcemia in animals?

(2) What are the mechanisms underlying hypercalcemia-indueced cardiac dysfunction?

(3) What are functional and metabolic changes in different animal models of hypercalcemia? What tests and parameters are required for determination of these changes?

（赵丽梅　赵　颖）

# Chapter 3　Acid-base Disturbance

### ［Course Experiment］: Metabolic Acid-base Disturbance in Rabbits

(selected from: LIU J X. Experiments in physiology and pathophysiology［M］. Hangzhou: Zhejiang University Press,2012. )

**1. Basic studies on the establishment of animal models for acid-base disturbance by direct injection of hydrochloric acid and sodium bicarbonate**

➤ JAVAHERI S, DE HEMPTINNE A, VANHEEL B, et al. Changes in brain ECF pH during metabolic acidosis and alkalosis: a microelectrode study[J]. J Appl Physiol Respir Environ Exerc Physiol, 1983,55(6):1849 – 1853.

➤ FRANS A, CLERBAUX T, WILLEMS E, et al. Effect of metabolic acidosis on pulmonary gas exchange of artificially ventilated dogs[J]. J Appl Physiol, 1993,74 (5):2301 – 2308.

➤ STENGL M, LEDVINOVA L, CHVOJKA J, et al. Effects of clinically relevant acute hypercapnic and metabolic acidosis on the cardiovascular system: an experimental porcine study[J]. Crit Care, 2013,17(6):R303.

➤ LÓPEZ I, AGUILERA-TEJERO E, ESTEPA J C, et al. Role of acidosis-induced increases in calcium on PTH secretion in acute metabolic and respiratory acidosis in the dog[J]. Am J Physiol Endocrinol Metab, 2004,286(5):E780 – 785.

➤ ANG R C, HOOP B, KAZEMI H. Brain glutamate metabolism during metabolic alkalosis and acidosis[J]. J Appl Physiol, 1992,73(6):2552 – 2558.

➤ PAVLIN E G, HORNBEIN T F. Distribution of $H^+$ and $HCO_3^-$ between CSF and blood during metabolic alkalosis in dogs[J]. Am J Physiol, 1975,228(4):1141 – 1144.

➤ LEMIEUX G, KISS A L, LEMIEUX C, et al. Renal tubular biochemistry during acute and chronic metabolic alkalosis in the dog[J]. Kidney Int, 1985,27(6):908 – 918.

➤ NISHIO I. Changes in respiratory system resistance and reactance following acute respiratory and metabolic alkalosis in dogs[J]. J Anesth, 1996,10(4):282 – 288.

**2. Case reports and clinical studies**

➤ JURISIC D, SAMARDZIC J, HRECKOVSKI B, et al. Massive necrosis of the upper gastrointestinal tract with acute gastric perforation and metabolic acidosis after hydrochloric acid (HCl) ingestion[J]. Zentralbl Chir, 2011,136(3):289 – 290.

➤ LINFORD S M, JAMES H D. Sodium bicarbonate abuse: a case report[J]. Br J Psychiatry, 1986,149:502 – 503.

➤ MENNEN M, SLOVIS C M. Severe metabolic alkalosis in the emergency department [J]. Ann Emerg Med, 1988,17(4):354 – 357.

➤ GREEN S, SIEGLER J C. Empirical modeling of metabolic alkalosis induced by sodium bicarbonate ingestion[J]. Appl Physiol Nutr Metab, 2016,41(10):1092 – 1095.

➤ ZOLADZ J A, SZKUTNIK Z, DUDA K, et al. Preexercise metabolic alkalosis induced via bicarbonate ingestion accelerates $VO_2$ kinetics at the onset of a high-power-output exercise in humans[J]. J Appl Physiol, 2005,98(3):895 – 904.

Questions:

(1) What are changes of blood gas in rabbits with metabolic acid-base disturbances?

(2) What experimental indexes can be used to determine the development of metabolic acidosis or alkalosis in animals?

(3) When animals or humans develop metabolic acidosis or alkalosis, what changes are induced in respiratory and circulatory systems? What are the underlying mechanisms?

［**Extended Experiments**］

**1.　Animal models and clinical studies on exercise，diet，drugs/compounds and disease-related metabolic acidosis**

➤ ROBERGS R A, GHIASVAND F, PARKER D. Biochemistry of exercise-induced metabolic acidosis［J］. Am J Physiol Regul Integr Comp Physiol, 2004, 287（3）: R502 – 516.

➤ DILGER R N, BAKER D H. Excess dietary L-cysteine causes lethal metabolic acidosis in chicks［J］. J Nutr, 2008, 138（9）: 1628 – 1633.

➤ SAFIRSTEIN R, GLASSMAN V P, DISCALA V A. Effects of an NH$_4$Cl-induced metabolic acidosis on salt and water reabsorption in dog kidney［J］. Am J Physiol, 1973, 225（4）: 805 – 809.

➤ SABBOH H, BESSON C, TRESSOL J C, et al. Excess casein in the diet is not the unique cause of low-grade metabolic acidosis: role of a deficit in potassium citrate in a rat model［J］. Ann Nutr Metab, 2006, 50（3）: 229 – 236.

➤ PHAM A Q, XU L H, MOE O W. Drug-induced metabolic acidosis［J］. F1000Res, 2015, 4（F1000 Faculty Rev）: 1460.

➤ MIRSKY I A, NELSON N, ELGART S. Diabetic acidosis and coma in the monkey ［J］. Science, 1941, 93（2424）: 576.

➤ LÓPEZ-CAYUQUEO K I, CHAVEZ-CANALES M, PILLOT A, et al. A mouse model of pseudohypoaldosteronism type Ⅱ reveals a novel mechanism of renal tubular acidosis ［J］. Kidney Int, 2018, 94（3）: 514 – 523.

➤ HARRIS A N, GRIMM P R, LEE H W, et al. Mechanism of hyperkalemia-induced metabolic acidosis［J］. J Am Soc Nephrol, 2018, 29（5）: 1411 – 1425.

➤ WAGNER C A. Metabolic acidosis: new insights from mouse models［J］. Curr Opin Nephrol Hypertens, 2007, 16（5）: 471 – 476.

**2.　Animal models of metabolic alkalosis caused by operation and diet**

➤ GINGERICH D A, MURDICK P W. Experimentally induced intestinal obstruction in sheep: paradoxical aciduria in metabolic alkalosis［J］. Am J Vet Res, 1975, 36（5）: 663 – 668.

➤ HULTER H N, TOTO R D, ILNICKI L P, et al. Metabolic alkalosis in models of primary and secondary hyperparathyroid states ［J］. Am J Physiol, 1983, 245（4）: F450 – 461.

➤ BORKAN S, NORTHRUP T E, COHEN J J, et al. Renal response to metabolic alkalosis induced by isovolemic hemofiltration in the dog［J］. Kidney Int, 1987, 32（3）: 322 – 328.

➤ WESSON D E. Augmented bicarbonate reabsorption by both the proximal and distal nephron maintains chloride-deplete metabolic alkalosis in rats［J］. J Clin Invest, 1989, 84（5）: 1460 – 1469.

➢ SMITH D F, LUNN D P, ROBINSON G M, et al. Experimental model of hypochloremic metabolic alkalosis caused by diversion of abomasal outflow in sheep[J]. Am J Vet Res, 1990,51(11):1715 – 1722.

➢ LEVINE D Z, IACOVITTI M, HARRISON V. Bicarbonate secretion in vivo by rat distal tubules during alkalosis induced by dietary chloride restriction and alkali loading [J]. J Clin Invest, 1991,87(5):1513 – 1518.

➢ PRADERVAND S, WANG Q, BURNIER M, et al. A mouse model for Liddle's syndrome[J]. J Am Soc Nephrol, 1999,10(12):2527 – 2533.

Questions:

(1) What are the mechanisms underlying the development of metabolic acid-base disturbances in various experimental models?

(2) How similar in pathogenesis and symptoms is between various animal models and clinical metabolic acid-base disturbances?

(郑　栋　赵丽梅)

# Chapter 4　Fever

## [ Extended Experiments ]

**1. New or old perspectives on fever**

➢ WALTER E J, HANNA-JUMMA S, CARRARETTO M, et al. The pathophysiological basis and consequences of fever[J]. Crit Care, 2016,20(1):200.

➢ HARDEN L M, KENT S, PITTMAN Q J, et al. Fever and sickness behavior: friend or foe? [J]. Brain Behav Immun, 2015,50:322 – 333.

➢ BECKER J H, WU S C. Fever—an update[J]. J Am Podiatr Med Assoc, 2010,100 (4):281 – 290.

➢ BERNHEIM H A, BLOCK L H, ATKINS E. Fever: pathogenesis, pathophysiology, and purpose[J]. Ann Intern Med, 1979,91(2):261 – 270.

**2. Literatures on effects of fever on the central nervous system**

➢ BURKE S, HANANI M. The actions of hyperthermia on the autonomic nervous system: central and peripheral mechanisms and clinical implications[J]. Auton Neurosci, 2012, 168(1 – 2):4 – 13.

➢ DIETRICH W D, BRAMLETT H M. Hyperthermia and central nervous system injury [J]. Prog Brain Res, 2007,162:201 – 217.

➢ SMINIA P, HULSHOF M C. Hyperthermia and the central nervous system[J]. Prog

Brain Res, 1998,115:337 – 350.

**3. Clinical studies on thermotherapy**

➤ WALTER E J, CARRARETTO M. The neurological and cognitive consequences of hyperthermia[J]. Crit Care, 2016,20(1):199.

➤ DIETRICH W D, BRAMLETT H M. Hyperthermia and central nervous system injury [J]. Prog Brain Res, 2007,162:201 – 217.

➤ TISHIN A M, SHTIL A A, PYATAKOV A P, et al. Developing antitumor magnetic hyperthermia: principles, materials and devices [J]. Recent Pat Anticancer Drug Discov, 2016,11(4):360 – 375.

Questions:

(1) What kind of experiments can you design to study fever? How can it be carried out?

(2) What models and techniques can be used to study the mechanisms of CNS symptoms caused by fever?

(3) What patients can be treated with thermotherapy? What are the potential mechanisms underlying the treatment of tumor with hyperthermia?

(孙丽娜)

# Chapter 5    Stress

## [Course Experiment]: Effects of Stress on Behavior, Learning and Memory in Mice

(selected from: WANG J Z, QIAN R Z. Experimental instructions for pathophysiology [M]. Beijing:People's Medical Publishing House,2017. )

**1. Early preclinical studies and reviews on pathogenesis**

➤ MITCHELL D, OSBORNE E W, O'BOYLE M W. Habituation under stress: shocked mice show nonassociative learning in a T-maze[J]. Behav Neural Biol, 1985,43(2): 212 – 217.

➤ DE WIED D, CROISET G. Stress modulation of learning and memory processes[J]. Methods Achiev Exp Pathol, 1991,15:167 – 199.

➤ BANGASSER D A, SHORS T J. Critical brain circuits at the intersection between stress and learning[J]. Neurosci Biobehav Rev, 2010,34(8):1223 – 1233.

➤ LUKSYS G, SANDI C. Neural mechanisms and computations underlying stress effects on learning and memory[J]. Curr Opin Neurobiol, 2011,21(3):502 – 508.

**2. Population studies**

➢ KALISH H I, GARMEZY N, RODNICK E H, et al. The effects of anxiety and experimentally-induced stress on verbal learning[J]. J Gen Psychol, 1958,59(1):87 – 95.

➢ DOWD S B. Stress in clinical learning：a transactional approach[J]. Radiol Technol, 1985,56(3):154 – 158.

➢ PAUL M, BELLEBAUM C, GHIO M, et al. Stress effects on learning and feedback-related neural activity depend on feedback delay[J]. Psychophysiology, 2020, 57 (2):e13471.

➢ CARVALHEIRO J, CONCEIÇÃO V A, MESQUITA A, et al. Acute stress impairs reward learning in men[J]. Brain Cogn, 2021,147:105657.

Questions：

（1）What indicators can be used to determine the stress response in experimental animals?

（2）What are the mechanisms underlying effects of acute stress on the learning ability in experimental animals? Are they also involved in acute stress-associated human learning disorders?

（3）How to determine effects of stress associated neurohumoral reactions on the learning ability in both animals and humans?

## ［Extended Experiments］

**1. Studies on depression**

In recent years, due to the increasing incidence, depression has become one of the most common mental diseases. The pathogenesis of depression is closely related to stress. Followed are some literatures on experimental methods and pathogenesis of depression.

➢ HAO Y, GE H, SUN M, et al. Selecting an appropriate animal model of depression [J]. Int J Mol Sci, 2019,20(19):4827.

➢ MÉNARD C, HODES G E, RUSSO S J. Pathogenesis of depression：insights from human and rodent studies[J]. Neuroscience, 2016,321:138 – 162.

➢ CZÉH B, FUCHS E, WIBORG O, et al. Animal models of major depression and their clinical implications[J]. Prog Neuropsychopharmacol Biol Psychiatry, 2016,64:293 – 310.

➢ PLANCHEZ B, SURGET A, BELZUNG C. Animal models of major depression： drawbacks and challenges[J]. J Neural Transm (Vienna), 2019,126(11):1383 – 1408.

**2. Studies on heat shock proteins**

Heat shock proteins (HSPs) are one of the first discovered stress proteins in cells, and their expression levels are directly related to the strength of stress. HSPs can effectively enhance the anti-injury ability of cells and thereby have nonspecific protective effects on cells. Followed are a list of research literatures on heat shock proteins.

➢ JACOB P, HIRT H, BENDAHMANE A. The heat-shock protein/chaperone network and multiple stress resistance[J]. Plant Biotechnol J, 2017,15(4):405 – 414.

➢ CHEN B, FEDER M E, KANG L. Evolution of heat-shock protein expression underlying adaptive responses to environmental stress[J]. Mol Ecol, 2018,27(15): 3040 – 3054.

➢ GARBUZ D G. Regulation of heat shock gene expression in response to stress[J]. Mol Biol (Mosk), 2017,51(3):400 – 417.

➢ BEERE H M, GREEN D R. Stress management-heat shock protein-70 and the regulation of apoptosis[J]. Trends Cell Biol, 2001,11(1):6 – 10.

**3. Studies on psychosomatic disorder**

With stimulation of social-psychological factors, psychosomatic disorder, a psychological condition that leads to physical symptoms, gradually increase. Psychosomatic diseases are closely related to long-term or excessive stress on the body. Followed are some literatures on psychosomatic disorder.

➢ PETRIE J R, GUZIK T J, TOUYZ R M. Diabetes, hypertension, and cardiovascular disease: clinical insights and vascular mechanisms[J]. Can J Cardiol, 2018,34(5): 575 – 584.

➢ BOONE J L. Stress and hypertension[J]. Prim Care, 1991,18(3):623 – 649.

➢ HAMMEN C. Stress and depression[J]. Annu Rev Clin Psychol, 2005,1:293 – 319.

➢ BURGESS C. Stress and cancer[J]. Cancer Surv, 1987,6(3):403 – 416.

➢ ZILAEE M, SHIRALI S. Heat shock proteins and diabetes[J]. Can J Diabetes, 2016, 40(6):594 – 602.

Questions:

(1) What kind of acid-base balance disorder may develop in response to stress? Please design an experiment to prove your idea.

(2) What animal can be used to induce stress? How to evaluate the state of stress in animals?

(3) What are the regulatory mechanisms involved in cellular stress responses? How to test these cellular changes in a lab?

(4) Please try to design an experiment to figure out the relationship between stress and psychosomatic disorders.

(孙丽娜)

# Chapter 6    Hypoxia

## [Course Experiment]: Different Types of Hypoxia in Mice

(selected from: XIE K M, WANG G Q, JIANG X H, et al. Functional experimental science[M]. Beijing: Higher Education Press,2014.)

### 1. Preclinical and clinical studies on the metabolic changes of hypotonic hypoxia

➢ LENFANT C, WAYS P, AUCUTT C, et al. Effect of chronic hypoxic hypoxia on the $O_2$-Hb dissociation curve and respiratory gas transport in man[J]. Respir Physiol, 1969,7(1):7 – 29.

➢ HONIG A. Electrolytes, body fluid volumes and renal function in acute hypoxic hypoxia [J]. Acta Physiol Pol, 1979,30(18 Suppl):93 – 125.

➢ KOZNIEWSKA E, WELLER L, HÖPER J, et al. Cerebrocortical microcirculation in different stages of hypoxic hypoxia[J]. J Cereb Blood Flow Metab, 1987,7(4):464 – 470.

➢ DANNENBERG R, KLIMA S. Effects of short-term hypoxic hypoxia on the sodium and potassium homoeostasis in humans[J]. Biomed Biochim Acta, 1989,48(2 – 3):S274 – 278.

➢ MANKOVSKAYA I N, LYABAKH K G. Oxygen transport to muscular tissue under adaptation to hypoxic hypoxia[J]. Adv Exp Med Biol, 1999,471:295 – 306.

➢ LU G, DING D, SHI M. Acute adaptation of mice to hypoxic hypoxia[J]. Biol Signals Recept, 1999,8(4 – 5):247 – 255.

➢ JONES J G, BAKEWELL S E, HENEGHAN C P, et al. Profound hypoxemia in pulmonary patients in airline-equivalent hypoxia: roles of $V_A/Q$ and shunt[J]. Aviat Space Environ Med, 2008,79(2):81 – 86.

➢ PETRASSI F A, HODKINSON P D, WALTERS P L, et al. Hypoxic hypoxia at moderate altitudes: review of the state of the science[J]. Aviat Space Environ Med, 2012,83(10):975 – 984.

### 2. Preclinical and clinical studies on the pathogenesis of hemic hypoxia

➢ WESTPHAL R G, AZEN E A. Experimental enterogenous cyanosis and anaemia[J]. Br J Haematol, 1972,22(5):609 – 616.

➢ BAUMEL I P, PITTERMAN A, PATEL G, et al. Mechanisms underlying potentiation of barbiturate action by sodium nitrite in the mouse: the role of methemoglobin-induced hypoxia[J]. J Pharmacol Exp Ther, 1974,188(2):481 – 489.

➢ BRADBERRY S M, GAZZARD B, VALE J A. Methemoglobinemia caused by the accidental contamination of drinking water with sodium nitrite [J]. J Toxicol Clin Toxicol, 1994,32(2):173 – 178.

➢ LEE S S, CHOI I S, SONG K S. Hematologic changes in acute carbon monoxide intoxication[J]. Yonsei Med J, 1994,35(3):245 – 251.

➢ GABRIELLI A, LAYON A J. Carbon monoxide intoxication during pregnancy: a case presentation and pathophysiologic discussion, with emphasis on molecular mechanisms [J]. J Clin Anesth, 1995,7(1):82 – 87.

➢ LEE A C, OU Y, LAM S Y, et al. Non-accidental carbon monoxide poisoning from burning charcoal in attempted combined homicide-suicide[J]. J Paediatr Child Health, 2002,38(5):465 – 468.

➢ SKOLD A, COSCO D L, KLEIN R. Methemoglobinemia: pathogenesis, diagnosis, and management[J]. South Med J, 2011,104(11):757 – 761.

**3.   Case reports on histogenous hypoxia and related preclinical studies**

➢ BAIN J T, KNOWLES E L. Successful treatment of cyanide poisoning[J]. Br Med J, 1967,2(5554):763.

➢ PIANTADOSI C A, SYLVIA A L, JÖBSIS F F. Cyanide-induced cytochrome a, a3 oxidation-reduction responses in rat brain *in vivo*[J]. J Clin Invest, 1983, 72 (4): 1224 – 1233.

➢ JEEVARATNAM K, VIDYA S, VAIDYANATHAN C S. In vitro and in vivo effect of methyl isocyanate on rat liver mitochondrial respiration[J]. Toxicol Appl Pharmacol, 1992,117(2):172 – 179.

➢ ABOUL-ENEIN F, LASSMANN H. Mitochondrial damage and histotoxic hypoxia: a pathway of tissue injury in inflammatory brain disease? [J]. Acta Neuropathol, 2005, 109(1):49 – 55.

➢ BERLING I, BUCKLEY N A, MOSTAFA A, et al. 2-Methyl-4-chlorophenoxyacetic acid and bromoxynil herbicide death[J]. Clin Toxicol (Phila), 2015,53(5):486 – 488.

Questions:

(1) What's the difference among mechanisms involved in distinct types of hypoxia?

(2) What are the defects in the induction of hemic hypoxia by CO produced via the reaction of formic acid with concentrated sulfuric acid? How to improve it?

(3) In addition to potassium cyanide, what else can be used to induce histogenous hypoxia? Please briefly describe underlying mechanisms and rescue methods.

(4) What kind of water-electrolyte disorder and acid-base imbalance may develop under hypoxia?

## 〔Extended Experiments〕

**1. Literatures on the central nervous alterations in hypoxia**

➢ CERVÓS-NAVARRO J, SAMPAOLO S, HAMDORF G. Brain changes in experimental chronic hypoxia[J]. Exp Pathol, 1991,42(4):205 – 212.

➢ HIRANO S, HASEGAWA M, KAMEI A, et al. Responses of cerebral blood volume and oxygenation to carotid ligation and hypoxia in young rabbits: near-infrared spectroscopy study[J]. J Child Neurol, 1993,8(3):237 – 241.

➢ GOLAN H, HULEIHEL M. The effect of prenatal hypoxia on brain development: short-and long-term consequences demonstrated in rodent models[J]. Dev Sci, 2006,9(4):338 – 349.

➢ ADHAMI F, LIAO G, MOROZOV Y M, et al. Cerebral ischemia-hypoxia induces intravascular coagulation and autophagy[J]. Am J Pathol, 2006,169(2):566 – 583.

➢ RODRIGO J, FERNÁNDEZ A P, SERRANO J, et al. The role of free radicals in cerebral hypoxia and ischemia[J]. Free Radic Biol Med, 2005,39(1):26 – 50.

➢ DEKOSKY S T, KOCHANEK P M, VALADKA A B, et al. Blood biomarkers for detection of brain injury in COVID-19 patients[J]. J Neurotrauma, 2021,38(1):1 – 43.

**2. Reviews on oxygen therapy**

➢ CHOUDHURY R. Hypoxia and hyperbaric oxygen therapy: a review[J]. Int J Gen Med, 2018,11:431 – 442.

➢ ALLARDET-SERVENT J, SICARD G, METZ V, et al. Benefits and risks of oxygen therapy during acute medical illness: just a matter of dose! [J]. Rev Med Interne, 2019, 40(10):670 – 676.

➢ TRETTER V, ZACH M L, BÖHME S, et al. Investigating disturbances of oxygen homeostasis: from cellular mechanisms to the clinical practice[J]. Front Physiol, 2020, 11:947.

➢ FISCHER I, BARAK B. Molecular and therapeutic aspects of hyperbaric oxygen therapy in neurological conditions[J]. Biomolecules, 2020,10(9):1247.

➢ JIANG B, WEI H. Oxygen therapy strategies and techniques to treat hypoxia in COVID-19 patients[J]. Eur Rev Med Pharmacol Sci, 2020,24(19):10239 – 10246.

➢ SEN S, SEN S. Therapeutic effects of hyperbaric oxygen: integrated review[J]. Med Gas Res, 2021,11(1):30 – 33.

Questions:

(1) How do cells adjust oxygen balance *in vivo*?

(2) What is the adaptive regulation of brain in hypoxia? What are the mechanisms involved?

(3) What are side effects of oxygen therapy? What are the mechanisms involved?

(孙丽娜)

# Chapter 7　Shock

## ［Course Experiment］—Hemorrhagic Shock in Rabbits

（selected from：XIE K M, WANG G Q, JIANG X H, et al. Functional experimental science［M］. Beijing：Higher Education Press,2014. ）

### Reviews on animal models of hemorrhagic shock

➢ FÜLÖP A, TURÓCZI Z, GARBAISZ D, et al. Experimental models of hemorrhagic shock：a review［J］. Eur Surg Res, 2013,50(2)：57 – 70.

➢ MOOCHHALA S, WU J, LU J. Hemorrhagic shock：an overview of animal models ［J］. Front Biosci (Landmark Ed), 2009,14(12)：4631 – 4639.

➢ LOMAS-NIERA J L, PERL M, CHUNG C S, et al. Shock and hemorrhage：an overview of animal models［J］. Shock, 2005,24 (suppl 1)：33 – 39.

Questions：

（1）What parameters can be used to determine the onset of shock in this rabbit model?

（2）In addition to rabbits, what other animals can be used to induce hemorrhagic shock?

（3）Please analyze the advantages and disadvantages of various experimental animals for induction of hemorrhagic shock.

## ［Extended Experiments］

### 1.　Animal models of anaphylactic shock

➢ BARSAN W G, HEDGES J R, SYVERUD S A, et al. A hemodynamic model for anaphylactic shock［J］. Ann Emerg Med, 1985,14(9)：834 – 839.

➢ HIEDA Y, KAGEURA M, HARA K, et al. An experimental model of death from anaphylactic shock with compound 48/80 and postmortem changes in levels of histamine in blood［J］. Forensic Sci Int, 1990,45(1 – 2)：159 – 169.

➢ GREENBERG M I, ROBERTS J R, KRUSZ J C, et al. Endotracheal epinephrine in a canine anaphylactic shock model［J］. JACEP, 1979,8(12)：500 – 503.

### 2.　Animal models of septic shock

➢ LILLEY E, ARMSTRONG R, CLARK N, et al. Refinement of animal models of sepsis and septic shock［J］. Shock, 2015,43(4)：304 – 316.

➢ VILLA P, GHEZZI P. Animal models of endotoxic shock［J］. Methods Mol Med, 2004,98：199 – 206.

Questions:

(1) What are the mechanisms underlying the development of anaphylactic and septic shock in animals, respectively?

(2) What are the advantages and disadvantages of all animal models in the extended experiments?

(赵丽梅)

# Chapter 8    Disturbances of Hemostasis

## [Course Experiment]: Disseminated Intravascular Coagulation in Rabbits

(selected from: WANG J Z, QIAN R Z. Experimental instructions for pathophysiology [M]. Beijing: People's Medical Publishing House, 2017.)

**1. Early preclinical studies and the latest review on the pathogenesis**

➤ MENACHE D, BEHRE H E, ORTHNER C L, et al. Coagulation Factor IX concentrate: method of preparation and assessment of potential *in vivo* thrombogenicity in animal models[J]. Blood, 1984, 64(6): 1220 – 1227.

➤ HARRISON J, ABILDGAARD C, LAZERSON J, et al. Assessment of thrombogenicity of prothrombin complex concentrates in a porcine model[J]. Thromb Res, 1985, 38(2): 173 – 188.

➤ LEVI M, SIVAPALARATNAM S. Disseminated intravascular coagulation: an update on pathogenesis and diagnosis[J]. Expert Rev Hematol, 2018, 11(8): 663 – 672.

**2. Case reports**

➤ OHGA S, SAITO M, MATSUKAZI A, et al. Disseminated intravascular coagulation in a patient with haemophilia B during factor IX replacement therapy[J]. Br J Haematol, 1993, 84(2): 343 – 345.

➤ EDWARDS R L, RICKLES F R, CRONLUND M. Abnormalities of blood coagulation in patients with cancer. Mononuclear cell tissue factor generation[J]. J Lab Clin Med, 1981, 98(6): 917 – 928.

Questions:

(1) What are the etiologies and mechanisms of DIC in this experimental model?

(2) In addition to the parameters in the teaching materials, what parameter can better indicate the progress of DIC?

(3) Are there any other animal models of DIC?

[Extended Experiments]

**1. DIC induced by sepsis and tissue factor**

➤ SUGA Y, KUBO A, KATSURA H, et al. Detailed exploration of pathophysiology involving inflammatory status and bleeding symptoms between lipopolysaccharide- and tissue factor-induced disseminated intravascular coagulation in rats[J]. Int J Hematol, 2021,114(2):172 – 178.

➤ SOERENSEN K E, OLSEN H G, SKOVGAARD K, et al. Disseminated intravascular coagulation in a novel porcine model of severe Staphylococcus aureus sepsis fulfills human clinical criteria[J]. J Comp Pathol, 2013,149(4):463 – 474.

**2. Reviews on the relevance of animal models to human DIC**

➤ ASAKURA H. Classifying types of disseminated intravascular coagulation: clinical and animal models[J]. J Intensive Care, 2014,2(1):20.

➤ BERTHELSEN L O, KRISTENSEN A T, TRANHOLM M. Animal models of DIC and their relevance to human DIC: a systematic review[J]. Thromb Res, 2011,128(2):103 – 116.

Questions:

(1) What are the differences among DIC in different diseases?

(2) What is the relevance of animal models to human DIC?

(3) What therapeutic strategy for DIC is indicated by the current preclinical research?

(刘立民    赵丽梅)


# Chapter 9    Ischemia-reperfusion Injury


[Course Experiment]: Ischemia-reperfusion Injury of Rat Heart

(selected from: WANG J Z, QIAN R Z. Experimental instructions for pathophysiology [M]. Beijing: People's Medical Publishing House,2017. )

**1. Previous preclinical studies and reviews on myocardial ischemia reperfusion**

➤ MURRY C E, JENNINGS R B, REIMER K A. Preconditioning with ischemia: a delay of lethal cell injury in ischemic myocardium[J]. Circulation, 1986,74(5):1124 – 1136.

➤ FRANK A, BONNEY M, BONNEY S, et al. Myocardial ischemia reperfusion injury: from basic science to clinical bedside[J]. Semin Cardiothorac Vasc Anesth, 2012,16

（3）:123 – 132.

**2. Case reports**

➢ TANAKA K, SATO N, YASUTAKE M, et al. Clinical course, timing of rupture and relationship with coronary recanalization therapy in 77 patients with ventricular free wall rupture following acute myocardial infarction[J]. J Nippon Med Sch, 2002,69(5): 481 – 488.

➢ TANAKA R, NAKAMURA T, KUMAMOTO H, et al. Detection of stunned myocardium in post-reperfusion cases of acute myocardial infarction[J]. Ann Nucl Med, 2003,17(1):53 – 60.

Questions:

（1）What cardiac changes are associated with ischemia-reperfusion injury?

（2）What should be done to reduce ischemia-reperfusion injury?

（3）Is the ischemia-reperfusion injury reversible or irreversible? Why?

## [Extended Experiments]

**1. Intestinal ischemia-reperfusion injury**

➢ GONZALEZ L M, MOESER A J, BLIKSLAGER A T. Animal models of ischemia-reperfusion-induced intestinal injury: progress and promise for translational research[J]. Am J Physiol Gastrointest Liver Physiol, 2015,308(2):G63 – 75.

**2. Renal ischemia-reperfusion injury**

➢ SHIVA N, SHARMA N, KULKARNI Y A, et al. Renal ischemia/reperfusion injury: an insight on *in vitro* and *in vivo* models[J]. Life Sci, 2020,256:117860.

**3. Cerebral ischemia-reperfusion injury**

➢ MA R, XIE Q, LI Y, et al. Animal models of cerebral ischemia: a review[J]. Biomed Pharmacother, 2020,131:110686.

**4. Pulmonary ischemia-reperfusion injury**

➢ FARD N, SAFFARI A, EMAMI G, et al. Acute respiratory distress syndrome induction by pulmonary ischemia-reperfusion injury in large animal models[J]. J Surg Res, 2014, 189(2):274 – 284.

➢ FERRARI R S, ANDRADE C F. Oxidative stress and lung ischemia-reperfusion injury [J]. Oxid Med Cell Longev, 2015,2015:590987.

**5. Hepatic ischemia-reperfusion injury**

➢ YANG W, CHEN J, MENG Y, et al. Novel targets for treating ischemia-reperfusion injury in the liver[J]. Int J Mol Sci, 2018,19(5):1302.

➢ ZHOU J, CHEN J, WEI Q, et al. The role of ischemia/reperfusion injury in early hepatic allograft dysfunction[J]. Liver Transpl, 2020,26(8):1034 – 1048.

Questions:

（1）What are the general and organ-specific mechanisms of ischemia-reperfusion injury?

（2）What are the organ-specific indexes of ischemia-reperfusion injury?

（3）What are the prevention strategies for the ischemia-reperfusion injury in humans?

（刘立民　赵丽梅）

# Chapter 10　Cardiac Insufficiency

## 〔Course Experiment〕: Pulmonary Embolism-Induced Acute Right-sided Heart Failure

（selected from: XIE K M, WANG G Q, JIANG X H, et al. Functional experimental science〔M〕. Beijing: Higher Education Press, 2014. ）

### 1. Case reports

➤ SHARMA M, SUERO-ABREU G A, NEUPANE R, et al. Role of phosphodiesterase-5 inhibitors in acute right ventricular failure due to pulmonary embolism〔J〕. Am J Case Rep, 2019, 20:1144 − 1147.

### 2. Literatures on animal models of right-sided heart failure

➤ GUPTA S C, VARIAN K D, BAL N C, et al. Pulmonary artery banding alters the expression of $Ca^{2+}$ transport proteins in the right atrium in rabbits〔J〕. Am J Physiol Heart Circ Physiol, 2009, 296(6):H1933 − 1939.

➤ ANDERSEN A, FEEN D, ANDERSEN S, et al. Animal models of right heart failure 〔J〕. Cardiovasc Diagn Ther, 2020, 10(5):1561 − 1579.

Questions:

（1）What indicators and signs can be used to determine the development of acute right-sided heart failure in animals?

（2）What are the mechanisms underlying the development of pulmonary embolism-induced acute right-sided heart failure?

（3）Besides the rabbit, what other experimental animals can be used to induce acute right-sided heart failure?

（4）What other methods can be used to induce right-sided heart failure?

## 〔Extended Experiments〕: Left-sided Heart Failure

### Literatures on animal models of left-sided heart failure

➤ LIU Y H, YANG X P, NASS O, et al. Chronic heart failure induced by coronary artery ligation in Lewis inbred rats〔J〕. Am J Physiol, 1997, 272(2):H722 − 727.

➤ MAGID N M, OPIO G, WALLERSON D C, et al. Heart failure due to chronic experimental aortic regurgitation[J]. Am J Physiol, 1994,267(2):H556 – 562.

➤ SABBAH H N, STEIN P D, KONO T, et al. A canine model of chronic heart failure produced by multiple sequential coronary microembolizations[J]. Am J Physiol, 1991, 260(4):H1379 – 1384.

➤ WEINHEIMER C J, LAI L, KELLY D P, et al. Novel mouse model of left ventricular pressure overload and infarction causing predictable ventricular remodelling and progression to heart failure[J]. Clin Exp Pharmacol Physiol, 2015,42(1):33 – 40.

➤ COPS J, HAESEN S, DE MOOR B, et al. Current animal models for the study of congestion in heart failure: an overview[J]. Heart Fail Rev, 2019,24(3):387 – 397.

➤ RIEHLE C, BAUERSACHS J. Small animal models of heart failure[J]. Cardiovasc Res, 2019,115(13):1838 – 1849.

➤ SILVA K, EMTER C A. Large animal models of heart failure: a translational bridge to clinical success[J]. JACC Basic Transl Sci, 2020,5(8):840 – 856.

Questions:

(1) What large and small animals can be used to induce left-sided heart failure? What are the advantages and disadvantages of each animal model?

(2) What methods can be used to induce chronic left-sided heart failure?

(3) What models of heart failure are better in simulations of pathological conditions in humans?

(赵丽梅)

# Chapter 11　　Pulmonary Insufficiency

## [Course Experiment]: Pulmonary Ventilatory Disorders in Rabbit

(selected from: XIE K M, WANG G Q, JIANG X H, et al. Functional experimental science[M]. Beijing: Higher Education Press,2014.)

### Case reports and reviews on pathogenesis

➤ GEORGE R B, HERBERT S J, SHAMES J M, et al. Pneumothorax complicating pulmonary emphysema[J]. JAMA, 1975,234(4):389 – 393.

➤ REES P J, HAY J G, WEBB J R. Acute exacerbation of upper airway obstruction in acromegaly[J]. Postgrad Med J, 1982,58(681):429 – 430.

➤ RAJU P, MANTHOUS C A. The pathogenesis of respiratory failure: an overview[J]. Respir Care Clin N Am, 2000,6(2):195 – 212.

Questions:

(1) How to classify the obstructive hypoventilation according to the location of blockage? What kind of obstructive hypoventilation is induced in the current experiment? What kind of dyspnea is associated with obstructive hypoventilation in the current experiment?

(2) What are the mechanisms of obstructive hypoventilation induced by partial cross-clamping of an endotracheal tube?

(3) What are the changes of BP, respiration and sinus reflex in rabbits with obstructive hypoventilation? What's the underlying mechanisms?

(4) What are the causes of restrictive hypoventilation? What are the specific mechanisms of restrictive hypoventilation in the current experiment?

(5) What are the changes of BP, respiration and sinus reflex in rabbits with severe restrictive hypoventilation? What's the underlying mechanisms?

## [Extended Experiments]

### 1. Basic and clinical studies on COPD and respiratory failure

➢ SERBAN K A, PETRACHE I. Mouse models of COPD[J]. Methods Mol Biol, 2018, 1809:379 – 394.

➢ JONES B, DONOVAN C, LIU G, et al. Animal models of COPD: what do they tell us? [J]. Respirology, 2017,22(1):21 – 32.

➢ O'DONNELL D E, MILNE K M, JAMES M D, et al. Dyspnea in COPD: new mechanistic insights and management implications[J]. Adv Ther, 2020,37(1):41 – 60.

### 2. Basic and clinical studies on ARDS and respiratory failure

➢ AEFFNER F, BOLON B, DAVIS I C. Mouse models of acute respiratory distress syndrome: a review of analytical approaches, pathologic features, and common measurements[J]. Toxicol Pathol, 2015,43(8):1074 – 1092.

➢ D'ALESSIO F R. Mouse models of acute lung injury and ARDS[J]. Methods Mol Biol, 2018,1809:341 – 350.

➢ GOH K J, CHOONG M C, CHEONG E H, et al. Rapid progression to acute respiratory distress syndrome: review of current understanding of critical illness from COVID-19 infection[J]. Ann Acad Med Singap, 2020,49(3):108 – 118.

Questions:

(1) What are the mechanisms of respiratory failure in the experimental models of COPD and ARDS, respectively?

(2) What parameters are used to determine the development of respiratory failure in the experimental models of COPD and ARDS, respectively?

(3) What pathogenesis of respiratory failure is still not clear in the experimental models of COPD and ARDS, respectively?

（孙晓东　孙丽娜）

# Chapter 12　Hepatic Insufficiency

[Course Experiment]：Hepatic Insufficiency in the Rabbit

(selected from：XIE K M, WANG G Q, JIANG X H, et al. Functional experimental science[M]. Beijing：Higher Education Press,2014. )

**Case reports and animal models on hepatic encephalopathy**

➢ FENTON J C, KNIGHT E J, HUMPHERSON P L. Milk-and-cheese diet in portal-systemic encephalopathy[J]. Lancet, 1966,1(7430):164 – 166.

➢ RUSSELL D M, KELLER F S, WHITAKER J N. Episodic confusion and tremor associated with extrahepatic portacaval shunting in cirrhotic liver disease [J]. Neurology, 1989,39(3):403 – 405.

➢ LEE Y L, PANG S, ONG C. Non-cirrhotic hyperammonaemia：are we missing the diagnosis? [J]. BMJ Case Rep, 2020,13(3):e233218.

➢ MARDINI H, RECORD C. Pathogenesis of hepatic encephalopathy：lessons from nitrogen challenges in man[J]. Metab Brain Dis, 2013,28(2):201 – 207.

➢ DEMORROW S, CUDALBU C, DAVIES N, et al. 2021 ISHEN guidelines on animal models of hepatic encephalopathy[J]. Liver Int, 2021,26.

Questions：

(1) What are the mechanisms underlying effects of epinephrine on BP and breathing? Please compare effects of epinephrine between the way of intravenous administration into the margial ear vein versus the mesenteric superior vein, and analyze differences between them.

(2) What's the pathogenesis of hepatic encephalopathy (HE) in the current rabbit model? Why sodium bicarbonate should be added in preparation of the ammonium chloride mixture for induction of HE?

(3) What are the changes of BP and breathing in the rabbit with HE? What's the underlying mechanisms?

(4) Why do rabbits with complete and insufficient functions require different amounts of ammonium chloride mixture for induction of HE?

[Extended Experiments]

**Hepatic encephalopathy：animal models, pathogenesis and clinical perspectives**

➢ MULLEN K D, BIRGISSON S, GACAD R C, et al. Animal models of hepatic encephalopathy and hyperammonemia[J]. Adv Exp Med Biol, 1994,368:1 – 10.

➢ DEMORROW S, CUDALBU C, DAVIES N, et al. 2021 ISHEN guidelines on animal models of hepatic encephalopathy[J]. Liver Int, 2021,41(7):1474 – 1488.

➢ WEISSENBORN K. Hepatic encephalopathy: definition, clinical grading and diagnostic principles[J]. Drugs, 2019,79(Suppl 1):5 – 9.

➢ GONZÁLEZ-REGUEIRO J A, HIGUERA-DE LA TIJERA M F, MORENO-ALCÁNTAR R, et al. Pathophysiology of hepatic encephalopathy and future treatment options[J]. Rev Gastroenterol Mex (Engl Ed), 2019,84(2):195 – 203.

Questions:

(1) What scientific questions can be addressed using animal models of hepatic encephalopathy?

(2) What are the advantages and disadvantages of animal models in studying hepatic encephalopathy?

(孙晓东　孙丽娜)

# Chapter 13　Renal Insufficiency

## [Course Experiment]: Acute Toxic Renal Failure of Rabbit

(selected from: WANG J Z, QIAN R Z. Experimental instructions for pathophysiology [M]. Beijing: People's Medical Publishing House, 2017.)

### 1.　Early preclinical studies

➢ HSU C H, KURTZ T W, ROSENZWEIG J, et al. Renal hemodynamics in $HgCl_2$-induced acute renal failure[J]. Nephron, 1977,18(6):326 – 332.

➢ HSU C H, KURTZ T W, WELLER J M. The role of tubular necrosis in the pathophysiology of acute renal failure[J]. Nephron, 1976,17(3):204 – 214.

➢ STACCHIOTTI A, BORSANI E, RODELLA L, et al. Dose-dependent mercuric chloride tubular injury in rat kidney[J]. Ultrastruct Pathol, 2003,27(4):253 – 259.

### 2.　Case reports

➢ MURPHY M J, CULLIFORD E J, PARSONS V. A case of poisoning with mercuric chloride[J]. Resuscitation, 1979,7(1):35 – 44.

➢ LAI K N, PUGSLEY D J, BLACK R B. Acute renal failure after peritoneal lavage with mercuric chloride[J]. Med J Aust, 1983,1(1):37 – 38.

➢ DHANAPRIYA J, GOPALAKRISHNAN N, ARUN V, et al. Acute kidney injury and disseminated intravascular coagulation due to mercuric chloride poisoning[J]. Indian J

Nephrol, 2016,26(3):206-208.

Questions:

(1) What are the mechanisms underlying the development of acute renal failure in the course experiment?

(2) Besides the indexes used in the current experiment, what else is better in determining the progression of acute renal failure?

(3) What experimental animals can be used to induce acute toxic renal failure? What differences are in disease course of different experimental animals?

## 〔Extended Experiments〕

**1. Animal models of acute renal injury caused by sepsis**

➤ DEJAGER L, PINHEIRO I, DEJONCKHEERE E, et al. Cecal ligation and puncture: the gold standard model for polymicrobial sepsis? [J]. Trends in Microbiology, 2011, 19(4):198-208.

**2. Animal models of acute renal injury caused by ischemia and reperfusion**

➤ HESKETH E E, CZOPEK A, CLAY M, et al. Renal ischaemia reperfusion injury: a mouse model of injury and regeneration[J]. J Vis Exp, 2014,(88):51816.

➤ WEI Q, DONG Z. Mouse model of ischemic acute kidney injury: technical notes and tricks[J]. Am J Physiol Renal Physiol, 2012,303(11): F1487-1494.

**3. Animal models of acute renal injury caused by unilateral ureteral obstruction**

➤ BANDER S J, BUERKERT J E, MARTIN D, et al. Long-term effects of 24-hr unilateral ureteral obstruction on renal function in the rat[J]. Kidney Int, 1985,28(4): 614-620.

➤ CHEVALIER R L, FORBES M S, THORNHILL B A. Ureteral obstruction as a model of renal interstitial fibrosis and obstructive nephropathy[J]. Kidney Int, 2009,75(11): 1145-1152.

➤ UCERO A C, BENITO-MARTIN A, IZQUIERDO M C, et al. Unilateral ureteral obstruction: beyond obstruction[J]. Int Urol Nephrol, 2014,46(4):765-776.

**4. Animal models of acute renal injury caused by drug**

➤ HOLDITCH S J, BROWN C N, LOMBARDI A M, et al. Recent advances in models, mechanisms, biomarkers, and interventions in cisplatin-induced acute kidney injury[J]. Int J Mol Sci, 2019,20(12):3011.

➤ PABLA N, DONG Z. Cisplatin nephrotoxicity: mechanisms and renoprotective strategies[J]. Kidney Int, 2008,73(9):994-1007.

➤ MATSUI K, KAMIJO-IKEMORIF A, SUGAYA T, et al. Renal liver-type fatty acid binding protein (L-FABP) attenuates acute kidney injury in aristolochic acid nephrotoxicity[J]. Am J Pathol, 2011,178(3):1021-1032.

➤ WU J, LIU X H, FAN J J, et al. Bardoxolone methyl (BARD) ameliorates aristolochic acid (AA)-induced acute kidney injury through Nrf2 pathway[J]. Toxicology, 2014, 318:22 − 31.

➢ WEN X Y, PENG Z Y, LI Y J, et al. One dose of cyclosporine A is protective at initiation of folic acid-induced acute kidney injury in mice[J]. Nephrol Dial Transplant, 2012,27(8):3100 − 3109.

➢ GENG Y Q, ZHANG L, FU B, et al. Mesenchymal stem cells ameliorate rhabdomyolysis-induced acute kidney injury via the activation of M2 macrophages[J]. Stem Cell Res Ther, 2014,5(3):80.

Questions:

(1) What differences in pathogenesis of acute renal failure are among different models?

(2) What indexes can be used to determine the acute renal injury in different models?

(3) Why should we construct different models of acute renal injury, and what is the clinical significance of these models?

(郑 栋 赵丽梅)

# Chapter 14　Brain Dysfunction

## [Extended Experiment] Effects of Ethanol on Learning and Memory in Mice

**Preclinical & clinical studies and reviews**

➢ BRADY M L, ALLAN A M, CALDWELL K K. A limited access mouse model of prenatal alcohol exposure that produces long-lasting deficits in hippocampal-dependent learning and memory[J]. Alcohol Clin Exp Res, 2012,36(3):457 − 466.

➢ SPEAR L P. Effects of adolescent alcohol consumption on the brain and behaviour[J]. Nat Rev Neurosci, 2018,19(4):197 − 214.

➢ BRUMBACK T, CAO D, MCNAMARA P, et al. Alcohol-induced performance impairment: a 5-year re-examination study in heavy and light drinkers [J]. Psychopharmacology (Berl), 2017,234(11):1749 − 1759.

➢ LOHESWARAN G, BARR M S, ZOMORRODI R, et al. Impairment of neuroplasticity in the dorsolateral prefrontal cortex by alcohol[J]. Sci Rep, 2017,7(1):5276.

Questions:

(1) In addition to the methods shown in the above literatures, what else can be employed to measure learning and memory?

(2) What indexes can be used to measure the learning and memory of animals in this experiment?

（3）What are the classifications of learning and memory? What kind of learning and memory is changed by ethanol?

（4）What diseases can induce the impairment of learning and memory?

（5）What learning and memory tests are used by clinical doctors?

（单立冬）